Mc...   *y*
and imm...   *r*
techn...   *y*

The production and
application of rodent
and human monoclonal antibodies

LABORATORY TECHNIQUES IN BIOCHEMISTRY AND MOLECULAR BIOLOGY

Volume 23

Edited by

P.C. van der VLIET — *Department for Physiological Chemistry, University of Utrecht, Utrecht*

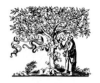

ELSEVIER
AMSTERDAM · LONDON · NEW YORK · TOKYO

MONOCLONAL ANTIBODY AND IMMUNOSENSOR TECHNOLOGY

The production and application of rodent
and human monoclonal antibodies

Ailsa M. Campbell

Department of Biochemistry,
University of Glasgow,
Glasgow G12 8QQ,
U.K.

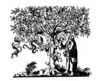

1991
ELSEVIER
AMSTERDAM · LONDON · NEW YORK · TOKYO

ISBN 0-444-81412-4 (pocket edition)
ISBN 0-444-81413-2 (library edition)
ISSN 0-7204-4200-1 (series)

Published by:
ELSEVIER SCIENCE PUBLISHERS B.V.
P.O. BOX 211
1000 AE AMSTERDAM
THE NETHERLANDS

Sole distributors for the U.S.A. and Canada:
ELSEVIER SCIENCE PUBLISHING COMPANY, INC.
655 AVENUE OF THE AMERICAS
NEW YORK, NY 10010
U.S.A.

Library of Congress Card No. 85-647011

Printed in the Netherlands on acid-free paper

Preface

This book is the successor to a book in the same series entitled Monoclonal Antibody Technology, published in 1984. Even at that time it was apparent that unrealistic projections were being made for a useful but not omnipotent technology. The main problem is, and has always been, that it is possible to obtain invaluable monoclonal antibodies as reagents, and also to obtain useless ones. The skill lies in the selection of high affinity Mabs by a method which is close to the final use and far too many research strategies have concentrated on quantity (numbers of positive clones) rather than quality. It has often been distressing to see the technique abused by those who do not appreciate the importance of affinity and native antigen presentation.

The basic method for Mab production remains unchanged and fusion and cloning methods are close to those used 10 years ago. The main changes relate to the methodology of selection and use. In the early 1980s people sought Mabs to simple soluble proteins and there is now a vast library of Mabs to abundant proteins such as lysosyme, all with no application. In contrast, there is an increasing interest in Mabs to cell membrane proteins and these are scarcely ever produced by the generation of Mabs to denatured proteins or peptides, since epitopes are usually conformational. Thus selection techniques have changed.

Too many researchers fail to understand that a monoclonal antibody is not necessarily monospecific. I have emphasised this point heavily in various sections of the book. A good Mab is usually monospecific unless slammed up against the wall of an ELISA plate against molar amounts of irrelevant antigen in which case it may give a slight signal. A bad Mab will cross-react with a wide range of antigens. The methods of obtaining the former are detailed.

This book has a slight bias towards Mabs directed to supposed tumour antigens. I have been astonished by the frequency with which Mabs to uncharacterised antigens have been used, to predictably little effect in 'tumor therapy', especially as the adverse side effects of a mouse Mab are considerable (Section 1.9). Almost all these Mabs are to high density structural antigens which, in the light of modern understanding of oncogene product function, are irrelevant to tumour progression. This tendency is unfortunate, since far better Mabs could be made in the light of modern knowledge of the nature of tumour progression.

The book also covers the concepts behind the emerging biosensor techniques (Chapter 12). Frankly, having made my way through the mystiques of the systems, I was surprised by their primitive low detection limits despite their cost and cumbersome nature. It would appear that there has been a breakdown in communications between Mab technologists and electrochemical or opto-electronic engineers where the latter group have assumed that antibodies have exquisite specificity and no cross-reactive potential and the former have failed to disabuse them of this fact. In terms of classic detection systems, for my own work, I am now proceeding to use enzyme-linked chemiluminescent detection systems and an instant camera.

I have also covered the gene cloning strategies for Mabs and again have found that many of the complex systems, once understood and applied, are unsuitable for Mab production. In particular, PCR generated variable gene libraries (Section 9.6) are technically unsound for reasons stated in the text. However, other aspects of genetic manipulation involving PCR are very exciting and the prospect of immortalising human Mab responses by PCR of early unstable, but high affinity clones seems to have immense potential. Tobacco plants and alfalfa looping moths notwithstanding, the best expression system is still a myeloma cell.

I have included a section on Mab patents which I particularly enjoyed investigating. The fact that the original Kohler-Milstein fusion procedure was not patented means that no financial concern or company promotes it. I should like to do so. It is still the best way of making a good Mab.

Ailsa Campbell
January 1991.

Acknowledgements

I should like to thank Celia Cannon, Pat Ferry, Souravi Ghosh, Lorraine Haynes and Delyth Wong in particular.

I should also like to acknowledge help from Munir Alam, Peggy Anderson, Rob Butcher, Flora Campbell, Magnus Campbell, Sue Christie, Bill Cushley, Bertil Damato, Chris Darnborough, Morag Davidson, Fiona Durie, Alan Hughes, Janet Jones, Moira McCann, Tom Mathieson and Ian Ramsden.

Abbreviations

ATR	Attenuated total reflectance
EBV	Epstein-Barr virus
ELISA	Enzyme-linked immunosorbent assay
FCFD	Fluorescent capillary fill device
G band	Band visible on human chromosome with Giemsa
HAT	Hypoxanthine, aminopterin and thymidine
HAz	Hypoxanthine and azaserine
HT	Hypoxanthine and thymidine
IRS	Internal reflection spectroscopy
PAGE	Polyacrylamide gel electrophoresis
PEG	Polyethylene glycol
PBS	Phosphate-buffered saline
SDS	Sodium dodecyl sulphate
SPR	Surface plasmon resonance
TIRF	Total internal reflection fluorescence

Contents

Chapter 7. Alternative strategies for the immortalisation of antibody producing cells 205

Chapter 8. Selection and cloning 225

CHAPTER 1

General properties and applications of monoclonal antibodies

1.1. History of Mab technology

The monoclonal antibody era began in 1975 with a report in Nature by Kohler and Milstein entitled 'Continuous culture of fused cells secreting antibody or pre-defined specificity'. Prior to that time, immunologists had two types of lymphocytes available for study. The first was established immortalised B lymphocytes from mineral oil induced murine plasmacytomas. These secreted an antibody of unknown and irrelevant specificity. The second was short lived primary cultures of splenic B lymphocytes, many of which secreted a specific antibody of interest but only for 10–14 days. Kohler and Milstein (1975, 1976) reported that they could fuse these two cell populations to produce offspring with the desirable characteristics of both parent cells, i.e., the immortality of the plasmacytoma and the specific antibody secretion of the splenic B cells. The cell line which made such antibodies was termed a hybridoma. While they concluded their report with the statement 'Such cultures could be valuable for medical and industrial use' and notified the U.K. Medical Research Council of this potential, no patent was taken out on the basic technique prior to publication. Patent applications were less common in medical and biological research at that time in comparison to the 1990s. Given the size of the current Mab market in diagnostics, it is generally asserted that if a comprehensive patent had been taken out, the U.K. MRC would have a steady licence income from the technique which would greatly complement and probably exceed its current total annual budget.

In 1984, Kohler and Milstein together with Niels Jerne were awarded the Nobel Prize for Medicine for their contribution to the development of monoclonal antibodies.

Monoclonal antibodies (Mabs) caused a literature explosion in the late 1970s. They reached their peak in scientific fashion around 1983 to the point where scientists generating polyclonal antisera for a task clearly suited to such sera were obliged by funding institutions to incorporate Mabs into projects for which they were clearly unsuited. Inevitably many premature claims were made in both the diagnostic and therapeutic fields and as these failed to prove generally reproducible, the technique became established on a more realistic basis around 1987 as an invaluable method for making stable and consistent rodent antibodies for diagnostic purposes.

Therapeutic applications and other types of applications remain to be proven to have the immediate utility of the application in these diagnostic systems. However, advances made on more cautious and rational strategies, particularly those incorporating recombinant DNA technology, prove encouraging. In addition strategies for producing Mabs to cell surface proteins are now very much more sophisticated and involve more modern and complex selection techniques.

Fusion between cells is thought to be a natural biological process encouraged by some types of virus. It is advantageous to the virus to promote the fusion of a cell which it has exhausted with a second cell of similar lineage in order to be be able to continue growth without exposure to the antibody arm of the immune system. In addition, fusion with dissimilar cells, abrogates the need for a cell surface receptor for entry. Inactivated Sendai virus has been known to promote such fusion for more than two decades (Harris and Watkins, 1975) and more recently, the HIV virus has been shown to be able to promote fusion between CD4+ cells (Lifson et al., 1986). Currently, in the laboratory, fusion is achieved by the use of polyethylene glycol (Pontecorvo, 1976).

Fusion techniques have been used in the laboratory for many other purposes. They were instrumental, in earlier times, in determining the human chromosomal locations of the genes coding for various enzyme activities (Ruddle and Kucherlapali, 1974) and in determining the dominant or recessive nature of malignancy (Harris 1970; Croce and Kaprowski, 1974). In addition, lymphocyte fusions were undertaken prior to the original report of Kohler and Milstein (1975). Sincovics et al. (1970) fused virus specific lymphocytes together with tumour cells. Interspecies lymphocyte fusions were performed by Schwaber and Cohen (1973) and human fusions by Bloom and Nakamura (1984). The basic difference in the case of Kohler and Milstein (1975) was that the cell lines they generated by fusion, once cloned, were stable and could continue to secrete antibody indefinitely. Hindsight suggests that the cell line P3K which is the progenitor of all the mouse myeloma lines (Section 3.4) had rare and valuable properties in this respect.

1.2. Introduction to Mab technology

1.2.1. The basic methodology

Polyclonal antiserum consists of a wide variety of antibody molecules of different specificity and affinity (Fig. 1.1). Each time an animal is bled, it yields a different 'cocktail' of such antibodies as its immune response to the injected and environmental antigen alters and B cell clones emerge and recede. The same animal can yield a highly specific antiserum directed against the chosen antigen in one bleed and a poor antiserum in another. The animal also has a limited lifespan and prior to the days of Mab technology, the death of a single rabbit could cause major problems in a diagnostic laboratory.

There is an additional inter-animal variability among animals which cannot readily be inbred in the same way as small rodents can be inbred to yield pure strains with matching histocompatibility antigens (Section 3.4). While large 'outbred' animals such as rabbits, sheep and goats, can yield a large quantity of specific antibody, their response to antigen is variable and it was often necessary to immunise up to 30 animals to obtain a high-affinity antiserum.

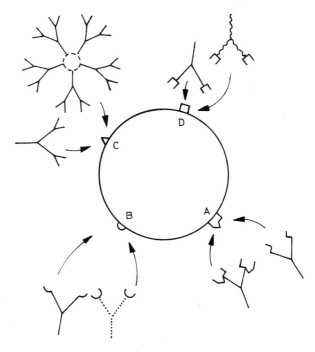

Fig. 1.1. The reaction of polyclonal antiserum with antigen. At epitope A are two antibodies of the same class but different specificities and affinities. At epitope B are two
antibodies of different subclass, specificity and affinity. At epitope C are two antibodies
of different class, one being an IgM, but of the same specificity and affinity (this is rare
– IgM antibodies are usually of lower affinity). At determinant D are two antibodies
of different subclass but the same specificity and affinity. In polyclonal serum the proportions of all these antibodies will vary with each animal and bleed. In monoclonal
antibody technology, each can be independently immortalised.

Inbred strains of mice or rats are readily obtained, since these can
be maintained economically in large numbers. One such inbred strain,
(Balb/c) is susceptible to the induction of plasmacytomas (myelomas)
in the peritoneal cavity by the injection of mineral oils. These cells
grow indefinitely in culture. Any antibody they make reflects the
unknown specificity of the original cell immortalised by the mineral
oil and is of no general interest. Subclones which secrete no antibody
can generally be selected.

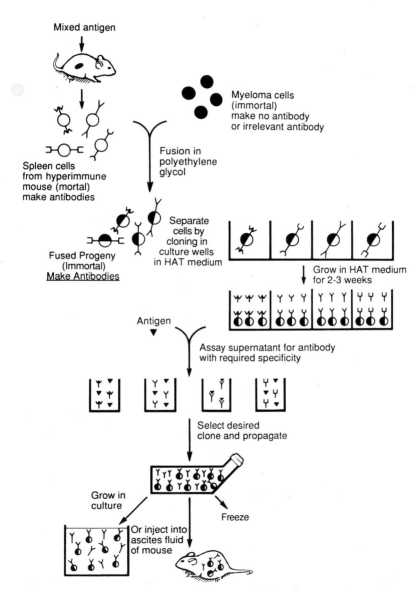

Fig. 1.2. The general procedure for monoclonal antibody production in rodents.

If these immortalised cells producing no antibody, or antibody of little interest, are then fused with the temporary population of spleen cells of a mouse responding to antigen (Fig. 1.2) then it is possible to freeze the optimal response of the spleen cells in time and isolate a series of hybridoma clones of immortalised cells which each individually produce any or all of the antibodies shown in Fig. 1.1.

Various additional technical requirements are essential components of the main process and these are discussed in succeeding chapters.

1.2.2. Comparison of monoclonal antibodies with conventional antiserum

Despite advances which can greatly reduce the cost of Mab production to simple antigens, it remains an expensive procedure in comparison to production of polyclonal antisera. It is only sensible to consider what advantages may therefore be realistically gained in the production of Mabs as opposed to polyclonal sera which can be absorbed against any known interfering antigens to give a good reagent for many purposes. Table 1.1 gives an overall comparison between the two strategies. The main feature of monoclonal antibodies which cannot be overemphasised, is that their quality is highly variable. In analogy with serum, it is possible to generate high-affinity monospecific Mabs but also low-affinity polyspecific Mabs. The skill in Mab technology lies in the selection of only those clones which secrete monospecific high-affinity antibodies. The more complex the antigen, the more skill is required for this task.

1.3. Specificity/affinity – the contribution of monoclonal antibody

1.3.1. The nature of the antibody-antigen reaction

All the classical work on antibody-antigen interactions, relates to the interaction of haptens, frequently cross-linked at high density to a

TABLE 1.1

Comparison between polyclonal antiserum and high- or low-affinity Mabs

	Polyclonal antiserum	Low-affinity Mab	High-affinity Mab
Determinants	Many	Several	One
Specificity	Highly polyspecific	Polyspecific	Monospecific
Affinity	Variable	Low	High
Contaminating immunoglobulin	High	Low	Low
Yield	High	Low	Low
Cost	Low	High	High
Standard nature	Variable with animal and bleed	Standard	Standard
Potential utility	Medium	Very low	Very high

protein and then assayed against the relevant antibody. Frequently, the subsequent kinetic or crystallographic analyses were on free hapten or hapten bound to a different protein. The antibody preparation itself was classically either a polyclonal one or a myeloma protein which chanced to bind the hapten at low affinity (e.g., Richards et al., 1975). The general applicability of such studies is clearly becoming limited as new information emerges on high-affinity protein – Mab contacts in cases where the Mab was specifically selected to bind that protein.

In the 1980s five detailed crystallographic studies were published showing, for the first time, exactly how a high-avidity Fab fragment of an IgG monoclonal antibody reacts with its antigen – three with lysosyome as antigen and two with influenza neuraminidase (Reviewed in Laver et al., 1990; Davies and Padlan, 1990). The data showed that the interaction was much more extensive than had previously been envisaged and emphasised the power of the innate immune system to mature a weak initial immune response to a high-affinity one involving over 90 contacts between 15–20 amino acids on a variety of structural loops of both molecules. None of the antibodies recognised 'linear' epitopes – a fact which has obvious implications in the generation of antibodies to peptides. These new observations made it clear that earlier conclusions from the myeloma/ hapten systems, suggesting that simple rules for Ab-Ag binding could be developed were naive. In reality, all forms of bonding mediating protein – protein interactions are used and possibly unfortunately, hydrophobic residues which can have less precisely predicted angles for protein engineering, form a major component. An additional, and highly relevant observation was that in the majority of these cases (Colman et al., 1987; Bhat et al., 1990), the antigen and possibly also the antibody, changes structure on interaction much as enzymes do with their substrates – in the nature of a handshake rather than a 'lock and key' mechanism.

1.3.2. A single monoclonal antibody can react with several dissimilar antigens

The above studies emphasise the fact that, while it is possible to produce high-affinity Mabs, it is possible to produce low-affinity ones where the variable region has 'spare capacity' to bind antigens with no similarity to the chosen one. Unfortunately, modern assay techniques make it all too easy to detect low-affinity contacts which do not reflect the immune response in the animal and, if immortalised, yield useless Mabs (Fig. 1.3). IgM Mabs are particularly likely to have this additional capacity to bind to irrelevant antigens because of their local high density of antibody binding sites (see Figs. 2.1, 2.4 and 2.5). With the occasional exception for precise use, IgM Mabs should always be regarded as unreliable and IgG Mabs should be selected (Section 2.2).

It is important to emphasise that a low-affinity Mab does not bind to **all** other antigens. There is simply a raised statistical chance of it being able to bind a much larger percentage of epitopes in irrelevant material, especially if this is presented at high density.

1.4. Specificity/affinity – the contribution of antigen

1.4.1. Avoiding making Mabs to similar antigens

This is self evident and essentially relies on the common sense of the investigator who, having selected conditions for obtaining only high-

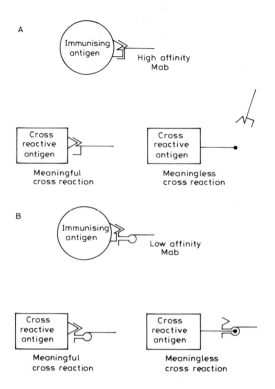

Fig. 1.3. The importance of making a high-affinity monoclonal antibody. (A) High-affinity (IgG) Mab binding to the original antigen at high-affinity. This Mab will usually only cross-react with other antigens which bear all or part of the original epitope. (B) Low-affinity (IgM) Mab which has poor contact with the original antigen. This Mab has spare capacity in its binding site and will cross-react with other antigens which bear no structural similarity to the original antigen.

affinity antibodies, must screen intelligently with all known potentially cross-reactive antigens and always be aware that another such antigen may be present in a complex mixture. If an antibody specific to an enzyme which shares structural motifs with another enzyme is required, then both enzymes should be cross-screened. If, for example, an antibody specific to isocitrate dehydrogenase is required, polyclonal serum will give significant but largely absorbable cross-reaction with lactate dehydrogenase. If the emerging Mabs from the fusion are selected to bind only to isocitrate dehydrogenase, then the final product will also do so and give a good reagent, superior to polyclonal antiserum.

If, however, the emerging Mabs from the fusion are selected without reference to other dehydrogenases, then there is a danger of producing Mabs which react with common protein motifs in the NAD binding site (Fig. 1.4). This Mab will cross-react to a much greater extent between all dehydrogenases than polyclonal antiserum raised against a single dehydrogenase where the polyclonal averaging effect will include binding to epitopes across the molecule. (It could, of course, be an excellent reagent for selecting a pool of dehydrogenases from an unknown mixture of enzymes if that is what is required – the important fact is to know what you want and select for it.)

1.4.2. High epitope density antigens

Antigens with regularly repeating structure tend to encourage low-affinity binding. Even IgG Mabs selected against a 'high epitope density antigen' (e.g., bacterial LPS, structural proteins, nucleic acids, or soluble proteins and peptides presented at too high a density on an

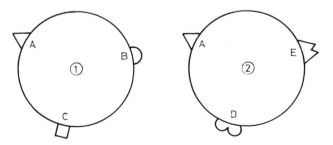

Fig. 1.4. The importance of intelligent selection procedures. (i) Largely dissimilar antigens. Antigens 1 and 2 are largely dissimilar but share epitope A. Polyclonal antiserum will cross-react only slightly between the two antigens. Mabs selected for binding to epitopes B and C or D and E will not cross-react. A Mab selected for binding to A will cross-react 100%.

ELISA plate), then they may also bind to irrelevant antigens. The critical factor is the local *molarity* of the epitope and antibody combining region. This vital area is further expanded in Chapter 2 where strategies for selecting only high affinity IgG Mabs are detailed.

1.4.3. Examples of bad Mabs

The doomsday scenario Mab is an IgM to an antigen such as DNA, actin, a polymeric carbohydrate antigen, or a peptide presented in molar amounts on a 'pin', selected on ELISA or dot-blot (Chapter 2). The true affinity of this Mab for the antigen is likely to be vanishingly low and the Mab may be expected to cross-react with a high percentage of other molecules tested including others in the group (e.g., the anti-DNA Mab will probably cross-react with the structural protein).

1.5. Specificity/affinity – the contribution of the assay system

Antibodies do not have a 'unique specificity' They are specific within a defined range of conditions. This is particularly relevant to 'epitope mapping' (Section 11.4) where an abnormally high concentration of an individual Mab is exposed to an artificially high concentration of peptides (inevitably on an ELISA assay which tends to amplify such non-specific interactions – Fig. 2.4) and occasionally shows an irrelevant, low-affinity binding to one of these. Forced up against the wall of an ELISA plate against molar concentrations of test reagent, even the best Mab may show very low-affinity binding but this will bear no relevance to its original eliciting epitope.

The final use of a Mab has to be maintained within the objectives of the laboratory throughout the production and test procedures. It is comparatively simple to demonstrate binding of any antigen to a host of Mabs on any assay system, but much more difficult to prove that the generated antibody has the required affinity and specificity profile for final intended use of the Mab (Chapter 2). A 'washing' (heterogeneous) assay will detect higher affinity (and higher specificity) Mabs and the more washes, the higher the affinity of Mab detected. A 'non-washing' (homogeneous) assay may give excellent results with the chosen antigen but show extensive cross-reactions. In applied terms, an antibody carefully isolated by ELISA assay to react with all forms of *Salmonella typhi* may well be of very little use as a probe to detect *Salmonella* in dubious duck liver pate if it is incorporated into a non-washing electrochemical immunosensor (Chapter 12), and an antibody carefully selected to bind only to tumour cells on an immunocytochemical assay may have limited application on injection into the human body if it should have even transient affinity for, say, the vast amounts of human cell surface antigens or structural proteins on the vascular epithelium which it will inevitably encounter on its journey to the tumour site.

1.6. Pooling of Mabs

Pooling of carefully selected Mabs may seem to be an illogical action but is not always so. Mabs are standard reagents whereas polyclonal serum is variable. While Mabs should never be pooled randomly, a defined pool of Mabs is a standard reagent which may be of value in several precisely defined situations.

1.6.1. Pooling of high-affinity Mabs to give comprehensive cover

Particularly in the case of viral isolates, or polymorphic (variable among individuals) antigens, a reagent which detects all forms including minor forms which may have been subject to mutation is required. Any individual Mab is at risk of being over-specific in this situation and therefore panels of Mabs, which should all be high affinity, can be used (Fig. 1.5).

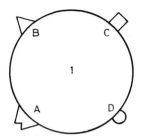 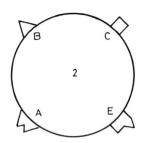

Fig. 1.5. The importance of intelligent selection procedures. (ii) Largely similar antigens. Antigens 1 and 2 are largely similar but differ in epitopes D and E. Polyclonal serum will cross-react extensively between the two and Mabs to A, B and C will cross-react 100%. However, Mabs to D and E will not recognise both antigens.

1.6.2. Pooling of high-affinity Mabs to further increase affinity

In certain highly defined cases where protein antigens are involved, pooling of high-affinity Mabs can increase affinity by mutual steric reinforcement and is reported to increase assay detectability limits (Ehrlich et al., 1982) (Fig. 1.6).

1.6.3. Pooling of Mabs to precipitate antigen

Precipitation of antigen requires a network of antibodies cross-linking with each other. With the exception of high epitope density antigens, Mabs rarely cross-link antigens sufficiently to precipitate by themselves, but will readily do so with the help of a second antibody (Section 11.2.4). While, in general, this use of a second antibody is preferable to using pools, judicious pooling can yield a precipitating Mab population.

1.6.4. Pooling of low-affinity Mabs to attempt to give a high-affinity reagent

Antigens for which a high-affinity Mab cannot be obtained (because they are high epitope density or because it is impossible to hyperim-

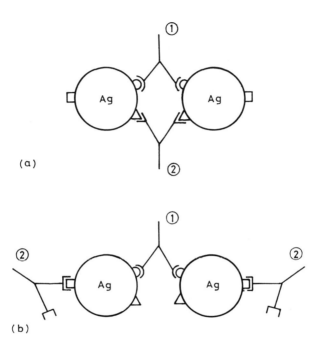

Fig. 1.6. Possible cooperative effects of Mabs. This occurs particularly in solution type assays. In (a) the geometry of each Mab-antigen complex is such that the two Mabs can act cooperatively stabilising the binding of each other. As a result the two Mabs together have a higher affinity than would be expected from a mixture. In (b) the position of the epitopes is such that cooperative binding does not occur.

munise with them) can be used to generate low-affinity Mabs which are then pooled. The basis of this is the theory of Talmage (1959) on the nature of polyclonal antibodies. In modern Mab terms, if it is impossible to be certain of a high-affinity Mabs, then pooling might provide a more reliable reagent. If selection processes fail to yield a high-affinity, high-specificity antibody but instead yields a panel of lower grade antibodies, then these may be pooled by the logic in Table 1.2. Unless the Mabs are very carefully selected, this can prove to be rather an expensive way of generating low-grade polyclonal antiserum.

TABLE 1.2

Last resort pooling strategy for polyspecific antibodies

Mab 1	Binds to antigens A, B and C
Mab 2	Binds to antigens A, D and E
Mab 3	Binds to antigens A, F and G
Mab 4	Binds to antigens A, H and I

An equal mixture of Mabs 1–4 binds predominantly to A.

1.7. The standard nature of Mabs

It is almost impossible to overestimate the value of the standard nature of Mabs. In a world increasingly subject to litigation, any final diagnostic system must be reliable and perform within the stated claims. The sheer variability of polyclonal antiserum makes it a very difficult reagent to use for this purpose. The fact that Mabs are continuously available as reliable reagents which always give the same data has made quality control systems very much easier to operate.

1.8. Yield and purity

Over the last few years there has been extensive research into methods of making Mabs in large amounts at minimal cost. These are discussed further in Chapters 9 and 10 and basically can be divided into categories according to requirements. The economical method of generating large amounts of Mab of limited purity is to do so in the ascites fluid of histocompatible mice. The preferred industrial method of generating large amounts has been bulk tissue culture, frequently in encapsulated or hollow fibre systems. Current strategies for generating large amounts involve expressing the cloned antibody genes in high producing eukaryote systems such as plants or baculoviruses. It should, however be strongly emphasised that only a very small number of Mabs are ever of the quality to merit production in such quantity.

1.9. Human monoclonal antibodies (HuMabs)

1.9.1. The requirement for human Mabs

There are two main perceived requirements for a human Mab. The first and financially the most important is for immunotherapy. Serotherapy in general has become less acceptable with the increasing understanding of blood borne diseases such as HIV and therapy with fully tested Mabs is much preferable. Mouse Mabs were originally thought to possibly be capable of filling this role. However, the requirement for human Mabs has become more clear as the extent of the toxic side effects of mouse Mab therapy have become apparent (see Section 1.12 below). In addition, mouse Mabs cannot be used in a continuous treatment regime as they are rejected by the human immune system. To some extent this has meant that 'partial responses' claimed for therapy of, say, tumours in man, cannot be truly evaluated since the logical clinical progression of giving a second dose of mouse Mab is precluded. In consequence, there are a large number of monoclonal antibodies recorded in the early literature claimed to have 'potential' which could not be further tested at the time because they were of murine origin.

The second requirement for human Mabs is to immortalise the specific human immune response. This may well overlap with the first requirement since the human immune response is considered to be more relevant than the rodent one for the generation of a reagent which may be useful in therapy. However, cases where the mouse response is known to be inappropriate and the genuine human response must therefore be immortalised include the case of rhesus antigens detailed below and also of the human HLA antigens. Since the mouse response to human HLA antigens is known to be dominated by a murine spectrum of antibodies to competing antigens which are foreign to mouse (but not man), mouse anti-HLA antibodies cannot be generated by conventional rodent techniques. Even known pure HLA antigens are seldom antigenic outwith their membrane context and injected purified from an SDS gel will give few useful typing antibodies. It is suggested that PCR (Chapter 9) of variable regions may yield new HLA typing reagents which detect at the genomic level. In the meantime current typing reagents for human HLA antigens are obtained from multiparous women or multiple blood transfusion recipients. The supply is variable in quality and quantity and 'tissue typing' of any individual incurs costs in excess of £ 200 (1991 prices) in the U.K. High-affinity, non-IgM isotype, human derived Mabs for HLA typing would therefore be extremely valuable reagents.

1.9.2. Background of HuMab 1980s developments

Human monoclonal antibody production has proved to be a very much more complex task than mouse Mab production. The reasons are given in Chapter 3 and relate to the difficulty of hyperimmunising humans with the relevant antigen and the lack of availability of a human cell line which gives stable fusions as does the P3K parent of all the mouse cell lines. In addition, in the case of human anti-tumour Mabs, a large number of polyreactive IgMs binding to common cytoskeletal proteins before the importance of screening on whole cells for IgG Mabs was fully appreciated (Section 2.6).

There are two basic current strategies. The first is to make 'genuine' human Mabs by transforming cells with Epstein-Barr Virus (EBV) and then stabilise them by repeated cloning or backfusion (Chapters 7 and 8). The second is to take a mouse Mab and 'humanise' it by attaching the constant chain regions of a human myeloma protein to the variable region of the mouse Mab (Morrison et al., 1984; Neuberger et al., 1985; Riechmann et al., 1988; LoBuglio et al., 1989; Hardman et al., 1989; Queen et al., 1990) (Chapter 9).

It is important to understand that the two techniques generate Mabs to different antigens and the former may be essential for some tasks (Fig. 1.7). Antibodies to the Rhesus antigens give the illustration. (The Rhesus antigen situation is however much more complex than described below and more advanced haematology or immunology texts should be consulted for more details.) Rh+ individuals are tolerised to the rhesus factor and do not respond to it. Rh− individu-

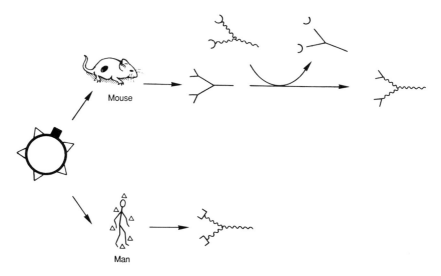

Fig. 1.7. The two strategies for human Mab production yield different Mabs. On the top line is the strategy for 'humanising' mouse Mabs. The mouse has responded to a major foreign human antigen which may not be the antigen to which a human Mab is required. On the bottom line, is a human, who sees the major antigen (triangle) as self and responds only to the minor antigen giving a 'genuine human' Mab to this minor antigen.

als only encounter the Rhesus factors in a faulty blood transfusion or, for women, if they give birth to an Rh+ child of the same ABO blood grouping. There is a requirement for human Mabs to give to Rh− mothers immediately after giving birth to ABO matched Rh+ infants to suppress the generation of anti-Rh antibodies in the mother, since such antibodies will cross the placenta and damage the second Rh+ child. However, human red blood cells injected into a mouse lead to a response which is dominated by antibodies to the human ABO blood group antigens. Thus, it is not possible to make Mabs to Rhesus factors in mice and the rare Rh− human volunteer carrying antibodies to the Rhesus factor is the only source. In consequence, groups working in the Rhesus area have persevered with the complex and unrewarding human technology and produced 'genuine' human Mabs (Melamed et al., 1987; Foung et al., 1987; Goosens et al., 1987; Kumpel et al., 1989a,b; Thomson et al., 1990).

In addition, several groups have produced 'genuine' human Mabs to tetanus toxoid (Kozbor and Roder, 1981; Boyd et al., 1984; Tiebout et al., 1984; Lanzavecchia, 1985). Both tetanus toxoid and Rhesus have the advantage that the human can be immunised and boosted to produce IgG antibodies (Section 3.6). In recent times, human Mabs from patients with high titres of common viral infections, notably HIV (Gorny et al., 1989; Robinson et al., 1990) and also CMV have also been obtained.

'Humanised' Mabs (Chapter 9) are different from 'genuine' human Mabs in that they detect the same antigens as the originally immunised mouse. Such antigens may not have been foreign to humans but are foreign to the mouse. Where the antigen is a well defined protein, the 'humanising' technology is potentially an immensely useful technique. However, where the antigen is not identified and characterised before 'humanising', there is a danger of producing 'humanised' Mabs which are not only useless, but also possibly harmful (by analogy with the Rhesus system above, this approach without previous knowledge, would yield Mabs to the ABO antigens which would damage the patient if applied in extensive therapy). It is possible that some of the 'humanised' Mabs to the high molecular weight carbohydrate material coating tumour cells may fall into this category.

1.9.3. Anticipated future developments

The availability of Polymerase Chain Reaction (PCR) makes it possible to consider generation of 'genuine' human Mabs by immortalising genuine human B lymphocyte responses at an early stage and at comparatively low cost. The various methods of approaching this are discussed in Section 9.6.

An even more artificial but potentially successful development of 'humanised' Mabs involves the grafting of variable regions with sequences involved in virus receptor recognition onto the constant regions of a human myeloma, thus creating an ideally and totally artificially designed HuMab (immunoadhesin – Capon et al., 1989). It is possibly unfortunate that such constructs, which have considerable potential to attack many other antigens successfully, have been designed largely to attack the HIV virus which is prone to immunological enhancement (Section 1.12.3). Immunological enhancement is a method by which a small compartment of the antibody response is believed to enable live virus to insert into host cells by virtue of binding to, and internalisation by, Fc receptors. It does not apply to the majority of viruses, to bacteria or to tumour cells and even for a single virus, does not apply to the majority of Mabs.

1.10. Chimaeric bifunctional monoclonal antibodies

Chimaeric antibodies which encompass rodent variable regions and human constant regions are regeants with considerable potential (Section 1.9 above). A second type of chimaeric hetero bifunctional antibody has been less successful to date for obvious reasons. This is either

(a) A Mab produced by a fusion of one Mab producing cell with another (for example a cell producing a Mab to specific antigen and a cell producing a Mab to an effector antigen). This can also be known as a 'quadroma'. Thus a Mab which has one arm specific for a tumour antigen and the other specific for an effector drug can be constructed. The presumed advantage is that, for in vivo therapy, the effector drug need not be administered until the antibody has localised within the target tissue and detrimental effects of non-specific binding will be avoided. The major disadvantage, dilution of specificity, will be apparent from inspection of Fig. 3.1 but in addition the magnification of bivalency is often lost (Section 2.2).

The technique may be developed further to create heterobifunctional 'humanised' Mabs in which the murine constant regions have been replaced by human constant regions and the two transfectomas produced have then been fused to yield humanised Mabs binding to two different antigens (Phelps et al., 1990).

(b) A double Mab may also be produced by chemical cross-linking between the constant chains of a Mab directed to a specific antigen to those of a Mab directed to an effector molecule or cell, thus retaining bivalence. The concept of any Mab-bound protein being lethal to the target cell now seems outdated in the light of modern knowledge of endocytosis and protein traffic within the cell. The alternative idea, of using such Mabs to artificially cross-link proteins and whole cells such as cytotoxic T cells, seems irrelevant in the current context of understanding of T cell recognition of antigen (Section 4.1).

1.11. Applications of Mabs – Diagnostic

1.11.1. Clinical diagnosis of soluble antigens

To a considerable extent, Mabs have replaced polyclonal antisera for this task in hospital laboratories. There are only two basic assay types — either double Mab 'sandwich' assays (Fig. 1.8) or single Mab la-

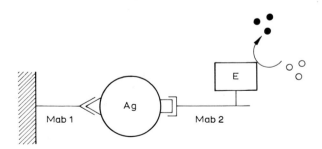

Fig. 1.8. The basic 'sandwich' assay for detection of antigen. One Mab attaches the antigen to a solid matrix while the other carries the detection system (in this case an enzyme). This is probably the best system for antigen detection. If one Mab binds irrelevant material, the other is unlikely to bind *the same* irrelevant material.

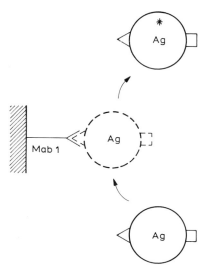

Fig. 1.9. The basic 'competition' assay. Antigen from the test sample replaces antigen attached to the detection system. The competition assay can also involve a Mab attached to the detection system being dislodged by a Mab attached to antigen from the sample. The same principles apply. This system is less precise than the sandwich system in Fig. 1.8 but the only one available for small antigens which cannot accommodate two high-affinity Mabs simultaneously.

belled antigen competition assays (Fig. 1.9). The former has the attractive quality of two different Mabs to distant epitopes on the molecule which minimises the chances of cross-reactivity with an irrelevant antigen. It also carries potentially lower 'detectability' limits (Section 2.1 and Ekins et al., 1989). The latter is more useful for small antigens where two independent Mab epitopes are unlikely to be available for steric reasons. The competition assay can also be replaced with labelled Mab rather than antigen but it remains a single Mab assay and therefore a lower quality assay than the sandwich one. (See also patent section 1.17.)

Entire volumes are written on the subject of immunoassay including two in this series (Tijssen, 1985; Chard, 1990). It is sufficient to refer the reader to the extent to which such books increasingly base the assay systems described on monoclonal rather than polyclonal systems. However, assay of Mabs is extensively covered in Chapter 2 of this book and includes application to the generation of Mabs to such antigens. In addition, the first generation immunological biosensors (Chapter 12) have tended to involve such comparatively simple antigens.

1.11.2. Diagnosis of pathogenic bacteria, viruses and parasites

This is again a situation in which Mabs have greatly simplified diagnosis. Bacterial, viral and parasitic isolates have been, and can continue to be, typed with much greater precision which allows disease spread to be mapped and epidemics to be detected and monitored with greater speed and efficiency. While the original motivation behind this was to identify blocking or protective antigens which might be useful in vaccine development strategies (Section 1.13), the diagnostic value has largely overtaken the potential therapeutic value.

1.11.3. Cell surface antigens and the CD system

The CD (Cluster Designation) system for identification of human cells of haemopoietic lineage is one of the most advanced demonstrations of the extent to which Mabs can be used to chart cell phenotype and differentiation status. The system is a result of international workshops which meet regularly to group together monoclonal antibodies produced in different laboratories with the same antigen recognition characteristics. This 'Cluster' of Mabs is then assigned a number according to the type of molecule identified by all the Mabs in the group. In consequence, the CD status of a molecule also defines the antigen itself. Such antigens not only define cell phenotype and lineage, but also the activation status of the cell bearing that phenotype and its possession of molecules with the ability to adhere to other cells through the LFA, ICAM and VLA family of adhesion molecules (Springer, 1990). At the 4th International Workshop in 1989 the number of antigens defined in this way rose to a CD value of 78, with many having newly discovered subsets so that the total number of defined molecules is now close to 100. In many ways this is one of the most sophisticated diagnostic uses of Mabs to date and there is, in principle, no reason why it should not also be possible to type other cell lineages in this manner. The clinical implications have been considerable. To give only three among a myriad of examples:

(1) The knowledge that the HIV virus infects helper T cells is as a direct result of the ability to generate Mabs which define its marker CD4 molecule and give the clinician consequent ability to monitor this disease.

(2) The immune status of localised lymphocyte deposits in a wide variety of diseases can be estimated. Thus the lymphocytes within a tumour, within a transplanted organ, or within arthritic joints can be assessed for phenotype and activation status with the relevant populations then being isolated and immortalised.

(3) Several CD antigens such as such as CALLA (CD9) and Campath (CDw52) have been target antigens for leukaemia therapy.

The full current CD designation can be found in Knapp et al. (1989) and a truncated version showing the best known is given in Table 1.3. It is worth noting that the CD system is almost exclusively addressed to cell surface glycoproteins. This reflects the extent to which live cells are used for FACS screening, the procedure preferentially recommended in this book for cell membrane proteins.

1.11.4. Diagnostic applications with cell surface antigens other than leucocyte cell surface antigens

Such cells have the potential for classification in a system such as the CD system described above. Technically, they present greater but nonetheless soluble problems. Many of the CD antigens were detected by Mabs generated from animals immunised with whole leucocyte cell populations, or purified membrane preparations. Whereas leuco-

TABLE 1.3

The CD classification of human leucocyte differentiation antigens

CD	Antigen	Location	Function where known
1a	49Kgp	Thy,B, Dend	
1b	45Kgp	Thy,B, Dend	
1c	43Kgp	Thy,B, Dend	
2	50Kgp	T	Rosette receptor, LFA-3 receptor
3	5 protein complex	T	Signal transduction for TCR
4	59Kgp	T helper	MHC Class II recognition
5	67Kgp	T,B subset	
6	90Kgp	T,B subset	
7	40Kgp	T	
8	32Kgp dimer	T cyto/sup	MHC Class I recognition
9	24K	prc-B, Mono, Plt	
10	90Kgp	pre-B	CALLA
11a	180Kgp	leucocytes	α-chain of LFA-1
11b	155Kgp	Mono, Gran, NK	C3b complement receptor
11c	150Kgp	Mono, Gran, NK	
13	150Kgp	Mono, Gran	
14	55Kgp	Mono, (Gran)	
15	CHO	Gran(mono)	
16	50-60Kgp	Gran, NK	Fc γ-receptor III
18	96Kgp	Leucocytes	β-chain for 11a, b and c
19	95Kgp	B cells	
20	35Kgp	B cells	
21	140K	B subset	EBV receptor, C3d receptor
22	135Kgp	B subset	
23	45Kgp	Activated B	Low-affinity IgE receptor
25	55Kgp	Activated T	TAC,Il-2 receptor, β-chain
28	44Kgp	T subset	
29	135Kgp	Broad	VLA beta
32(w)	40Kgp	Mono, Gran, B	Fc γ-receptor II
35	220Kgp	Gran, Mono, B	Complement Receptor I
45		Leucocytes	Leucocyte Common Antigen
45RA	220Kgp	T subset, B, Gran, Mono	
45RB		T subset, B, Gran, Mono	
45RO	180Kgp	T subset, B, Gran, Mono	
52(w)	21–28Kgp	Leucocytes	Campath I
54		Broad	ICAM-1
58	40–65Kgp	Leucocytes, epithelial	LFA-3
71	97Kgp	Growing cells	Transferrin receptor

CALLA = common acute lymphoblastic leukemias antigen; Dend = dendritic cells; gp = glycoprotein; Gran = granulocytes; ICAM = intercellular adhesion molecule; LFA = lymphocyte function antigen; Mono = monocytes; Plt = platelets; TCR = T cell receptor; Thy = thymocytes; VLA = very late antigen; w = workshop.

cytes grow freely in culture, most other cell types grow adherently in vivo and in vitro, secreting extracellular matrix material which is not generally very specific to cell phenotype. The material required to form these extracellular adhering matrices is highly antigenic and can dominate a fusion to the exclusion of the detection of cell surface proteins (see the analogy with rhesus antigens described in Fig. 1.7). Immunocytochemical assays distinguish poorly between Mabs to the matrix and Mabs to the cell surface proteins and the former again bias the panel of Mabs generated. Strategies which involve partial purification of genuine cell surface specific antigens to use for immunisation for Mab production are therefore likely to be necessary. Up until now, while the approaches involving partially purified membranes tend to lead to contamination with such immunodominant molecules, those involving SDS PAGE and other electrophoretic techniques tend to yield Mabs to denatured proteins, not detectable in the complex conformation adopted in cell membranes. Techniques which allow the isolation of pure membrane proteins without contamination or structural alteration are required.

With respect to intracellular proteins, adherent cells have a more complex range of cytoskeletal proteins to control their architecture than do lymphocytes. In the same way that the cell surface Mab population has been dominated by proteins to secreted matrices, so the intracellular Mab populations generated have been dominated by the major antigenic cytoskeletal proteins and it is likely that antigens purified free of these will be required before minor antigens can be detected. At the moment, interest has centred on the detection of known molecules such as oncogene products and growth factor or hormone receptors with Mabs made to the purified molecule. This approach has value, but does not detect new oncogene products, or growth factor and hormone receptors which may obviously be of interest. Unlike cell surface proteins, many of these may have a conformation which does not require membrane stabilisation. They are, however, present in very small amounts.

1.11.5. Diagnostics – personal kits

There is reported to be a massive potential market in the developed world for inexpensive personal diagnostic systems to be used by travellers or individuals who are likely to undergo hazardous experiences. The ideal end product is a personalised probe, possibly with a small reusable component, which can be used to test food, water or body secretions for a reliable and quick personal diagnosis by an untrained operator. Ideally for the 1980s obsession with personalised electronic gadgets, at any rate, such a probe should respond with an electronic noise or display on a small monitor. Pregnancy and ovulation diagnosis with Mabs have largely achieved this aim, although electronic attachments have proved unnecessary (Chapter 12). However, these particular detection systems are directed to protein samples in urine which is low in contaminating high molecular weight or particulate material in comparison to serum, secretions, whole cells, soil samples, foodstuffs etc. Detection of antibodies in these more complex samples at high resolution remains to be demonstrated for a personalised kit.

1.11.6. Diagnostics – forensic applications

These are extensive and, in addition to many of the viral, bacterial and diagnostic applications, include
(i) Detection of undeclared additives in food and drink.
(ii) Detection of irregular trace reagents in 'patent busting' products such as perfumes or whiskies from an illicit source.
(iii) Detection of small quantities of illicit drugs in medicines.
(iv) Detection of potentially explosive material.
It will be evident that these all involve trace antigens and require a highly monospecific IgG detecting system. This is often coupled to a thin layer chromatography system or a filter system which selectively concentrates antigen.

1.11.7. Diagnostics – immunoscintigraphy for in vivo tumour diagnosis

Mabs have been extensively employed in this clinical area, sometimes successfully (reviewed by Foon, 1989). This area, like the therapeutic Mab area, has been inhibited by individual research groups insisting on making and using only their own Mabs with inadequate external intellectual contact and thus assuming that all Mabs are monospecific in all environments (Sections 1.3 and 2.2). Indeed some notionally 'anti-tumour Mabs' were simultaneously claimed to be able to detect shed tumour antigen in blood for speedy tumour diagnosis while also being claimed to be able to localise the same tumours in the body. The fact that the two claims were incompatible was ignored and industrial companies were happy to take up both possibilities. Such multiple early claims damaged the anti-tumour Mab field with industrial managers and this is a pity as good Mabs have considerable diagnostic potential.

Mabs presented with an in vivo environment have a much wider challenge than on a slide of fixed tissue or an ELISA plate. Even the lowest affinity for, say, an ABO blood group antigen means that the Mab will be immobilised and internalised to the liver by the reticuloendothelial system because of the massive amount of ABO RBCs in the circulation (Section 1.9.2, above). Even the smallest affinity for an abundant protein lining the vasculatory system will lead to diffuse distribution because successive amounts of antibody will be diverted on the route to intended antigen (Section 1.5). These are likely contributors to the facts that the half life of human Mabs in patients is highly variable, and that in most patients a very small amount finally, if ever localises on the antigen, and often takes several days to do so. The current clinical requirements by many ethical committees for test in nude or SCID mice do not encompass the possibility of many of such non-obvious cross-reactions.

Most of the in vivo studies to date have used established mouse Mabs which are labelled with a gamma emitting isotope such as ^{111}-indium, ^{99}technicium or ^{123}iodine. In addition, ^{131}I is used for both imaging and potential therapy (see below). The basic principle is that such methods may be able to locate occult metastatic deposits not visible in the increasing variety of non-antibody based scanning methods such as CATscans and magnetic resonance imaging. Most of the data to date suggest that while the appropriate Mabs can locate tumour deposits in many patients, they do not do so in 100% of patients and in consequence they have to be used in conjunction with other scanning methods. It is possible that, as the importance of using high-affinity IgG Mabs rather than using the first Mab on offer becomes appreciated, single Mabs or even wider pools of Mabs will improve this success rate in the future. Given the increasing commercial pressure on health authorities not to indulge in high technology work without proven justification, it will be necessary for Mabs to be more closely evaluated.

1.12. Therapeutic applications

1.12.1. Introduction

In terms of both the commercial market and the media, the massive revolution caused by Mabs in basic diagnostic research and the commercial sector largely might not have taken place. It is the concept of the Mab as a 'magic bullet' , capable of obliterating an infectious agent or tumour which remains dominant. The general public interest in, and projected commercial market for, therapeutic Mabs is many orders of magnitude greater than for diagnostics. A patient can be diagnosed to have a disease with a few nanograms of antibody but if Mab treatment is a realistic possibility for his condition, he may require up to gram amounts for therapy. The slight irony for the Mab technologist is that high-affinity Mabs may well offer inexpensive and specific therapy but they have been somewhat abused by the haste of many sectors of the biotechnology industry to achieve a marketable reagent before their competitors and, in consequence, offering inferior reagents to the market.

To a considerable extent, the scientific community at all levels responded to the potential use of Mabs in the 1980s by producing new methods of increasing the yield of the already extensive range of anti-bodies to small soluble proteins such as hen eggwhite lysosyme (HEL), or keyhole limpet haemocyanin (KLH) in the mouse and, where human Mabs were involved, to tetanus toxin, justifying these as 'model systems'.

However, with the exception of bacterial toxins, relevant target antigens were (and are) presented on complex organisms such as viruses, bacteria and whole cells and such antigens present a much greater challenge than small soluble proteins both to the immune system and the Mab technologist seeking to produce high-affinity monospecific reagents.

1.12.2. Therapy for bacterial infection

Bacterial disease is not perceived as a major problem in the developed world where the major causes of death are malignancy or failures of the cardiovascular system, both being diseases of comparatively elder-ly people. In the developing world, bacterial infections form the main contribution to mortality, particularly infant mortality, but the devel-oping world cannot afford expensive new generation reagents such as Mabs. Development of Mab techniques for bacterial infections has largely centred on areas such as sporadic outburst of public panic in food poisoning or legionella exposure, and neutralisation of toxins (see below).

Bacteria, being generally extracellular parasites, are naturally at-tacked predominantly by the antibody arm of the immune response. Evidence for this comes from individuals who lack the ability to gen-erate antibodies and are consequently more susceptible to bacterial at-tack but can cope with viral infection. Given antibiotics, such individ-uals can lead comparatively normal lives and the prevalence of low cost antibiotics has made Mabs largely uncompetitive in this area. High affinity Mabs directed against bacterial cell surface antigens might well be superior, albeit at higher cost, if they were capable of being delivered in the right place. This last is important as the requirement for many anti-bacterial responses is highly localised in, for example, the gut where localised delivery of Mabs of the relevant class (usually IgA) and effector function may be necessary. However, the application of Mabs in this direction is obviously limited by the competition from comparatively inexpensive alternatives encompassing not only antibiotics but also other types of inexpensive therapy – for example rehydration therapy for cholera. The approaches of Mab technology thought to have commercial potential for the developed world tend therefore to be currently focussed on Mabs to bacterial toxins and in particular endotoxin of gram negative bacteria (discussed further with respect to patents in Section 1.17) which causes systemic septic shock in postoperative or burn damaged patients.

1.12.3. Therapy for viral infection

Viruses are not, in a normal primary infection, generally controlled by antibodies but rather by cytotoxic T lymphocytes. Viruses largely replicate within cells where they are inaccessible to the antibody arm of the immune response and can often move between cells by encouraging an exhausted infectious cell to fuse with a new one, thus remaining inaccessible to antibody.

The cytotoxic T lymphocytes which recognise and kill virus infected cells do not appear to detect the viral coat proteins. These coat proteins were frequently used to elicit and monitor antibody responses to candidate coat protein vaccines of the 1980s. Instead, however, many cytotoxic T cells recognise a peptide derived from internal viral proteins such as the matrix or nucleoprotein, presented in a groove on Class I MHC antigens (Bjorkman et al., 1987). Thus the major natural response to viral infection involves a different constituency of molecules, all inaccessible to antibody. It is important to realise that by asking antibodies to tackle a viral infection without the support of the T lymphocyte arm of the immune response, the clinician is asking them to perform outwith their natural role.

Viruses enter their target cells by virtue of the virus coat protein being able to attach to a normal cell surface molecule which it uses as a 'receptor'. A consequent Mab based strategy has been to replace the variable regions of the Mab heavy chain with virus receptor sequences by the use of recombinant DNA technology. Logically, such a molecule (termed an immunoadhesin) should have the ability not only to bind free virus, but also to neutralise it by the use of the classic mechanisms of antibody dependent cellular cytotoxicity (ADCC) via Fc receptors or by invoking the considerable amplification offered by the complement cascade. While some Mabs appear to be able to perform this function in vitro, they frequently lack the capacity to make an impact in the more complex in vivo situation.

In addition, it is worth noting that some Mabs may not only be merely ineffective in controlling virus infection but can also assist the virus in gaining entry to cells (Section 1.9.3). Anti-viral antibodies including Mabs are occasionally capable of enhancing, rather than repressing the immune response to antigen (Bolognesi, 1989; Robinson et al., 1990). Selection procedures must therefore exclude this population of Mabs.

1.12.4. Therapy for tumours

1.12.4.1. Background
Before considering the use of Mabs as anti-tumour reagents, it is relevant to appreciate the primitive nature of most traditionally employed chemical anti-tumour reagents. These are generally directed against the molecules involved in DNA replication. Cells in the body grow at different rates and naturally fast growing cells which are adversely affected by such therapy include cells which generate fresh skin and hair tissue, cells of the gut epithelium and cells of the lymphoid system. Patients undergoing chemotherapy, have intestinal malfunction, distressing cutaneous manifestations and, above all a severely compromised immune system. In consequence, a concerned clinician always looks for more specific reagents directed to a smaller constituency of cells, and in particular avoiding destruction of cells of the immune system. The ideal reagent is one which still encompasses the tumour cell population and which will also make higher and poten-

tially more effective dosages tolerable. Mabs would appear to be the natural reagent to perform such a function. However, the consequences of therapy with mouse Mabs are not insignificant and side effects include fever, rash, urticaria and (in the case of Mabs to cells of haemopoietic lineage) myelosuppression. Such side effects limit the dosage. In addition, mouse Mabs are frequently rejected so that a programme of continuous therapy is not practicable (reviewed by Foon, 1989).

1.12.4.2. Therapy of leukaemia or lymphoma

Leucocyte phenotype during developmental progression is now well charted by the CD system described in Section 1.11 above. In leukaemia, there is generally a predominance of a population of abnormal lymphoid cells bearing only one or two CD antigens. Logically, it should be possible to attack such cells with a Mab directed to the leukaemia cells bearing this CD antigen. Therapy can even be performed ex vivo by removing the bone marrow population and destroying the cells which carry the relevant CD antigen before returning it to the irradiated patient. In vivo for lymphomas where solid deposits of tumour accumulate within lymphoid organs, a similar strategy can be applied by continuous infusion of antibody. Such an approach has largely been unsuccessful, at least one of the reasons being detailed in Fig. 1.10. The bulk of the tumour does not represent the original 'clonogenic' cell, but rather an outgrowing population derived from this cell but bearing different CD antigens (Greaves, 1982). However, if a human Mab is used, it should in theory be possible to repeat the therapy routinely to remove the tumour bulk.

As a consequence of some of the difficulties occasioned by using a single stage specific CD antigen as therapeutic target, a totally new strategy may be adopted (Hale et al., 1988). If a CD molecule with a wide representation throughout the leucocyte population is chosen as the Mab target, the patient will be severely immunocompromised. However, such a condition will only be temporary so long as the CD target is not expressed on the human haemopoietic stem cells and the patient will experience few of the side effects of cytotoxic drugs on the

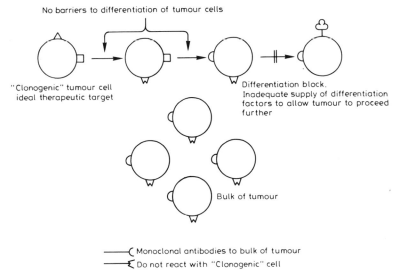

No barriers to differentiation of tumour cells

"Clonogenic" tumour cell
ideal therapeutic target

Differentiation block.
Inadequate supply of differentiation
factors to allow tumour to proceed
further

Bulk of tumour

Monoclonal antibodies to bulk of tumour
Do not react with "Clonogenic" cell

Fig. 1.10. Why Mab therapy fails. The bulk of the tumour has been generated from a small number of clonogenic cells which differentiate through several stages so that most of the cells in the tumour do not carry the relevant cell surface target molecules.

gut and skin. If the stem cells are unaffected by the Mab therapy, the immune system will regenerate within a few weeks. If, however, the stem cells are affected by the Mab therapy, the clinical outcome of such therapy will be poor. The final possibility is that the stem cells are themselves the clonogenic cell population, in which case therapy with Mabs is not a realistic possibility.

1.12.4.3. Therapy of solid tumours
Solid tumours present more complex problems. There are, as yet, few known cell surface lineage differentiation markers equivalent to the CD system of lymphoid cells. Such markers as are known (for example the EGF receptor) tend to be too widely distributed on normal cells to be a good therapeutic target. The greater number of attempts to date have been with mouse Mabs either alone, or attached to an isotope that emits localised destructive radiation such as [131]I. To re-

duce toxicity, rejection by the human immune system, and non-specific binding, the latter 'boosted' therapy is very often with the $F(ab)_2$ fragment (Fig. 9.2). There have been sporadic reports of complete responses and many of partial responses but the side effects can be considerable (see above) and the technique has not yet become firmly established in clinical programmes outside a small number of laboratories.

Therapeutic strategies have tended therefore to be based on the 'humanising' of mouse Mabs which themselves appear to detect poorly characterised tumour associated antigens. These carry the risk of all applications of such 'humanised' technology described in the rhesus example cited above (Section 1.9), i.e., being reactive with a natural 'self' antigen (Fig. 1.7). However, most reports of therapy of non-lymphoid tumours with human Mabs indicate that the adverse side effects experienced with mouse Mabs are greatly reduced or totally eliminated, although the tumour itself has not been reduced.

Most of the 'genuine human' Mabs to solid tumours were generated from blood B cells, assuming that a systemic response could be amplified. It is now clear that the peripheral blood B cell population is too diverse and polyspecific (Section 1.3) for such a task. New strategies are required for solid tumours. For example the IgG expressing B lymphocytes close to or integral to the tumour should be used (draining nodes, tumour infiltrating B cells etc).

1.12.5. Therapy for parasite diseases

This combines many of the problems in other types of therapy. Like tumour cells, parasites can regenerate if the source organism is not destroyed. In consequence, therapeutic Mabs are too expensive to contemplate on the vast scale in which such therapy would be required. Parasite diseases are common in underdeveloped countries which cannot afford expensive therapeutic techniques. Parasites are highly complex and parasite immunology remains in a comparatively primitive stage. This is clearly a situation where vaccination rather than therapy is the more appropriate prophylactic approach.

In consequence, there has been a search for protective or blocking antigens which might be useful in vaccine generation. The main problem with this approach is that it does not identify T cell epitopes. Classical parasitology has tended to identify diseases as 'T cell mediated' or 'B cell mediated' whereas modern understanding of the immune response suggests that both responses involve helper T cells detecting processed parasite antigen presented on host cells (See 1.13 below). Parasite immunologists have had to change strategy in light of the understanding that the antibody arm of the immune system is only a part of the total response.

1.13. Mabs in vaccine development strategies

1.13.1. Mabs as reagents to identify candidate vaccine molecules

As discussed above, in relation to parasites, Mabs can only identify part of the epitope involved in any vaccine, i.e., the B cell target epitope. Such concepts were superceded by the evidence that the immune response by cytotoxic T cells depends on a peptide of the antigen being presented in the 'groove' of Class I MHC molecules (Bjorkman et al., 1987) with clear indications that helper T cells operated by a similar mechanism involving Class II MHC antigens (Brown et al., 1988). Thus, any effective vaccine must also involve peptides presented to the immune system by MHC Class I antigens, and MHC Class II antigens (Chapter 4). Such peptides are particularly variable among the human population which has widely diverse MHC (HLA) antigens. In an outbred group of individuals infected with a virus, whether it be a herd of cattle, or a group of infected humans, any one individual may 'present' a 12–20 amino acid viral peptide derived from the viral matrix protein to cytotoxic T cells whereas another individual will present a totally dissimilar peptide from the viral nucleoprotein to cytotoxic T cells. It is assumed that the same process is likely to occur with helper T cell presentation by MHC class II antigens although different peptides will again be involved. As a result, recombinant DNA vaccines using a single peptide or protein identi-fied by a single Mab are of limited value and T cell epitopes covering all major Class I and Class II MHC binding peptides within the anti-gen must also be incorporated.

Mabs again have therefore more a research role in such cases. Mabs to major and minor MHC antigens are required to precipitate them and lead to the subsequent determination of which peptide is present in the groove. In addition, human EBV transformants from a wide range of patients provide immortalised B cell clones as highly efficient 'antigen presenting' systems for the study of the mechanism of antigen internalisation and processing.

1.13.2. Mabs alone as vaccines

The concept of Mabs themselves as vaccines was largely based on the 'anti-idiotype' theory (Fig. 1.11). This in turn was based on the notion that an antibody combining site could be used in immunisation to create a second antibody which was a mirror image of the antigen. This second antibody, being non-pathogenic, could, in theory, there-fore safely be used in large amounts to elicit an immune response to pathogens such as viruses or tumour cells. While most protein chem-ists have always viewed such concepts with a reaction ranging from cynicism to outright scorn, many papers were published on the area in the late 1980s. Most involved poor detection systems (largely de-tecting polyspecific IgM Mabs) and poor, if any, control experiments. It was probably not helpful that many of the target antigens were car-bohydrate in nature and susceptible to low-affinity binding. The strat-egy may yet work well with high-affinity Mabs to protein epitopes.

The knowledge of the nature of T cell recognition systems which involve a separate part of the antigen (Section 1.13.1 and 4.6) con-firms that such approaches were too simple. Additional evidence against this hypothesis was provided by the confirmation that all crys-tallographically defined antibody-antigen interactions (Section 1.3) involve induced fit and changes in antigen and antibody structure (Coleman et al., 1987; Bhat et al., 1990) so that simple jigsaw-puzzle

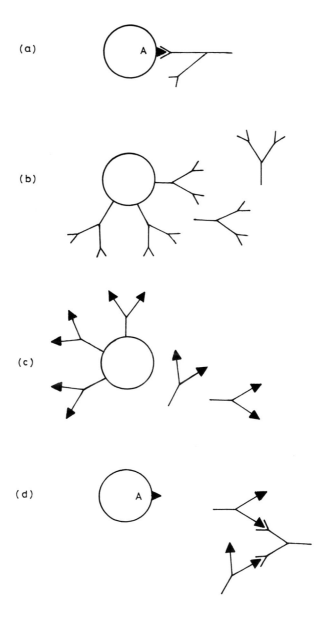

type attitudes were not experimentally sustainable. Finally, an antigen-Mab reaction and anti-idiotype-Mab reaction for the same Mab and antigen were shown to have unrelated recognition patterns (Bentley et al., 1990).

Many anti-idiotype observations remain to be resolved. Jerne shared the Nobel prize with Kohler and Milstein in 1984 for his theoretical description of a potential idiotypic network, but his contributions to immunology extend far beyond that. Personalities apart, accumulating evidence suggests that any specific mirror image of antigen and 2nd (anti-idiotype) antibody is, at least in monoclonal terms, serendipitous. On a practical point, while it is simple to obtain low-affinity polyspecific IgM Mabs from a mouse immunised with a mouse Mab, it is exceedingly difficult to obtain a high-affinity, non-cross-reactive IgG Mab. More rigorous experimental systems will be required to prove that the anti-idiotype approach is anything but a minor, low-affinity ripple, in the immune system.

1.14. Mabs as catalysts (abzymes)

This application of Mabs was first described in 1986 (Tramontano et al, 1986; Pollack et al., 1986) and the field has grown rapidly since (Reviewed by Shokat and Schultz, 1990; technical descriptions by Tramontano and Schloeder, 1989 and Pollack et al., 1989). The basic concept behind catalytic Mabs is that a Mab generated to a molecule or molecules which mimic the transition state between substrate and product may accelerate the reaction by forcing the substrate into a suitable conformation for conversion into product (Fig. 1.12). Where bimolecular reactions are involved, the antibody can bring the two molecules together to significantly increase their probability of inter-

---

←

Fig. 1.11. The anti-idiotype strategy. The concepts behind this are that a high-affinity Mab (b) may itself be used to immunise a mouse to give a Mab directed to the first Mab which is a 'mirror image' of the antigen (c). This Mab may then be used as a component of a non-pathogenic and therefore safe vaccine or as an inhibitor of autoimmune antibody binding (d).

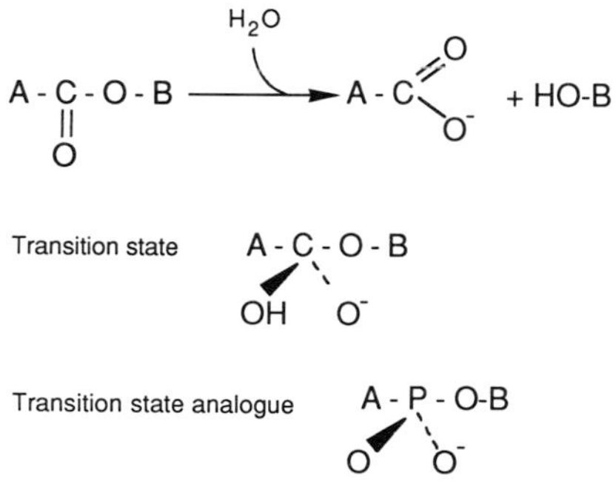

$$A - \underset{\underset{O}{\|}}{C} - O - B \xrightarrow{\overset{H_2O}{\curvearrowright}} A - C\underset{O^-}{\overset{O}{\diagup}} + HO\text{-}B$$

Transition state $A - \underset{OH \quad O^-}{C} - O - B$

Transition state analogue $A - \underset{O \quad O^-}{P} - O\text{-}B$

Fig. 1.12. Catalytic Mabs – simple example of ester hydrolysis. The enzyme catalyses the reaction by binding the unstable transition state analogue at high-affinity, thus forcing the reaction. A stable transition state analogue which mimics this intermediate can be formed with the pentavalent phosphorus atom as its central point.

action, potentially even orienting the reactive sites towards each other. As with enzymes, the Mab does not alter the equilibrium of the reaction but rather reduces the free energy requirement of the reaction to below that of the uncatalysed reaction. The efficiency of the Mab as catalyst is judged by the extent to which it can enhance the rate of the reaction over the background uncatalysed rate and enhancement figures as high as 10^6 have been reported.

This technology is at an early stage and early high-affinity extrapolations will inevitably be modulated by experience. The 'transition state analogue' antigens have to be attached to protein haptens (usually BSA and KLH) for both immunisation and assay. Emerging clones are usually not assayed for enzyme activity but only for binding to the intermediate complex since the amount of antibody is too small, and catalysis is too weak to allow sufficient product molecules to be detected within the assay period. Typical K_{cat} values of the early catalytic Mabs range from 0.01 to 10 min^{-1} which compares highly unfavourably with enzymes. One of the problems is the slow rate of product desorption (Benkovic et al., 1990) and this may be improved by alteration the structure of the transition state analogue. Newer techniques such as site directed mutagenesis (Section 9.4.4) to introduce potential catalytic groups (Baldwin and Schultz, 1989) or metal ion binding residues (Iversen et al., 1990) into the Mab together with or replacing the transition state strategy described above may greatly improve the efficiency of catalytic Mabs and the efficiency of their production. Probably the ideal method to improve catalytic efficiency would be to introduce the genes encoding antibody into a prokaryotic or eukaryotic system under conditions in which possession of the catalytic activity in question confers a selective growth advantage (Hilvert et al., 1988). Such a system would require to be able correctly to assemble the Mab, or at the least, its Fab fragment and this would usually require additional engineering of the antibody chains (Section 9.5).

1.15. Mabs in purification

Mabs can be utilised in immunoaffinity chromatography to purify small components from complex mixtures (Fig. 1.13). The section devoted to this is small because it is generally highly successful and now a standard technique (see Chapter 10). One of the most successful applications of affinity chromatography remains the purification of alpha interferon by Secher and Burke (1980). Starting with an antigen less than 1% pure, they were able both to immunise and screen with a complex mixture by using for the latter a bioassay which did not require pure antigen. They then used the resulting Mab to effect the final purification. The majority of antigens cannot readily be accommodated in a bioassay and so this particular elegant approach is restricted.

Immunoaffinity purification is a situation in which it is possible to consider using slightly lower affinity Mabs. One of the major problems with the use of polyclonal antisera for immunoaffinity purification has been the difficulty of eluting the bound antigen under conditions which do not denature it irreversibly and delicate antigens can be purified more readily by Mab technology. The use of lower affinity Mabs does, however, mean inevitably that some irrelevant material may be bound and the purification may only be partial.

The fine specificity of Mabs means that they may be used to purify

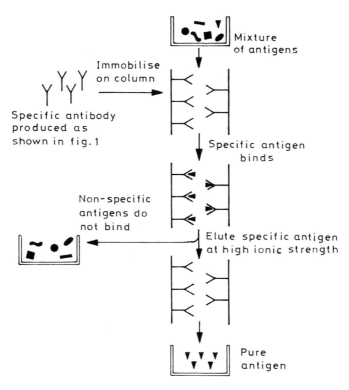

Fig. 1.13. The use of Mabs in purification of minor antigens in a complex mixture. This
works well only if the Mab is of high affinity.

closely related enantiomorphs (racemates) in a situation where chemical methods are generally non-selective. (Knox and Galfre, 1986.)

1.16. Mabs in basic immunological research

This book is not the appropriate vehicle to describe such a comprehensive area. However, it is worth noting that human hybridomas
are excellent vehicles for the study of antigen presentation (Reid and
Watts, 1990) since B cells are highly efficient presenters (Fig. 4.3) and

the relevant peptide presented in the MHC groove can then be immunoprecipitated with Mabs to MHC antigens. At the time of writing, Mabs to the T cell receptor variable regions also excite much interest. The T cell receptor is different in its variable regions from antibody in that there are a comparatively small number of V genes (Davis, 1988), with diversity being generated by D, J and N region variation. Thus antibodies to these V gene products can be used to study the clonality of a T cell response and also have the potential to be used in selective immunotherapy for autoimmune conditions (Sinha et al., 1990) or post transplant control of rejection. As in many other modern uses of Mabs, the requirement for Mabs to a membrane protein usually means that immunisation and screening require that the protein be presented in its membrane context.

1.17. Patent considerations for Mabs

Kohler and Milstein did not patent the basic mouse fusion technique, so, in principle, it can be used by any individual or company. However, almost all applications and variations on the technique have been filed in patent applications. This section gives a brief account of patent rules followed by an account of how they have been interpreted to date for monoclonal antibodies. The final advice given has to be taken in the context of the fluidity of the current legal interpretation of biotechnological patents.

1.17.1. The patent system

Patent rules were designed to deal with applications which relate to advancements in the design of simple items such as bicycles or (classically) mousetraps. These rules were based on the premise that an inventor who has a good idea, should be able to put his or her idea onto the market or into the public domain without it being immediately adopted by a large company or wealthy individual who would give the inventor no reward for his originality. By filing his invention with the patent office, the inventor could protect his device or process from exploitation and any individual or organisation which used or marketed the device would then be obliged to pay the inventor some form of royalty. This could either be in a lump sum, or a 'licence' awarded by the patentholder whereby he or she received a certain percentage of the profits of the individual or company exploiting the invention.

A patent gives the inventor rights for the sole exploitation of the invention for 17 years in the U.K. (20 in the U.S.A.).

Patent agents act as intermediaries between the individual inventor and the law and can give realistic advice as to whether an idea is worth filing for patent and how the wording may be used to encompass all potential future infringements.

The process became more commercial as science developed to the point of individual inventors becoming a rare group and large pharmaceutical companies have routinely filed patents for new drugs, new methods for making them and their potential new uses over the last 3 decades.

The biotechnology revolution, however, has meant that patent lawyers have had to adapt to new concepts and ideas, frequently referring these to higher courts.

1.17.2. Classic patent rules

These were based on an invention being novel, useful and non-obvious.

The possible use of inventions was based on five Sections

(i) New Processes – new ways of making a product – changing the traditional chemical or industrial route. Mab generation by recombinant DNA technology can obviously be adapted to fit this role.

(ii) New Machines – a new type of recording or videoing, electronically powered cigarette lighters, electric cars etc. Mab based biosensors might be included into this category.

(iii) New manufactures/articles of manufacture. Skid resistant motor tyres, wigs that look like normal hair etc. While there is clearly some overlap with category (i), human Mabs that carry mouse Mab features could be in this category.

(iv) New compositions of matter. Polyester fabric, a new glue etc. Mabs are not usually cited as being in this category but recombinant ones might be so classified.

(v) New uses of any of the above (i) to (iv), i.e., Using a venetian blind cleaner as a seed planter. Technically the original paper was directed to Sheep Red Blood Cells as antigen. Thus technically any other antigen might be classified as a 'new use'. However, catalytic Mabs might be the best example for this category as this is clearly a genuine new use.

One could make a justification for a Mab of any type in the context of most of the above criteria and many hopeful Mab technologists have done so.

1.17.3. Novelty and non-obviousness

The two further qualifications implicit in the patent application are novelty (i.e., not previously described) and non-obviousness (involving an inventive step). In Mab technology these tend to overlap with an emphasis on the latter. For example using a Mab to replace a polyclonal antibody in an established immunoassay system is not novel and it is obvious. However, altering the assay system to one which only works with Mabs (even if it is inferior to a polyclonal one) could be proposed as novel and, depending on the system employed, possibly non-obvious. Both in Mab technology and some aspects of recombinant DNA technology, it is this definition of 'non-obvious' that has been most frequently challenged.

1.17.4. Prior art

This relates to whether the key elements of novelty in a patent are in the 'public domain'. If they have been published, or presented at a meeting, or previously filed in another patent application, they are in the public domain. It is therefore important to file a patent application before undertaking any of these activities. The presentation of an idea in a grant application is usually not considered to be in the public domain as these are supposedly confidential. In some countries, however, it is possible to file a patent up to 1 year after publication.

Academics can use any technique under patent for research purposes as long as they do not sell their research for profit. Problems can occasionally arise when one academic uses an idea under patent to Company A and passes this idea to a colleague who works with Company B leading to legal action between the two companies. Academics in the biomedical area should all have an understanding of the rudimentaries of patent law and this is now incorporated in many undergraduate courses.

1.17.5. How some Mab patents have operated to date

(i) Immunoassay   The main application challenged in the courts to date has been the sandwich assay (Fig. 1.8). The dispute has been extensively covered by the scientific press (Ekins, 1989; Greene and Duft, 1990; Ekins, 1990). The essence of the dispute is that while a sandwich assay might be considered reasonably ' obvious', it was not a practicable immunoassay technique prior to the development of Mabs as the background was too high and antibodies in the detecting polyclonal antibody population could often dislodge those in the capture polyclonal antibody population. Hybridtech, a subsidiary company of Eli Lilly, filed a patent to cover this sandwich technique with any label – isotope, enzyme or fluorophor – on the second Mab. Two firms, Monoclonal Antibodies Inc and Abbott Laboratories Inc, produced sandwich type Mab kits for various antigens. In consequence, Hybridtech challenged for patent infringement. After lengthy legal proceedings, judgement was awarded in Hybridtech's favour and Abbott and Hybridtech are reported to have come to a private licensing arrangement. The definition of 'obvious' would appear to have been a key feature of this decision and in the US patent courts was interpreted to include 'people of ordinary skill.' Clearly a technique involving refinement in immunoassay is not obvious to people of ordinary skill among the general public.

This case has implications for anyone who uses a sandwich kit. The original patent rules could be interpreted so that even if an institution such as an industrial company or hospital generates a sandwich kit to use 'in house', they are technically infringing the patentholder's rights since they have copied his invention without giving him a percentage of profits. Fortunately, in practical terms, most firms do not, at least at the moment, consider the cost of litigation to be worth challenging 'in house' use.

(ii) Immunotherapy As has been indicated above, Mab therapy is still in its early stages. However, because the potential commercial market is much larger and the complexity of generation and application of therapeutic Mabs is much greater, conflicts over therapeutic use are likely to be a major battle for Mab technologists and to incur considerable legal costs. The major pilot dispute in this area relates to Mabs to bacterial endotoxin. This endotoxin is released by gram negative bateria infecting wounds or burns and is responsible for post operative shock and mortality. Antibiotics are ineffective once the toxin is released. The original patent filed by Xoma was broadly based and included both the possibility of human and mouse Mabs to endotoxin for treating affected individuals. Xoma have concentrated on producing mouse Mabs to the endotoxin. Centocor have, however, produced a human Mab to the same antigen and Xoma has filed for patent infringement. Given the additional complexities involved in generating human Mabs (Section 1.9 above and Table 3.2), and affinity and specificity considerations, such cases will severely strain the already over-worked patent offices in understanding the finer points of Mab expertise.

1.17.6. Mab technology already filed for patent

With the exception of the basic Kolher and Milstein technique, almost every conceivable method of making, improving, or using Mabs is already applied for in patent and thus in the public domain (but not issued with patent rights in most cases). Most large institutional (or city) libraries have access to the patent index of the World Patent Organisation and it is possible to do a conventional computer search using key words or phrases. Such a search with 'monoclonal antibodies' produces over 2000 entries and most are formed in the manner of 'The use of a monoclonal antibody from any mammalian species to Antigen X for the diagnosis and therapy of disease Y'. Most of these applications are pending and it remains to be seen whether they are considered 'obvious'.

Any application involving recombinant DNA is patented.

1.17.7. How to patent a new application of Mabs

(i) For Mab technologists working through an institution.

The best advice is obviously to approach a suitably qualified patent agent through the institution in which the technologist operates. Most U.K. universities give 50% of revenue (after costs) back to the inventor. However, if you are employed by them, they can negotiate with a contracting body for 'intellectual property rights'. In other words if, in carrying out contract work you develop a new idea, your employer and contractor must decide which of them owns it.

(ii) For Mab technologists wishing to file patents for their own personal ideas.

These individuals should first check their contracts of employment which may not contain clauses which forbid them from filing for patents in areas directly relevant to their employment. The filing of a patent incurs costs which are high to any personal budget but low to corporate budgets. For the European Patent Office first filing costs are in the region of 3000DM (Deutschmarks) at first filing. Annual renewal fees thereafter are approximately 2/3 of the filing fee. While exchange rates vary, the American Patent Office operates within similar financial ranges. In most countries, the filing and maintenance fees of a single patent is close to the annual cost of a foreign holiday or second hand car. It is still therefore possible for an individual to maintain a patent for a new use of Mabs which he or she believes to be original in the main developed countries where it may have a market (U.S.A.,

Japan, Israel, Australia and European countries both with and without the jurisdiction of the European Patent Office). If a patent is directed 3rd world application, it may be necessary to file individual patents with the appropriate offices of each of the relevant countries.

However, the major financial difficulty for the individual scientist comes in challenging the patent in the lawcourts of the appropriate country or ecomomic confederation when the patent is infringed by a larger institution. The costs of legal action have largely corrupted the intentions of the original patent legislation.

1.18. Buying a Mab

Commercially supplied Mabs are expensive as the companies involved seek to recoup development costs. In the 1980s, many companies purchased hybridomas for inclusion in their catalogues to extend their range but did this without regard to quality. A quick way of judging a company's repertoire is to judge whether they still offer IgM Mabs to DNA or actin. If they do, their quality control may be suspect.

In general, the operator should buy a Mab which is designed for a particular task identical or close to final use. An explanation of how the antibody has been assessed in a range of techniques should be available from the firm. The Mab technologist must then decide if the Mab will be suitable for the appropriate task. The field for the major antigens is highly competitive and most firms will readily offer a small free sample of a Mab to prove their quality. In general such Mabs are supplied as tissue culture supernatant and constitute a small proportion of the protein in the sample so it is not practical to consider direct labelling. Many firms also supply directly labelled Mabs and these are inevitably very expensive. If large amounts of any Mab are required for a project, then one should at least consider making the Mab 'in house'. However, by doing so, as discussed above, it is possible that one will be infringing a patent.

CHAPTER 2

Assay techniques

2.1. General assay requirements

This chapter is largely about screening for monoclonal antibodies. Inevitably, it also involves many concepts which are also relevant in their application.

2.1.1. Definitions and concepts

Many of the general terms used in immunoassay are confused in the diverse literature on the subject. Tijssen (1985), defining these terms for enzyme immunoassay, categorised the main definitions as:

(a) *Detectability* (or detection limit) defines the lowest level of detection of antigen which is detected by any assay system and whether it can detect to picomole, femtomole levels etc. This parameter is often quoted in research papers as sensitivity.

(b) *Sensitivity*, on the other hand is the change of signal with change in antigen concentration, i.e., if the antigen concentration is doubled, does the reading on the monitoring system double or quadruple? The latter is a more sensitive assay.

(c) *Precision* is the degree to which an assay system duplicates or where a standard curve of antigen concentration has minimal scatter.

(d) *Accuracy* is the extent to which the assay gives the correct result with respect to the theoretical result.

(e) *Specificity* refers to the degree of discrimination of the assay between positive and negative controls and this relates intimately to the affinity differences between these two.

These definitions are seldom correctly used but serve to emphasise the various parameters which control the utility of an assay. The jargon of the 1990s has added to the above, phrases such as

(f) *Signal/noise ratio*. This is generally used to describe the ratio of positive controls (serum or Mab) to negative ones (no antigen, no antibody etc). In practice, for a monoclonal antibody, it has most in common with (e) – specificity – above. While most people appreciate that with polyclonal serum there will be a variety of antibodies with varying cross-reactive potential and consequently a precise level of dilution at which this can be optimised, there tends to be an assumption that a Mab is a totally specific molecule giving only the correct signal. Thus any background reading is assumed to be created by contaminating molecules with unidentified non-specific, spurious binding properties. In reality, even the highest affinity monoclonal will bind at low affinity to a small proportion of the molecules in a complex mixture if it is faced by an overwhelming number of them in the absence of its main antigen (Fig. 1.3) while a poor affinity one can bind an extensive variety of irrelevant molecules. Many assay systems which claim to improve 'sensitivity' are complex and costly sandwich systems which simply amplify both specific binding and non-specific binding and are consequently of limited value.

For screening the priority is generally high specificity, i.e., high affinity for chosen antigen and low affinity for all others. The one possible exception to this may be catalytic antibodies where binding alone is not sufficient (see Section 2.10).

2.1.2. Technical requirements

The assay system is probably the most critical factor in the generation of a large panel of high-affinity monoclonal antibodies relevant to the envisaged application. The emerging clones secrete small amounts of antibody and early cloning of positive cells is a key factor in the production of successful long-term hybridomas. Since this is optimised by a highly specific, assay system with low detection limits, many of the techniques which work well with polyclonal antiserum are not optimal for screening. Additionally, many conventional assays such as those involving immunoprecipitation, depend on multiple epitopes on the antigen and these are ill suited for monoclonal antibody selection.

It is almost impossible to emphasise too often that the final use of the antibody should, wherever possible, determine the type of initial screening assay employed. If the final projected use is too complex to be employed for extensive screening, then the most sensible approach is to perform an initial screen with a specific, possibly irrelevant, assay and as soon as possible thereafter (possibly simultaneous to a first speculative cloning of good wells), a secondary check to make sure that the Mab behaves appropriately on the system intended for final use.

2.2. Theoretical considerations

2.2.1. The nature of the antibody–antigen interaction

The precise nature of the interaction of Mabs with large protein antigens is discussed in detail in Section 1.3.1. The relevant points to note are the epitopes characterised to date are all conformational rather than linear and that 'induced' fit where antigen and antibody both change in conformation to a greater or lesser degree in all cases. Both of these factors have implications for assay. The former means that peptides are generally unsuitable for generation and assay for high-affinity Mabs, the latter that assay systems involving rigidly immobilised antigen may fail to detect Mabs which participate in extensive induced fit interactions.

2.2.2. The kinetics of antibody–antigen interactions

The precise kinetics of antibody–antigen interactions for myelomas/ polyclonal antibodies with haptens are extensively analysed in several texts (Weber, 1975; Tijssen, 1985). There are few detailed published analyses of the parameters relating to a statistically large enough panel of Mabs to be know whether these conclusions are applicable to Mabs directed to complex protein epitopes.

The initial rate of association of an antibody with an antigen is described by the standard equation:

$$\text{rate of formation of product} = K_{ass}(\text{antibody})(\text{antigen})$$

and is defined in terms of $M^{-1}s^{-1}$. In the classical hapten studies, K_{ass} has been shown to remain remarkably constant among antibodies of all types at 10^7 to 10^8 $M^{-1}s^{-1}$.

At *screening*, the requirement is to detect tiny amounts of potentially useful antibody against comparatively large amounts of known antigen, i.e., $Ag > > Ab$.

For *application*, the most usual requirement is to detect tiny amounts of antigen within a complex mixture with a Mab which has already been established as a potentially useful reagent, i.e., $Ab > > Ag$.

The *antibody* concentration at first screening is very low indeed. The antibody secreted by 100 cells is being tested and these cells are largely concentrated on growth and division rather than antibody production, which is optimal in non-dividing cells (Chapter 10). Thus antibody concentration may be in the range 10^{-12} to 10^{-14} M.

Screening with antigen at high density always yields more positive results. Thus an ELISA plate with 100 ng of antigen will give fewer positives than a nitrocellulose blot with 100 μg (Section 2.6.1). If the first screening gives too many clones to handle, then the fusion can be rescreened at lower antigen density. If the concentration of antigen is unavoidably low – for example screening for a low-density cell surface protein, then it is advisable to use a comparatively long incubation time (Mason and Williams, 1980).

The dissociation rate of an antibody-antigen complex is defined by the equation:

$$\text{Initial rate of dissociation} = K_{diss}(\text{antibody} - \text{antigen})$$

It is defined in s^{-1}, i.e., the rate at which the Ab/Ag complex will dissociate in a single second. It is easier to visualise in half life ($0.69/K_{diss}$ – the time it takes for half the complex to dissociate). As with the association constant, this range was defined with haptens interacting with polyclonal antibodies.

With most antibody-antigen reactions, it is the dissociation rate that determines the final affinity of the antibody. This can vary over a wide range from 1000 s^{-1} (half life 7×10^{-4} s – a low-affinity antibody) to 0.001 s^{-1} (half life $7 \times 10^{+2}$ s – a high-affinity antibody) but is obviously very much lower than the association rate in order for the interaction to be observable in this first place. The dissociation rate is not only the most variable among different antibodies under a defined set of conditions but also the most variable in a single antibody with respect to environmental conditions such as pH, temperature etc. Thus, in any assay which involves washing (heterogeneous assay), the numbers of washes, method of washing (e.g., flushing versus immersion), and wash buffer, all contribute to the rate at which antibody dissociates from the relevant antigen as well as irrelevant antigen. The antibody which many people require has a long half life with chosen antigen and a short half life with all others.

The final affinity of the interaction is determined by the balance between the association and dissociation processes at equilibrium:

$$K_{eq} = (Ab - Ag)/(Ab)(Ag) = K_{ass}/K_{diss}$$

Affinity is therefore expressed usually in M^{-1} but there remains wide variation in how it is presented. If it is presented as K_D then it is the inverse of K_{eq} and equal to (Ab)(Ag)/(Ab − Ag), the units being M.

To check methods and data it is therefore advisable to compare your own antibody and method with respect to the methods used in determining affinity (Section 11.6) since frequently inappropriate methods have been used and published affinities have limited validity.

As emphasised above, for almost all applications of monoclonal antibodies, the higher the affinity, the better the antibody will perform the function for which it is being selected. The *avidity* of an antibody for an antigen is defined as the strength of the equilibrium interaction between antibody and antigen and is the parameter which is generally measured. The *true affinity* is the strength of interaction between a single antibody Fab and a single epitope and is seldom measured.

2.2.3. Additional considerations which affect basic kinetic equations

High affinity antibodies are not only desirable for their good binding but also for their superior specificity. As a general rule, the higher the true affinity of the antibody Fab for its epitope, the less likely the antibody is to form low-affinity contacts with dissimilar antigens. Several factors can affect the selection of such a high-affinity antibody.

(a) Antigen concentrations required for screening
While it is tempting to screen with large amounts of antigen bound to a solid support, and this procedure will indeed give more positive findings and lead to a larger number of hybridomas, the use of large amounts of antigen will bias the screening process towards the selection of a lower affinity antibody (Lehtonen and Viljanen, 1980; Pesce et al., 1978; Bruins et al., 1978). As the subcloning and expansion of large numbers of clones is an expensive and time consuming procedure, it is preferable to screen with comparatively small amounts of antigen, sufficient to give good positives for the system under test. If a fusion yields large numbers of positives, immediate rescreening at low antigen density (see above) is a very sensible tactic. This is also true for recombinant methods involving screening on filter paper (Section 9.6).

(b) Effects of antigen multivalence
Multivalent antigens are commonly materials such as structural or cytoskeletal proteins, bacterial cell surface carbohydrates (e.g., LPS on gram negative bacteria) and also autoantigens such as DNA. While these may be at apparently low concentrations in microgram terms, the local concentration of identical epitopes is extremely high. This pushes the reaction forward towards association and tends to give the incorrect assumption that the precise interaction is of the high-affinity type where in fact the actual contact points between antibody and antigen may be very limited. While this phenomenon in reverse has been

known for 20 years from the observation by Hornick and Karush (1972) that the polymerisation of haptens such as DNP increased their measured affinity for antibody by 1000 fold, its significance is not always appreciated. In this case, screening at low antigen density is of limited value, and the operator must simply be aware that the interaction may be of low avidity, and consequently also of poor specificity.

(c) Effects of antibody multivalence

The above considerations also apply to antibody multivalence. An IgG molecule, by virtue of the increased local interacting concentration provided by its bivalence can have an avidity 100 fold greater than that of a single Fab, and a decavalent IgM, can have an avidity 10^6 greater than its Fab. This means that the actual contacts between antibody Fab and antigen may, as in (b) above be weak and amplified by the polyvalence. This phenomenon occurs regularly with IgM Mabs which are frequently reported to be detected as participants in unexpected cross-reactions, sometimes reacting with 5 or more structurally dissimilar antigens (Casali and Notkins, 1989). Since they are also generally harder to purify and store, IgM antibodies are therefore generally to be avoided wherever possible and the most convenient way of doing this is to screen with detecting antibodies specific to the IgG γ-chain. Antibodies to the whole IgG molecule will detect IgM Mabs as well as IgG ones by virtue of their interaction with the constant portion of the light chain (Section 2.6.6).

It will be evident that an IgM Mab directed to a multivalent antigen is a very poor reagent indeed and liable to participate in numerous undesirable cross-reactions (Fig. 2.1)

(d) Washing (heterogeneous) versus non-washing (homogeneous) assays and their relevance to immunosensors

The most common type of method employed for screening emerging clones is undoubtedly washing assays such as ELISA or other solid-phase assays where once antibody has bound to antigen, the free material is washed away. In all these assays it is the signal/noise ratio (see above) which is important. The more the system is washed (for exam-

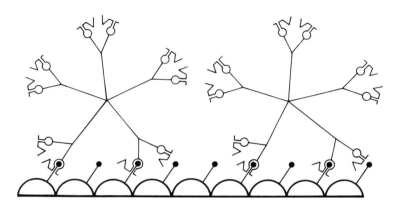

Fig. 2.1. Common undesirable cross-reaction to avoid. A low-affinity Mab (Fig. 1.3) selected on the chosen antigen, can cross-react giving apparently high-affinity binding on an irrelevant structure. The commonest case (low-affinity, high-antigen and antibody binding site density) is shown here. This is commonly experienced with IgM Mabs and polymeric antigens.

ple the use of the biotin streptavidin system (Section 2.6.7) involves an extra washing step) the lower the background will become but, unless the antibody has a very high affinity, the lower the foreground will also become. Conversely, attempts to gain extra detectability by amplifying the detection system, may also amplify the background signal of a low-affinity antibody.

Non-washing, homogeneous, methods are the ones in which low-affinity non-specific binding can be most readily demonstrated. Such methods including complement fixation and, in particular, agglutination, have been successfully employed for the generation of Mabs where the final use has been appropriate to that method. However, the chance of reaction with irrelevant background noise material is high. More recently many of the biosensor systems involving optical methods such as surface plasmon resonance have been developed and these are effectively non or low washing methods, i.e., the interaction between antibody and antigen is observed while free antibody or antigen remains nearby. Due to the kinetic factors governing the reaction, such assays detect very low-affinity contacts with irrelevant antigens in addition to the expected higher affinity contacts with the chosen antigen and many antibodies which appear to be specific against all tested antigens on washing assays, can in fact react with a wide variety of others when tested on a non-washing assay. It is particularly important for the Mab producer to understand and explain this to scientists involved in developing the electronic side of any immunosensor, or a great deal of money can be wasted (Chapter 12).

(e) Antibodies for in vivo use
In this particular situation, it is not possible for the antibody to be tested in its final use until long after first screening of primary clones, partly because of ethical considerations, but more pragmatically because of the sheer quantity required. This is possibly the ultimate field test since the Mab technologist has no control over the reaction conditions and the antibody, in moving through the body, encounters very large amounts of numerous antigens with which it may form minor contacts including serum proteins, common cell surface antigens and, in particular, extracellular structural proteins. While it is impossible to test an antibody for all the molecules that it may encounter, it would obviously be advisable to perform an early check that the Mab did not display even a weak interaction with high internal epitope density structural proteins such as the collagens.

The other convenient check to be performed at an early stage is whether the mouse Mab binds to human Fc receptors in the absence of antigen. In practice this is only a problem relating to highly specialised applications but has often been invoked as the theoretical reason for poor localisation of an antibody.

2.3. Practical screening in the lab

2.3.1. Numbers of assays

The numbers of plates to be used in initial fusions and in subsequent clonings is discussed later. In a typical conventional fusion procedure utilising 8 to 10×96 well plates, up to 1000 samples must be assayed in a short period of time. Each fusion is usually screened several times. Subcloning usually involves a further large number of assays. For this reason, in the early 1980s, solid-phase assays where the antigen was detected by ELISA or filter binding systems became the major method of screening for antigens since these are readily performed by a single operator in a short period of time. For those whose projected final use involves a washing type assay (Section 2.2.3 above) they give an excellent preliminary screening system. In more recent times, it has become apparent that such assays are inappropriate for many antigens of interest such as proteins on the inner or outer cell membrane or for antibodies whose final intended use is in a non-washing assay. The use of a probe designed to detect only a chosen isotype (usually IgG) greatly reduces the complexity of screening after the first step since it gives fewer positives of higher quality. If it is necessary to use a time consuming assay, it is quite possible to test only those wells in which an emerging clone is evident but even this will be a large number if the fusion is successful.

Recombinant methods tend to produce very large numbers of samples for assay and the limiting factor is the assay capacity of the relevant lab. These are further discussed in Section 9.6.4.

2.3.2. When to assay

In terms of clonal growth, the time of assay should be soon after clones are microscopically visible (5–10 days after a good fusion), again a few days later when the early clones are visible to the eye and new ones develop, and again a few days further on for the same reason. Screening should continue for two or three weeks as clones can emerge at different rates and good clones which secrete antibody are often slower to expand.

2.3.3. Conditions of assay

In general, yet again, these should be as close as possible to the final use. For example some Mabs have considerable pH dependence and a change of one pH unit can mean the difference between a positive and a negative (Fig. 2.2). Solid surfaces can grossly alter pH optima because of local charge effects, especially where hydrogen peroxide is involved in detection so that a Mab detected by agglutination may change in detectability on a solid surface. In addition, Mabs will obviously react differently when tested with enzyme probes optimal at differing pH values. If the final use will involve a variety of pH values, it is advisable to check at an early stage that the Mab has the capacity to react throughout this range. If in vivo use is contemplated, the screening temperature and pH should be appropriate and if use in the field is contemplated then the likely environmental range of both should be checked. If the Mab is to be used in the detection of biological material in, say, water samples, then the binding stage of the screening assay should be checked at low ionic strength. This is all self evident but infrequently performed at the early stages in many labs.

Where secondary biological detection systems are used (for example

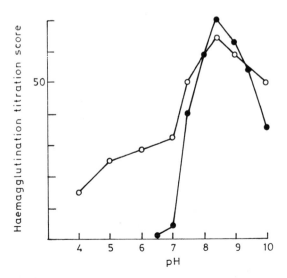

Fig. 2.2. pH dependence of a Mab directed to the human N blood group antigen. The serum polyclonal antibody can be detected at most pH values but the Mab is not detectable below pH 7. (Courtesy of Dr. Robin Fraser and Dr Angus Munro.)

in dot-blot or ELISA assays), then the proteins involved are relevant. For example alkaline phosphatase works better at higher pH values and horseradish peroxidasc at lower pH and temperature values (Section 2.6.7).

2.4. Antibody sampling

It has been emphasised in Section 2.2 that the amount of antibody available in the supernatant of a newly established hybridoma is small. Antibodies, like other proteins, will be adsorbed readily on surfaces of glass or synthetic materials despite the buffering effects of the serum in which the hybridomas are grown. Thus any assay system which involves multiple transfers from the tissue culture plate to the final assay is to be avoided. It is even technically possible to assay using short-term tissue culture in antigen coated plates thus avoiding any transfer at all but this is obviously not practical for emerging clones which require further culturing.

The other main consideration is to keep the tissue culture plate sterile while removing the sample. It is largely this consideration that made the many types of sampling device which appeared on the market in the early 1980s impractical. Most laboratories sample using multichannel micropipettes with autoclavable tips.

2.5. Types of assay

It is difficult to classify the possible types of assay for hybridomas without consideration of the relevant antigen and the final use. The condition of the antigen (formaldehyde fixed, radiolabelled, bound to other molecules, relative accessibility on or within cells) should be as close as possible to final use. While historically cellular assays were the first to be used for hybridoma detection (Kohler and Milstein, 1975), in more recent years solid-phase assay systems have become by far the most common. Biological assays are the least common. More recent assays have emerged with the growth the Fluorescent Activated Cell Sorter (FACS) population throughout laboratories so that this once specialised technique is now in comparatively common use.

2.6. Solid-phase assays

The solid-phase assay system is widely used largely because of its ability to handle very large numbers of samples in a short period of time. It can be adapted to accommodate complex antigens such as bacteria and whole cells (although the latter is not recommended (Section 2.6.2)). The growth in the use of ELISA (Enzyme Linked Immuno-Sorbent Assay) and dot- or slot-blot assays in particular has been logarithmic since the first reported use by Engvall and Perlman in 1971 (reviewed in Engvall and Pesce, 1982). All aspects of enzyme immunoassay are covered in Tijssen (1985). The basis of this type of assay is shown Fig. 2.3. In the ELISA, dot-blot, or (more rarely) radioactive

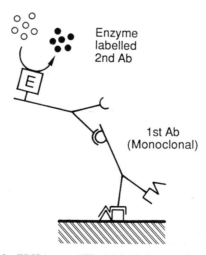

Fig. 2.3. The basis of the ELISA assay. The Mab binds to antigen attached to a solid surface and is then detected by a second (polyclonal) antibody preparation directed to the non-variable regions of the Mab.

binding assay, the antigen is bound to a specially coated 96 well plate or a paper support and incubated with the supernatant containing the monoclonal antibody. A second anti-mouse IgG antibody coupled to enzyme or radioisotope is then used to detect the first.

2.6.1. The nature of the solid support

The chemical nature of the solid support may be glass (Engvall and Perlman, 1971), nylon (Hendry and Herrman, 1980), Sepharose, cellulose (Giallongo et al., 1982 ; King and Kochoumian, 1979), cyanogen bromide or DBM activated paper (Lehtonen and Viljanen, 1980), or nitrocellulose paper (Hawkes 1986). The physical nature can be balls (Ziola et al., 1977), rings (Lehtonen and Viljanen, 1980), beads of varying capacity (Giallongo et al., 1982; Henry and Herrman, 1980), and discs or sheets of paper. However, the majority of assays are performed in two systems The first is with a solid-phase support which is in the form of a 96 well polystyrene or polyvinyl plate. The plates are generally coated with material which encourages the binding of the antigen. Manufacturers are generally elusive about the precise chemical nature of the plate and coating. This type of plate is marketed by all the major manufacturers and the performance may vary widely under assay conditions. Some give good positives with sera from immunised animals but also high background with negative serum and in any preliminary test of the plates it is the signal to noise ratio that should be evaluated. While it has been emphasised that maximum detectability is necessary for early screening, the plates contribute substantially to the cost of hybridoma production and more economical ones of slightly lower quality are frequently employed. It is advisable to test a range of papers in your own laboratory with your own antigen and test serum and most manufacturers will happily part with trial samples in exchange for your data.

The other main solid support used for screening is nitrocellulose or other types of paper (see Stott 1989 for a review). Nitrocellulose binds protein at higher density than most ELISA plates (Table 2.1). Antigen can either be dotted on the paper (dot-blot) or may be held in a

96 compartment manifold giving the same effect as an ELISA plate. If the antigen is streaked in a line, or a manifold which streaks antigen in a line is used, the system is referred to as a 'slot-blot'. ELISA and dot-blot on nitrocellulose, being the commonest systems are the solid-phase protocols described in detail. A very small amount of antigen can be dotted at high density on nitrocellulose and this technique is steadily gaining ground where rare antigens are involved. It is also the technique of choice where recombinant DNA methodology is used, largely because the operators are familiar with it.

It is important to note that a *high capacity for protein is not necessarily desirable* (Section 2.2.3). For almost all uses a high-affinity Mab is required and while screening with large amounts of protein may give *quantitatively* more positive results (nitrocellulose commonly detects more positive clones than ELISA), the *quality* of the extra positives may be poor and the operator will simply go to additional trouble subcloning large numbers of poor clones. Low affinity Mabs are all too readily isolated from solid-phase screening and also tend to cross-react on solid-phase screening (Fig. 2.4).

2.6.2. *Attachment of antigen*

Soluble antigens such as proteins, nucleic acids and carbohydrate (including bacterial polysaccharides and lipopolysaccharides) can be passively adsorbed onto the solid support of an ELISA plate or paper. If the antigen is a pure soluble protein then it is usually coated with 100 μl of a solution of 1–10 μg/ml. More is not usually advisable and may be detrimental. An ELISA plate has limited capacity and excess antigen may leach from it taking the bound test Mab with it while for both ELISA and nitrocellulose, excess antigen will bias the selection in favour of low-affinity Mabs (Section 2.2.3). Affinity is generally artificially increased on solid-phase assays in any case and ELISA assays are susceptible to the detection of irrelevant cross-reactions (Fig. 2.4). Early ELISA assays used high pH values to bind antigen to solid phase and this is the reason that many protocols still suggest unexpectedly high pH values for binding. With modern solid supports

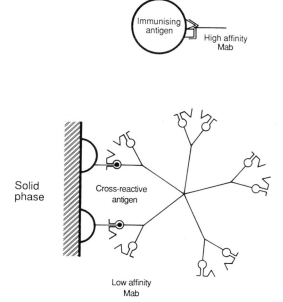

Fig. 2.4. Solid phase assays can encourage the production of low-affinity Mabs. In effect, the original soluble antigen has been made into a polymeric antigen by fixation on the plate in two dimensions and at high density. In screening, this can yield low-affinity Mabs (for assay of a Mab selected under stringent conditions, it can amplify the detection system).

this is quite unnecessary and it is better practice to bind at the pH value of the subsequent assay procedures.

Binding a protein to a solid phase can denature it so some extent, as can be shown by loss of enzyme activity (Berkowitz and Webert, 1981). This can also be true of both ELISA plates and nitrocellulose, the latter being largely a hydrophobic binding system (van Oss et al., 1987). Where immunological activity is relevant this may lead to the selection of Mabs which bind to epitopes not available in the native protein structure. Consequently it is sometimes possible for antibodies to be selected by solid-phase binding assay and be found unreactive in liquid phase assay (Miller et al., 1983). Nucleic acid molecules also appear to be susceptible to this and many anti-DNA Mabs selected on ELISA perform poorly in solid-phase assays (Eilat, 1986). In general, lipids do not perform well on solid-phase assays. It is possible to bind lipid to an ELISA plate by drying it down from a chloroform/ethanol solution but a high-affinity IgG Mab to a lipid is not a realistic aim as they are naturally poor antigens.

Many solid-phase assays are now performed with particulate material such as chromosomes, viruses, parasites or whole cells. There are two basic ways of attaching these to ELISA plates. They can either be put on in a suspension and dried down, or put on in a suspension and centrifuged down. Either way there is no covalent attachment and an obvious risk that during the subsequent detection procedures, some of the material will be lost. However, the system has been successful for many groups. Bacteria generally behave fairly well in such systems however and can be coated at around 10^7 or fewer cells/well. Early protocols involved fixation procedures for cellular material on ELISA plates involving glutaraldehyde with or without polylysine (Heusser et al., 1981) but these are probably unnecessary.

Despite the foregoing, i.e., the fact that it is technically possible to select a Mab to a cellular antigen on ELISA, it is not usually advisable to use such a crude screening system. A low-affinity antibody may bind at high concentration to a major constituent of the cells, particularly if this constituent has a repetitive structure (Fig. 2.1). In the case of, say, a gram negative bacteria, the dominant antigen on the plate will be lipopolysaccharide (LPS) and should one want a Mab to a protein component, it would be advisable to screen with protein only, or a mutant which lacks the ability to make LPS. The situation is even more complex with whole cells as antigen. They may look intact on the ELISA plate but the membrane will inevitably be breached at some points sufficient to allow the passage of the antibody into the cell. This means that cellular ELISA assays have tended to yield Mabs only reactive with major cellular components such as cytoskeletal proteins. Fig. 2.5 shows one example where a low-affinity IgM Mab binding a cytoskeletal protein may be misinterpreted by assay as binding to a membrane – the distinction is important where immunoscintigraphy or therapy is contemplated (Sections 1.11 and 1.12). If the re-

quired Mab is to react with an intracellular protein such as an oncogene product, then some degree of prior purification from the
dominant proteins is necessary. If the Mab is required to bind to an
antigen on the outside of the cell membrane, then it is advisable to
screen *live* cells either by ELISA methods (Section 2.7), by fluorescence microscopy with live cells, staining as for FACS, or by FACS
itself (Section 2.8).

2.6.3. Blocking of remaining sites on the solid support

Most solid supports adsorb proteins non-specifically as discussed in
Section 2.6.1. It is evident that they will also absorb antibody if this
is not prevented by use of a blocking reagent. Mab containing tissue
culture supernatants already have a considerable amount of irrelevant
protein if the hybridomas have been grown in foetal calf serum
(Chapter 5) and therefore, with ELISA plates, blocking is not usually
too critical. With nitrocellulose membranes, given their high capacity
for protein, good blocking is essential and more blocker is used. Some
of the common blocking reagents are listed in Table 2.1. The most effective are the non-ionic detergents such as Tween 20 but these can
be too effective, removing antigen and promoting the dissociation of
weakly bound antibody (see Section 2.2.2 on kinetics). Low levels of
Tween are also frequently incorporated into subsequent washes. Each
antibody-antigen system has its individual optimal blocking conditions.
The suggested system used in this book is either Blotto or BSA with
0.05% Tween in ELISA washes and 0.1% Tween in dot-blot washes.

2.6.4. Storage of antigen-bound solid supports

Most antigen bound ELISA plates can be stored at 4°C for several
weeks. 0.02% (w/v) azide is included to avoid bacterial contamination
and the plates are stored in blocking buffer to avoid antigen desorption. This is washed off *immediately* before use. If the second antibody
is labelled with peroxidase it should be noted that azide inhibits this
and must be removed in the washing. Dried antigen bound to nitrocel-

TABLE 2.1
Blocking methods

Buffer	Comment
ELISA	
1% BSA (10 mg/ml)	Used to be thought to be needed pure No longer so BUT Must have no bovine IgG if Protein A involved
5% Blotto (50 mg/ml skimmed dried milk)	Cheap, usually low background Has to be homogeneous suspension
0.2% Gelatin (2 mg/ml)	Low on non-specific binding Expensive if pure
1% (v/v) non-specific serum	Variable with antigen No good with protein A or G detection
Dot-blot	
3% BSA (10 mg/ml)	Used pure to achieve standard assay. Hence comparatively expensive Must have no IgG if Protein A involved
5% Blotto (50 mg/ml skimmed dried milk)	Cheap, usually low background Has to be homogeneous suspension Can block plate washer nozzles
0.1–0.5% Tween 20% (v/v)	Harsh – can remove protein/disrupt binding Cheap. Paper can be stained for protein.
10% (v/v) non-specific serum (Goat, sheep, horse)	Variable with antigen No good with protein A or G detection

lulose may be stored for months, between two sheets of 3-mm filter paper, wrapped in Clingfilm at 4°C.

2.6.5. Incubation with antigen

Many of the factors dictating the incubation time with the antigen

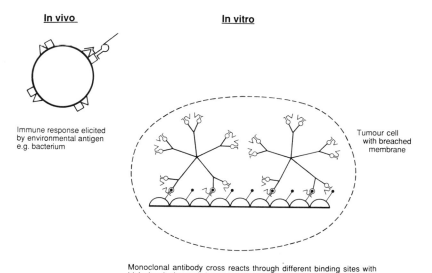

In vivo

In vitro

Immune response elicited
by environmental antigen
e.g. bacterium

Tumour cell
with breached
membrane

Monoclonal antibody cross reacts through different binding sites with
high density intracellular material and is incorrectly identified as having
been elicted by tumour.

Fig. 2.5. Screening on whole cells must be with intact cells. The antibody population
is dominated by low-affinity Mabs. These can bind at low affinity to irrelevant structures with high epitope density (Fig. 1.3). Thus a Mab to an environmental antigen can
be misinterpreted as cell specific if it can penetrate the membrane and bind at low affinity to structural proteins with the cell.

have already been discussed in detail in Sections 2.2. and 2.3. The
assay with the serum of the immunised animal can be used at 30 or
60 minutes but it is preferable to use a longer time for initial Mab
screening. Generally people either put the supernatants onto the prepared plates or papers immediately after checking the clones at the
start of the day and develop the assay at the end, or they incubate
overnight. A simple practical point, often overlooked by the operator,
is that the same areas of solid support should be covered by antigen,
blocker and Mab. Adding a different volume of any of the three in
a different way may give unexpected results.

2.6.6. The nature of the second antibody

The bound Mab is usually detected with a second, polyclonal (and it *should* be polyclonal to detect all murine IgG epitopes) antibody directed against the constant regions of the mouse immunoglobulin. Covalently linked to this second antibody can be either an isotope or, more usually, an enzyme with a chromogenic substrate. Sheep, rabbit or goat anti mouse IgG antibodies linked to enzyme are usually used to detect murine hybdridomas. These are simple to make in principle (although the products have highly variable quality) and in consequence the marketing of enzyme labelled second antibodies is a highly competitive field. It is also a volatile one – a firm which was supplying excellent second antibodies can produce ones of lower quality a few months later. Firms which market additional equipment (e.g., flow cytometers) will often offer these at reduced cost in return for a commitment to buy their Mabs in order to undercut those of their competitors who only make antibodies, and there is a possibility of the large equipment firms overtaking the small high-quality producers so that there will be a reduction in the current range of good reagents at low price. Should this happen, Mab technologists will be better advised to make their own (Protocol 12.2 and 12.3). At the time of writing, purchase of antibodies for screening is convenient for most people.

Table 2.2 gives a guide to how to read the catalogues, and for simplicity, uses goat but it could be rabbit, rat etc. The main importance is the use of outbred animals to avoid the repertoire gaps common in inbred strains.

The main obvious message of Table 2.2 is that an antibody raised against the IgG class can (and in practice does) detect a large number of IgM antibodies. These are low avidity and polyspecific and seldom useful as a reagent (Section 2.2.2). They are able to do this by reaction with the constant region determinants of the γ or κ light chains. While these seem to be a small section of an antibody, the fact that IgMs bind more readily and have 10 of such chains to offer to the second antibody, means that one detects as many positive IgMs as IgGs using an antibody directed to the whole IgG molecule . The protocols de-

TABLE 2.2
Technical descriptions of second antibodies

Description	What it means
Goat* anti-mouse immunoglobulin (Also called goat anti-mouse Ig**)	Polyclonal antiserum obtained from goat(s) immunised with a crude preparation of mouse antibodies. This will detect all isotypes, and be biased towards the selection of IgG and IgM Mabs
Goat anti-mouse IgG**	Polyclonal antiserum obtained from goat(s) immunised with purified mouse IgG. This will also detect all isotypes and be biased towards the selection of IgG and IgM Mabs
Goat anti-mouse IgG** – affinity purified	Polyclonal antiserum obtained from goat(s) immunised with purified mouse IgG and then further purified by affinity absorption to mouse IgG so that it only contains antibodies reactive with mouse IgG (unlike the above two examples where there will also be antibodies to whatever environmental pathogens the goat has recently encountered). This will also detect all isotypes including IgM Mabs
Goat anti-mouse IgG. γ-Chain specific	Polyclonal antiserum obtained from goat(s) immunised with the constant region of purified mouse γ-chain. Fc or anti-mouse IgG adsorbed free of light chain reactivity. *This one really is IgG specific.*

* For goat, read also rabbit, sheep, horse etc – any outbred strain.
** Do not confuse Ig (immunoglobulins of all classes) with IgG.
It is also possible to buy such antibodies pre-absorbed against human IgG for use with human tissues or cells which may contain or secrete this.

scribed here therefore use antibodies to the γ-chain only. If IgA or IgE Mabs are specifically required then it is advisable to use alpha or epsilon specific probes and to adopt an immunisation or tissue selection strategy which will favour them (Chapter 4).

An alternative strategy to using second antibodies for screening is to use the heavily marketed, enzyme or radiolabelled Protein A or Protein G (See Table 10.2 for detailed specificities). These have the attractive feature that they are unreactive with IgM. At the screening stage, Protein A is generally good for detecting all subclasses of

human IgG, poor for most rat IgGs, and best for mouse IgG2a and
IgG2b. Thus in a mouse fusion it may bias the repertoire of clones
selected towards these isotypes. Since they lie to the right of IgG1 and
IgG3 on the isotype switch profile (see Section 4.1), these isotypes are
of higher average affinity and may offer a positive advantage. The
only problem might occur where a carbohydrate antigen unattached to
protein has been used since this will lead to a predominantly IgM and
IgG3 response in the mouse which will be poorly detected by Protein
A. While Protein G may prove to be an equally good or better reagent, there are still limited amounts of data available on its use for
screening.

2.6.7. Enzymes used in screening ELISA/dot-blot assays

The enzyme linked to the second antibody has to have certain qualities. It must be able to be purified in large amounts from a simple
source, and has to have active groups which allow it to link readily
to antibodies without loss of enzyme or antibody activity. Ideally, it
should have a high turnover number under assay conditions. It must
be robust and not susceptible to denaturation at room temperature
or on storage. It has to be able to generate coloured soluble (ELISA)
and insoluble (dot-blot) products from inexpensive colourless soluble
substrates. As a result of largely commercial evolutionary pressures,
involving such considerations, only three enzymes are now generally
used for colour development with second antibody and one of these
three (β-galactosidase) is rarely used. ELISA involves a water soluble
product located in the appropriate well of the ELISA plate and quan-
titated by visual and spectrophotometric methods. Dot- (or slot-)blot
screening involves a water insoluble product, which locates close to
the antigen on an immunoblot or on immunocytochemistry. Variations on ELISA involve either fluorescent or chemiluminescent substrates which require specialised detection devices. These substrate
systems lower the detectability limits of the enzyme itself but do not
necessarily lower the signal/noise ratio for a low-affinity antibody.
The use of these and other enzymes together with their use for ELISA

TABLE 2.3
Substrates and assay conditions for detection enzymes

Horseradish peroxidase
Notes: (i) All substrates require fresh H_2O_2
(ii) Too much H_2O_2 inhibits the reaction
(iii) Several substrates are carcinogenic/mutagneic

SOLUBLE SUBSTRATES (ELISA)
(i) OPD (*o*-phenylenediamine)
Mild carcinogen. Absorbs 492 nm
0.04 mg/ml in 0.05 M Na citrate, 0.15 M Na phosphate, 0.01% H_2O_2, pH 6.0.
Stop with 1 M H_2SO_4.

(ii) TMB (3,3′,5,5′-tetramethylbenzidine)
Absorbs (acid) 450 nm.
80 μg/ml TMB in 0.1 M Na acetate, 0.01% H_2O_2, pH 5.8
Stop with 1 M H_2SO_4. Blue colour turns yellow.

(iii) ABTS (2.2′-azinodi(3-ethylbenzthiazoline sulphonate))
Aborbs 410 and 650 nm
1 mM in 0.05 M Na citrate, 0.15 M Na phosphate, 0.01% H_2O_2.
Stop with 1.5 mM NaN_3 in 0.1 M citric acid

CHEMILUMINESCENT SUBSTRATES (CAN BE USED ON ELISA OR BLOT)
Luminol/iodophenol. pH optimum of chemiluminescence is 8.5; 0.2 mg/ml luminol,
0.5 mg/ml iodophenol, 0.01% H_2O_2 in 0.1 M Tris, pH 8.5.

INSOLUBLE SUBSTRATES (DOT-BLOT)/IMMUNOCYTOCHEMISTRY
(All stopped by washing slide or paper)
(i) 4-chloro-1-naphthol. Stock solution 3 mg/ml of 4-chloronaphthol in methanol.
Dilute with 5 volumes PBS and add H_2O_2 to 0.01%.
Blue/black ppt. Soluble in alcohol and organic solvents.

(ii) DAB (3.3′-diaminobenzidine tetrahydrochloride) *Carcinogen.*
6 mg in 10 ml 0.05 M Tris/HCl, 0.1 M NaCl, pH 7.6, 0.01% H_2O_2
More sensitive when used with 0.03% (w/v) $NiCl_2$ or $CoCl_2$ (filter any precipitate)
Brown ppt. Insoluble in alcohol or organic solvents.

(iii) AEC (3-amino-9-ethylcarbazole)
Make stock 0.4% (w/v) in dimethylformamide or DMSO. Use 0.7 ml of this in 10 ml
0.1 M Na acetate, pH 5.2, 0.02% H_2O_2. Filter if necessary.
Red ppt. Soluble in alcohol. Fades in light.

TABLE 2.3 *(continued)*

Alkaline phosphatase (intestinal)
Notes: (i) Bacterial alkaline phosphatase has a lower pH optimum and requires different assay conditions
   (ii) Do not use phosphate in the buffer at any stage of an assay employing this enzyme
   (iii) All reactions can be stopped with 0.1M EDTA
   (iv) Levamisole (1 mM) can be used to inhibit endogenous enzyme activity in some tissues before staining.

SOLUBLE SUBSTRATE (ELISA)
pNPP (*p*-nitrophenyl phosphate)
Absorbs at 405 nm. 1 mg/ml in 10 mM diethanolamine 0.5 mM $MgCl_2$, pH 9.5.

CHEMILUMINESCENT SUBSTRATE (CAN BE USED ON ELISA OR BLOT)
Adamantyl-1,2-dioxetane phosphate (AMPPD)

FLUOROGENIC SUBSTRATE
4-MU-P (4-methylumbelliferyl phosphate).
0.1 mM in 10 mM diethanolamine 0.5 mM $MgCl_2$.
Excite at 360 nm. Read at 450 nm.

INSOLUBLE SUBSTRATES (DOT-BLOT/IMMUNOCYTOCHEMISTRY)
(i) BCIP/NBT (5-bromo-4-chloroindolyl phosphate/nitro blue tetrazolium).
Stock solutions of (a) 0.5 g NBT in 10 ml 70% dimethylformamide
(b) 1.0 g BCIP in 10 ml 100% dimethylformamide
Just before use add 66 μl each of (a) and (b) to 10 ml 0.1 M Tris, 0.1 M NaCl, 5 mM $MgCl_2$, pH 9.5. Bluish purple.

(ii) NABP/FR (naphthol-AS-MX-phosphate/Fast red)
Stock solution of 10 mg/ml naphthol-AS-MX-phosphate. Add 0.2 ml to 9.8 ml 0.1 M Tris-HCl, 0.1 M NaCl, pH 8.5. Immediately before use, dissolve 10 mg Fast red TR is this.
Red ppt. Soluble in alcohol and organic solvents.

(iii) NABP/NF (Naphthol-AS-BI phosphate/New fuschin)
All solutions fresh
Solution (a) 0.2 ml 5% New Fuschin in 2 M HCl added to 0.5 ml 4% sodium nitrite. Shake.
Add 100 ml 0.05 M Tris, pH 9
Solution (b) 50 mg naphthol-AS-BI-phosphate in 0.6 ml dimethylformamide.
Mix (a) and (b), filter if necessary.
Red ppt. Insoluble in alcohol or organic solvents.

TABLE 2.3 *(continued)*

β-Galactosidase

SOLUBLE SUBSTRATE (ELISA)
ONPG-(*o*-nitrophenyl-D-galactopyranoside)
7 mg/ml in PBS, 1 mM MgCl$_2$, 10 mM mercaptoethanol, pH 7.5.
Stop with 2 M Na$_2$CO$_3$. Read at 410 nm.

FLUOROGENIC SUBSTRATE
4-MU-GAL (4-methylumbelliferyl-D-galactopyranoside)
Stock solution of 1% in dimethyl formamide. Dilute 0.34 ml with 100 ml PBS, 1 mM
MgCl$_2$, 0.1% BSA
Stop with 1 M glycine/NaOH, pH 10.3
Excite at 360 nm, read at 450 nm.

INSOLUBLE SUBSTRATE
BCIG (5-bromo-4-chloro-3-indolyl-D-galactoside)
Dissolve 10 mg BCIG in 0.5 ml dimethylformamide. Add 0.25 ml to 10 ml PBS, 1 mM
MgCl$_2$, 3 mM potassium ferricyanide.
Purple ppt. Insoluble in alcohol or organic solvent.

---

only is comprehensively reviewed in Tijssen (1985). The enzymes and their substrates are described below and in Table 2.3.

(i) The earliest was *alkaline phosphatase* (usually from calf intestine or *E. coli*), a dimeric zinc containing enzyme with subunit molecular weight 80,000–85,000. The calf intestine alkaline phosphatase (see Fernley, 1971 for a detailed description) has an optimum pH of 10.3 and is assayed in diethanolamine buffer. The *E. coli* alkaline phosphatase (see Reid and Wilson, 1971 for a detailed description) has a pH optimum of 8 and is assayed in Tris buffer. Magnesium (or manganese or calcium) chloride is generally recommended during use although such divalent cations have been reported to be unnecessary in these buffers (Bergmeyer, 1974). Both enzymes are strongly inhibited by phosphate and should on no account be used with phosphate present either during incubation with substrate, or in preliminary washes, since trace amounts left over will be inhibitory. The substrate itself should be pure and not contain free phosphate. This enzyme has a fairly wide variety of substrates, all the main ones being non-carcinogenic. For ELISA, the usual one is *p*-nitrophenyl phosphate (NPP) and for dot-blot assays, the usual one is 5-bromo-4-chloroindolyl phosphate together with nitro blue tetrazolium (BCIP/NBT). More recently, the chemiluminescent substrate adamantyl-1,2-dioxetane phosphate (AMPPD) has been described (Voyta et al., 1988).

Alkaline phosphatase has very little carbohydrate and has to be linked to antibodies by means of glutaraldehyde and similar reagents which bind to basic amino acids and consequently may alter or reduce either antibody or enzyme activity (especially since histidine is required for activity). In addition, glutaraldehyde cross-linking tends to give very large heterogeneous complexes (Section 12.7). There is reported endogenous activity in many cells and tissues which can be inhibited by incubation with 0.1 mM levamisole in the second antibody preparation and washing before substrate is added. While this endogenous activity may be a problem in immunocytochemical assays, it does not usually affect ELISA assays on intact live cells or immunoblots on purified proteins. Alkaline phosphatase gives good results for both soluble and insoluble assays, and can be adapted readily to field use. For screening, it is generally more expensive than peroxidase and if a low pH is required, or the antigen to be screened is heavily phosphorylated, it would obviously be inappropriate.

A more complex alkaline phosphatase assay called APAAP, analogous to the PAP assay described below for peroxidase is occasionally described. It increases signal but also noise and has limited utility.

(ii) The enzyme in commonest recent use has been *horseradish peroxidase* (HRP) (molecular weight 44,000). Prior to the full advance of recombinant DNA technology, this enzyme was the most economical to make or buy. It detects optimally in the lower pH range (5–7). The active site contains iron in a porphyrin ring and in consequence the enzyme is inhibited by substances such as cyanide or azide (the latter being frequently used as an anti-bacterial agent in preparations of antibody or antigen). Most preparations of HRP have a substantial amount of carbohydrate and these can be linked by periodate to the carbohydrate residues in the constant region of an antibody, leaving the variable region unaffected. As there are limited amounts of carbohydrate on an antibody, there is also less chance of creating unwieldy and insoluble multimolecular complexes. HRP has a very wide range of substrates but many of these are carcinogenic in the Ames test for bacterial mutagenesis. For example, DAB (diaminobenzidine) should only be worked with under strictly controlled conditions and in many countries the group leader may violate Health and Safety legislation and lead to legal action against the host institution if it is not used according to the legislative requirements of the country in which the work is conducted. The hydrogen peroxide (H_2O_2) component of the substrate is the most difficult to control since it must be freshly prepared, tends to behave abnormally at solid surfaces, and deteriorates rapidly in assay buffer. This, together with the mutagenic properties of many other substrates, limits the field use of HRP. It is, however, highly suitable for laboratory use by trained personnel, for screening emerging clones, for antibodies better suited to a lower pH range, and for use with heavily phosphorylated antigens.

Peroxidases also have many substrates with chemiluminescent products which may be converted by photoelectric processes into electronic data (Chapter 12). Horseradish peroxidase has a variety of chemiluminescent substrates of which the most commonly used is luminol. The system had limited value because of the short duration of light emission until the discovery of various compounds which were able to both enhance the signal and prolong its duration. The best known among these enhancers are D-luciferin (Whitehead et al., 1983) and 4-iodophenol (Laing, 1986; Schneppenheim and Rautenberg, 1987). In consequence, a conventional ELISA assay may be converted to one which yields light rather than colour and this light can be detected by a monitoring system and converted into a signal. This is the basis of the Amerlite system marketed by Amersham International. Immunoblots may also be developed by this system followed by a few minutes exposure to X-ray film. Chemiluminescent assays are extensively described by a variety of authors in a substantial volume of the Journal of Bioluminescence and Chemiluminescence (Volume 4, 1989).

Peroxidase forms the main component of a complex called PAP (peroxidase–antiperoxidase) described originally by Sternberger (see

Sternberger, 1979 for review) and was widely used with polyclonal rabbit antiserum in the 1970s. It has translated poorly to the mouse or rat monoclonal assay systems. The basis of this technique is the use of an non-covalently linked peroxidase-antibody complex from the appropriate species which improves detectability but may also raise background. The sequence of the sandwich is

Solid phase _ Ag _ mouse Mab _ excess rabbit antimouse IgG _ mouse peroxidase-anti peroxidase complex _ substrate.

(iii) *β-galactosidase* (subunit molecular weight 115,000, active enzyme molecular weight 460,000) from *E. coli* is claimed to be active through a wider pH range than the above two and this could increase screening range if pH considerations do not restrict final use. It had a brief spurt of popularity when immunocytochemists working on tissue sections interpreted their high backgrounds as being due to endogenous activity of the other two enzymes. The large active form is a less robust enzyme of comparatively low stability, and there are now so many other interpretations for high backgrounds in immunocytochemistry that it has largely fallen into minor use in the laboratory. Its instability makes it comparatively impractical for any form of field work.

Other enzymes such as glucose oxidase or urease, both of which have projected applications in the immunosensor field, have failed to penetrate the market for mass screening antibodies for reasons of purification cost, substrate cost, lack of suitability for cross-linking, lack of stability etc.

The relevant substrates for all three are listed in Table 2.4 with references for those requiring greater detail.

Whether these conjugates are made in the laboratory or bought from commercial sources, they should be stored in aliquots at $-20°C$. There are also several systems involving the use of Biotin, which has an affinity of 10^{15} M^{-1} for the egg white protein, avidin or its bacterial equivalent, streptavidin. Biotin is chemically cross-linked to amino groups on the antibody (Protocol 12.4) and, if these are critical to binding, may reduce their affinity. For assay, the second antibody is biotinlylated and the colour reaction is then developed with either avidin or streptavidin cross-linked to enzyme. These systems give low backgrounds but involve an extra washing step and so give low fore-grounds – as ever, it is a question of signal to noise ratio and the more washes, the less the noise and the less the signal. Biotinylated antibod-ies carry an advantage in a large lab working with rat, human and mouse systems in that, if second antibody is biotinylated in all cases, the detection system can be common.

It is possible to amplify the signals from these or other enzymes by creating complex assay systems with further layers of enzyme and antibody to create a very sensitive system indeed (e.g., the PAP assay described above). All depend on the original antibody remaining bound while sequential layers are added to the tail of material at-tached to it. This seldom improves the signal/noise ratio if the basic attachment to specific antigen is low affinity (see Section 2.2.2). Either the background reading rises with the foreground, or the antibody is dissociated from specific antigen as well as non-specific by all the washing steps involved. Such assays are also expensive and inconven-ient for screening, which has to be done in a short period of time.

2.6.8. Radioactive detection systems

In these, the second antibody or protein A is linked to an isotope such as ^{125}I. The ELISA plate or nitrocellulose paper can then be autora-diographed or the wells or spots can be cut out and counted in a scin-tillation counter. Such screening methods have largely fallen out of use, being more expensive, time consuming, and environmentally haz-ardous. However, in cases where the final product monoclonal anti-body will be used in radioimmunoassay, they can be used for a second-ary screen. This can still be encountered where small molecules such as drugs and steroids are the antigen but are largely being replaced by the above antibody-linked enzyme chemiluminescent assays.

2.6.9. Washing

It will be evident that throughout solid-phase assays based either on microtitre plates or on nitrocellulose, there are washing steps required to remove unbound antigen, unbound blocker, unbound material from the hybridoma supernatant, unbound second antibody or Protein A etc. All antibodies have a finite dissociation rate from antigen (Section 2.2.2) and the more post binding washing steps there are, the more both signal and background will be reduced. In screening, this is difficult, as one has limited opportunity to find the most suitable conditions to select an (as yet) uncharacterised antibody which may be of considerable use as a sensor under different conditions. Essentially you are looking for optimal signal/noise ratio conditions related to final use without being able to play with these parameters as you would with the finallystabilised Mab.

On the mechanical side, poor washing may give false positives and over-zealous washing may give false negative results. Instruments which wash ELISA plates are readily available commercially and their theoretical main advantage is to give standard washing. However, if their jets are blocked or wrongly angled, they can be unhelpful. Probably the ideal way of 'hand' washing an ELISA mictrotitre plate is to immerse it totally, at an angle, over a defined period of time, smoothing out air bubbles over any well as you do so. Then give it a quick wrist flick over a sink and hammer it dry on a wad of paper towels. It is essential not to leave residual washing buffer in any well as this will dilute the subsequent reagent. One can also use a polythene bottle with a wide necked tube to flush out each well but one must maintain a standard pressure over all the wells on the plate.

Washing nitrocellulose paper is much more straightforward procedure and the paper only has to be gently agitated in the buffer. A laboratory gel shaker can be used for this but the time and volume involved will affect the result so should be kept standard with any deviations from routine being noted.

The washing buffer depends on the blocking system. For ELISA microtitre plates a routine buffer such as PBS is used with a small amount of non-ionic detergent (0.05% Tween 20). For paper, because it has a greater tendency to absorb irrelevant material, more detergent and/or additional blocking proteins are also usually incorporated.

2.6.10. Detection of signal

Most ELISA assays are read in spectrophotometers adapted for microtitre plates, available from all main suppliers. This is an excellent method for obtaining printed results for computerised storage and removes the subjective element, particularly if positive and negative controls are included. Where detailed quantitative analysis is required, as opposed to a discrimination between positive and negative, it is essential. However, for screening, It is a comparatively expensive piece of equipment and positive samples are in fact, always visible by eye. Specialised equipment is required for the detection of fluorescent products (Fluoroscan) and chemiluminescent substrates are either detected in a liquid scintillation counter with the coincidence counting mode switched off, by autoradiography or by luminometers which are now rapidly increasing in availability and, since they require no light input and only light measurement, may in future be avilable at low cost and size.

No equipment is necessary for dot-blots on a nitrocellulose base where the blot itself can be retained or photographed. If a printed record is required, or a detailed quantitative analysis is being undertaken, then the membrane can be made transparent by soaking in glycerol/water (Hawkes, 1986) if the product is soluble in organic solvents, or organic solvents such as xylene if it is not, and scanning on a transmission densitometer (Palfreyman et al., 1988). In screening, positives can be detected by eye. In addition, if a chemiluminescent substrate is used (Table 2.3) then the dots can be visualised on X-ray film (Schneppenheim and Rautenberg, 1987).

2.7. Protocols for solid-phase assays

There is no point in doing a fusion with an animal which has a low serum titre. In addition, it is obviously necessary to test the detection limits, sensitivity and reproducibility of the chosen screening assay. The methods described relate *only* to large amounts of purified protein antigen, to a readily used blocking reagent and to screening for IgG Mabs only. Most people now work with more complex antigens and are advised to read previous and subsequent sections.

2.7.1. Whether to use ELISA or dot-blot

For any new project, the investigator is strongly encouraged to try both procedures with immune serum prior to fusion.

For a pure protein, the main difference is the concentration of screening antigen which may be achieved (Section 2.2.2). The local concentration on a dot-blot protocol as described below can be very high indeed if purity, solubility and availability allow it. This means that it may be possible to detect more weak positives in emerging clones (although these may subsequently be shown to be of low affinity, and the density and presentation of screening antigen is most unlikely to be similar). Dot-blots also use very little serum/culture supernatant and can be sampled daily and tested at several antigen concentrations. The antigen is simply prepared on sheets of paper and the appropriate number of small squares are cut out (squared off nitrocellulose paper can even be purchased). With an ELISA plate, in contrast, it is common to use only a few of the 96 wells. Dot-blotting is therefore generally very much less expensive.

With the same concentration of antigen and antibody and all other factors with the exception of the nature of the final product (soluble versus non-soluble), being taken into consideration, ELISA is undoubtedly a more sensitive system with lower detection limits. It is also better for particulate antigens which attach poorly to nitrocellulose or other membranes giving erratic results, since nitrocellulose paper, unlike an ELISA plate, is not amenable to comparatively uniform centrifugation. ELISA provides a standard readout which can be stored and computerised. This is also possible for dot-blots with scanning densitometry but the technique is labour intensive and skilled.

Protocols 2.1 and 2.2 give the operator an opportunity to compare these for the appropriate antigen and serum before deciding which screening method best suits them.

PROTOCOL 2.1: ELISA ASSAY FOR ANTISERUM TITRE OF IgG ANTIBODIES
TO PURE PROTEIN ANTIGEN

Materials

(a) *Hardware* 2×96 well ELISA plates. One for the test serum and one for the control. An 8 channel multipipetter is also preferable. Optional extras are an ELISA platewasher and a platereader.

(b) *Antigen* (20 ml at 10 μg/ml). See later for impure/ expensive antigens.

(c) *First antibody* Pre-immune serum from the same animal or one of the same strain and age. Immune serum from an animal boosted intravenously 7–10 days (*not* 4 days) before bleeding (see Chapter 4).

(d) *Blocking reagent* 10 mg/ml bovine serum albumin (BSA) in PBS containing 0.05% Tween 20.

(e) *Second antibody* HRP labelled anti-mouse IgG, γ-chain specific (Sigma, Amersham, Dako or other company). In general, 1 ml of antiserum is supplied and recommended use is at a dilution of around 1 in 1000. For this, stock is diluted to 10 ml with PBS containing 0.5% BSA, and stored in 500 μl aliquots in 1 ml polytubes at $-20°$C. Dilute 200 μl of this stock to 20 ml with PBS containing 0.5% BSA just before assay. This is enough for two ELISA plates.

(f) *Substrate* Stock solution of 8 mg/ml 3,3′,5,5′-tetramethylbenzidine in DMSO (can be stored for up to 1 month in the dark). Just before use, for each ELISA plate, add 0.1 ml of this to 9.9 ml of 0.1 M Na acetate, pH 5.8, containing 0.01% H_2O_2 (0.32 μl/ml of stock 30% solution). It is important that the H_2O_2 be added *immediately* before use.

(g) *Stopping reagent* 1 M sulphuric acid (14 ml concentrated sulphuric acid diluted with 486 ml distilled water)

Procedure

(i) Prepare 2.5 ml each of solutions of pure antigen at 10, 1 and 0.1 μg/ml, (diluted in PBS containing *no* protein). (Do not exceed this amount of antigen. See later for impure and particulate antigens).

(ii) Microtitre plates generally have 96 wells labelled A–H and 1–12. For both ELISA plates, put 100 μl of the solution containing 10 μg/ml of antigen into all wells of Row A and B, 100 μl of the solution containing 1 μg of antigen into rows C and D, 100 μl of the solution containing 0.1 μg of antigen into rows E and F and the buffer which contained the antigen into rows G and H. Pipette accurately and into the centre of the well. Cover with clingfilm and leave for 1–2 hours at room temperature.

(iii) Wash the plate with PBS 0.05% Tween 20. Either use a plate washer or gently immerse the plate in buffer at an angle stroking to to eliminate bubbleholes over any well. Flick out the washing buffer and hammer dry hard over a wad of paper towels until the towels show no fluid stain. If you leave any fluid, it will give your poor duplication.

(iv) To all wells on the plate, add 100 μl blocking reagent. Pipette accurately and into the centre of the well. You want to block a similar area to the one you coated with antigen. Incubate for a minimum of one hour. Flick out and wash as before.

(v) Prepare serial dilutions of specific antiserum starting with 2 ml at 1 in 100 in PBS, 0.5% BSA (Tube 1). Prepare 10 tubes labelled 2–11 each with 1 ml PBS, 0.5% BSA. Take 1 ml from tube 1 and add it to Tube 2, mix, remove 1 ml and add this to Tube 3, mix, remove 1 ml and add it to tube 4 and so on. Tube 2 will then be at 1/200, Tube 3 at 1/400 and so on with Tube 11 being finally at 1/102,400.

Do precisely the same with the pre-immune serum.

(vi) To the Test ELISA plate add 100 μl of the 1/100 dilution of specific antiserum (Tube 1) to all wells in column 1, 100 μl of the 1/200 (Tube 2) to all wells in column 2, 100 μl of the 1/400 dilution into all wells in column 3 and so on, finally puting 100 μl from tube 11 into column 11 (1/102,400). To all wells in column 12 add 100 μl of PBS, 0.5% BSA.

Do precisely the same with the dilutions of pre-immune serum on the control ELISA plate.

Cover with clingfilm and incubate for a minimum of 1 hour. Flick off and wash as before.

(vii) Add 100 μl of second antibody to all wells on both plates. Incubate for a minimum of 1 hour. Flick off and wash as before.
(viii) Add 100 μl substrate solution to each well of both plates. Incubate 10–20 minutes. A pale blue colour indicates a positive sample.
(ix) Stop the reaction by the addition of 50 μl stopping reagent. Positives now appear yellow.
(x) Read at 450 nm in a multiscan spectrophotometer or inspect by eye.

To interpret your results, examine the data with respect to the following points:

(a) In general, the controls should be low (all of the control plate, column 12 and rows G and H on the test plate), if not, there may be an excess of second antibody or substrate.

(b) The duplication should be good. A1 = B1, A2 = B2 etc. When a fusion is performed, there is frequently not enough antibody to check duplication so complete confidence in this is essential. Poor duplication indicates a lack of standard washing and/or pipetting.

(c) The titre of the immune serum in comparison to the pre-immune. Wells A5 and B5 on the test plate (1/1600) should give a strong colour compared to wells A5 and B5 on the control plate. In a good serum, this will also be true for later wells, e.g., A8 and B8 (1/12800). The titre at which the test plate is above the control plate is the serum titre of the animal, i.e., if wells A7 and B7 are significantly higher in test than control, then the titre is 1/6400. It is not advisable to do a fusion if the serum titre is not over 1/1000.

(d) The titre can then be checked with the three concentrations of substrate to see if it is the same with 1μg on antigen on the plate (A and B) as with 0.1 (C and D) and 0.01 (E and F). If it is substantially better with the larger amount and one can afford enough antigen to do so, then it is better to screen with it. If it is only slightly better, and the antigen is expensive in cost or labour, then it may be better to screen with the smaller amount. You may obtain fewer positive clones, but they will all be of high affinity.

(e) Work out exactly what this has cost you and compare the cost of a dot-blot (Protocol 2.3), which has used less antigen at higher local concentration.

PROTOCOL 2.2: ELISA ASSAY FOR SCREENING OF A MOUSE FUSION FOR IgG ANTIBODIES

Materials

(a) *Hardware* 10×96 well ELISA plates (assuming the fusion is in 10×96 well culture plates – adjust accordingly). Sterile tips. An 8 channel multipipetter is also preferable. Optional extras are an ELISA platewasher and a platereader.

(b) *Antigen* (100 ml at 1 μg/ml). See later for impure/ expensive antigens.

(c) *Fusion plates* to be sampled in a sterile hood and fed with fresh medium *immediately* after sampling. 100 ml complete medium.

(d) *Blocking reagent* 100 ml of 10 mg/ml bovine serum albumin (BSA) in PBS containing 0.05% Tween 20.

(e) *Second antibody* HRP labelled anti-mouse IgG, γ-chain specific (Sigma, Amersham, Dako or other company). In general, 1 ml of antiserum is supplied and recommended use is at a dilution of around 1 in 1000. For this, stock is diluted to 10 ml with PBS containing 0.5% BSA, and stored in 0.5–1.0 ml aliquots in 1 ml polytubes at $-20°$C. Dilute 1 ml of this stock to 100 ml with PBS containing 0.5% BSA just before assay. This is enough for ten ELISA plates.

(f) *Substrate* Stock solution of 8 mg/ml 3,3′,5,5′-tetramethylbenzidine in DMSO (can be stored for up to 1 month). Just before use, for each ELISA plate, add 0.1 ml of this to 9.9 ml of 0.1 M Na acetate, pH 5.8, containing 0.01% H_2O_2 (0.32 μl/ml of stock 30% solution). It is important that the H_2O_2 be added *immediately* before use.

(g) *Stopping reagent* 1 M sulphuric acid (14 ml concentrated diluted with 486 ml distilled water).

Procedure

(i) Coat the ELISA plates with 100 μl/well of antigen, cover with clingfilm and leave for 1–2 hours at room temperature.

(ii) Wash the plate with PBS 0.05% Tween 20. Either use a platewasher or gently immerse the plate in buffer at an angle stroking to eliminate bubbleholes over any well. Flick out the washing buffer and hammer dry hard over a wad of paper towels until the towels show no fluid stain.

(iii) To all wells on the plate, add 100 μl blocking reagent. Pipette accurately and into the centre of the well. You want to block a similar area to the one you coated with antigen. Incubate for a minimum of one hour. Flick out and wash as before.

(iv) Sample 100 μl from each fusion well using a multipipette with sterile tips. It is not necessary to change tips between each well. Feed the fusion plates with fresh medium. Cover the assay plates with clingfilm and incubate for 2 hours or overnight.

(v) Add 100 μl of second antibody to all wells. Incubate for a minimum of 1 hour. Flick off and wash as before.

(vi) Add 100 μl substrate solution to each well of both plates. Incubate 10–20 minutes. A pale blue colour indicates a positive sample.

(vii) Stop the reaction by the addition of 50 μl stopping reagent. Positives now appear yellow.

(viii) Read at 450 nm in a multiscan spectrophotometer or inspect by eye.

Attend to the following points

(a) The control wells which only contained myeloma cells should give a low reading. More relevant are the wells which only contained spleen cells. These will often give quite a high reading at early screening stages as the spleen cells themselves will continue to secrete antibody for about 10 days. A well can only be scored as positive if it is above these controls.

(b) If there are too many positives to clone, wash the plates twice more and return to step (vi). The highest affinity Mabs will remain attached.

(c)   The positive wells should be checked with the original tissue culture plates to examine the size of the clone producing the antibody. If there are enough cells, they should be cloned as soon as possible (Chapter 8)

(d)   The tissue culture plate should be re-screened after 3–4 days.

2.7.2. ELISA assay for impure protein antigen

The utility of this depends on exactly how impure the antigen was, whether the materials contaminating it were also present in the immunising mixture and if so whether they were immunodominant. It is advisable to check the serum as described in protocol 2.1 above before proceeding, using more antigen to coat the ELISA plate. If you requires a Mab directed to a protein which comprised only 1% of both immunising and screening materials you are unlikely to obtain a satisfactory antibody on a solid-phase assay and an assay relevant to the biological function of the antigen is indicated. (Live cells by FACS, biological function blocking assays – see later.) Sometimes, however, there is a fairly minor contamination of a preparation. For example it is often difficult to obtain proteins from serum or cells grown in it totally free of albumin and cell membrane proteins often have trace contaminating cytoskeletal proteins. If the protein is only slightly impure, then a screening check against the major impurity (usually common and readily available in bulk) should be performed by either a second ELISA against the contaminating protein or an immunoblot at an early stage.

2.7.3. ELISA for bacterial antigens

ELISA can be performed with whole bacteria (100 μl at 10^8/ml) which are either centrifuged onto the ELISA plate at $1000 \times g$ for 5 minutes or dried down onto the ELISA plate at stage (ii) above. Centrifugation at later stages of the assay is not usually necessary.

Most bacteria are coated with material with a regular structure which frequently contains much carbohydrate (e.g., LPS in gram negative bacteria, exosporium coats in spores of gram positive bacteria). If you immunise and assay (or even just assay) with whole bacteria, you will obtain antibodies to these components and not internal bacterial proteins (see Section 4.18.2 for strategies relating to these antigens). FACS assay (Protocols 2.5 and 2.6) is sometimes applicable to bacterial antigens but bacteria can be readily agglutinated by antibodies and in these cases FACS is unsuitable.

2.7.4. ELISA for cellular antigens

If a whole cell was used as immunising antigen, or an autologous response is being tested within an affected individual, it should be noted that the response to a minor protein is likely to be weak and obscured by the response/non-specific binding to the major proteins. All methods for fixing cells to ELISA plates make the cells permeable and in consequence are of no use unless an antibody to cytoskeletal or nuclear structural proteins are required (Fig. 2.5). These have limited utility and those that have appeared regularly in the literature and in commercial catalogues have largely been by-products of programmes designed to produce Mabs to cell surface antigens. If an IgM detecting probe is used, the spectrum of positive responses will be dominated by non-specific IgM Mabs to common structural proteins. If an IgG specific probe is used as recommended, no high-affinity positive clones will be obtained.

Almost all applications of cellular antigens involve cell surface proteins detectable on live cells. It is possible to use live cells on ELISA (10^4/well), centrifuging the plate at $600 \times g$ for 5 minutes at each stage. Inevitably, some cells will be permeabilised by the process. This is less important at the later stages of assay when the controls will indicate whether or not non-specific binding is occurring, but will lead to non-specific binding at the antibody absorption stages. If you have access to a FACS (Protocols 2.5 and 2.6) then it is a better method.

PROTOCOL 2.3: DOT-BLOT ASSAY FOR ANTISERUM TITRE OF IgG
ANTIBODIES TO PURE PROTEIN ANTIGEN

Materials

(a) *Hardware* Nitrocellulose paper (0.45 μ). Soft pencil. Accurate
    micropipetter. Circular rocker type lab shaker for washing
    (gentle but not vigorous – available in most labs where recombin-
    ant DNA work is being undertaken).
    Manifolds which hold the paper during the assay can also be pur-
    chased but offer little advantage using an unnecessary amount of
    material and giving limited advantage. They also tend to leak.
(b) *Antigen* (200 μl at 100 μg/ml). See later for impure/ expensive
    antigens.
(c) *First antibody* Pre-immune serum from the same animal or one of
    the same strain and age. Immune serum from an animal boosted
    intravenously 7–10 days (*not* 4 days) before bleeding (see Chapter 4).
(d) *Blocking reagent* 10 mg/ ml bovine serum albumin (BSA) in PBS
    containing 0.1% Tween 20.
(e) *Second antibody* HRP labelled anti-mouse IgG, γ-chain specific
    (Sigma, Amersham, Dako or other company). In general, 1 ml of
    antiserum is supplied and recommended use is at a dilution of
    around 1 in 1000. For this, stock is diluted to 10 ml with PBS
    containing 0.5% BSA, and stored in 0.5–1.0 ml aliquots in poly-
    tubes at $-20°$C. Dilute 100 μl of this stock to 10 ml with PBS
    containing 0.5% BSA just before assay.
(f) *Substrate* Stock solution 3 mg/ml of 4-chloronaphthol in meth-
    anol, stored for up to 1 month in a dark bottle. Dilute with 5
    volumes PBS and add H_2O_2 to 0.01%. It is important that the
    H_2O_2 be added *immediately* before use.

Procedure

(i) Wear gloves – nitrocellulose binds protein very readily. Rule off
5×5 mm squares on the sheet of nitrocellulose paper with a blunt

graphite pencil while the paper is slightly damp, resting the nitrocellulose on clean filter paper. Cut off two sections of this, each containing
12 across by 8 down squares and label them rows A–H (1–8) and columns (1–12) to give the equivalent of the two ELISA plate in protocol
2.1. Cut off the top left hand corner so that you know the orientation
of the paper.

(ii) Prepare 200 μl each of solutions of pure antigen at 100, 10, and
1 μg/ml, (diluted in PBS containing no protein). (Note that this is a
higher antigen concentration than is used for ELISA in protocol 2.1.)

(iii) For each sheet, pipette 2 μl of the solution containing 100 μg /ml
of antigen into the centre of all squares in Row A and B, 2 μl of the
solution containing 10 μg of antigen into all squares in rows C and
D, 2 μl of the solution containing 1 μg of antigen into all squares in
rows E and F and the 2 μl buffer which contained the antigen into
squares in rows G and H. Pipette accurately and into the centre of
the square. It is possible to allow the paper(s) to dry out to flexibility
but not to the point of being brittle.

(iv) Wash the paper(s) for at least 1 hour by putting it (them) in a suitably sized *very clean* plastic container (the type of container which
holds an ELISA plate is particularly useful) with sufficient PBS 0.05%
Tween 20 to cover it (them) – 5 ml for a 15 cm/30 cm/2 cm container
– more for a larger one, covering this container with lid or clingfilm
and rocking either by hand or on laboratory devices sold for this purpose.

Alternatively, one can obtain a commercial polythene bag sealer
and a roll of polythene, and make a customised container, containing
suitable volume for each set of squares.

(v) Incubate the papers in blocking reagent for 2 hours with washing
in the same containers and manner as that used for washing.

(vi) Prepare serial dilutions of specific antiserum starting with 200 μl
at 1 in 100 in PBS, 0.5% BSA (Tube 1). Prepare 10 tubes labelled 2–11
each with 100 μl PBS, 0.5% BSA. Take 100 μl from tube 1 and add
it to Tube 2, mix, remove 100 μl and add this to Tube 3, mix, remove
100 μl and add it to Tube 4 and so on. Tube 2 will then be at 1/200,
Tube 3 at 1/400 and so on with Tube 11 being finally at 1/102,400.

Do precisely the same with the pre-immune serum.

(vii) To precisely the same central position in each spot, add 2 μl of the 1/100 dilution of specific antiserum (Tube 1) to all wells in column 1, 100 μl of the 1/200 (Tube 2) to all wells in column 2, 2 μl of the 1/400 dilution into all wells in column 3 and so on, finally putting 2 μl from tube 11 into column 11 (1/102,400). To all spots in column 12 add 2 μl of PBS, 0.5% BSA.

Do precisely the same with the dilutions of pre-immune serum on the control piece of nitrocellulose. Incubate for a mimimum of one hour in humidified conditions, on no account allowing the paper to dry out. Wash as before.

(viii) Incubate the paper(s) in 2nd antibody (2 ml/cm^2) for 1 hour with rocking. Then wash as before.

(ix) Incubate the strips in 5–10 ml substrate solution. Positives are dark blue/purple. Stop the reaction by washing in distilled water.

(x) Inspect by eye and/or photograph. The colour is stronger when the paper is wet.

To interpret your results, examine the data with respect to the following points

(a) In general, the controls should be low (all of the control paper, column 12 and rows G and H on the test paper), if not, there may be an excess of second antibody or substrate.

(b) The duplication should be good. A1 = B1, A2 = B2 etc. When a fusion is performed, there is frequently not enough antibody to check duplication so complete confidence in this is essential. Poor duplication indicates a lack of standard exposure to washing and/or pipetting reagents.

(c) The titre of the immune serum in comparison to the pre-immune. Spots A5 and B5 on the test paper (1/1600) should give a strong colour compared to spots A5 and B5 on the control paper. In a high-titre serum, this will also be true for later spots, e.g., A8 and B8 (1/12800). The titre at which the test paper is above the control paper is the serum titre of the animal, i.e., if spots A7 and

B7 are significantly higher in test than control, then the titre is 1/6400. It is not advisable to do a fusion if the serum titre is not over 1/1000.

(d) The titre can then be checked with the three concentrations of substrate to see if it is the same with 0.2 μg on antigen on the paper (A and B) as with 0.02 (C and D) and 0.002 (E and F). If it is substantially better with the larger amount and one can afford enough antigen to do so, then it is better to screen with it. If it is only slightly better, and the antigen is expensive in cost or labour, then it may be better to screen with the smaller amount. One may obtain fewer positive clones, but they will all be of high affinity.

(e) Work out exactly what this has cost and compare the cost with ELISA which has used more dilute antigen over a wider area.

PROTOCOL 2.4: DOT-BLOT ASSAY FOR SCREENING A MOUSE FUSION FOR IgG ANTIBODIES TO PURE PROTEIN ANTIGEN

Materials

(a) *Hardware* Nitrocellulose paper (0.45 μ). Soft pencil. Accurate micropipetter. Circular rocker type lab shaker for washing (gentle but not vigorous – available in most labs where recombinant DNA work is being undertaken).
Manifolds which hold the paper during the assay can also be purchased but offer little advantage using an unnecessary amount of material and giving limited advantage. They also tend to leak.

(b) *Antigen* (2 ml at 10 μg/ml). See later for impure/ expensive antigens

(c) *Fusion plates* To be sampled in a sterile hood. This protocol is for 10 × 96 well fusion plates.

(d) *Blocking reagent* 10 mg/ml bovine serum albumin (BSA) in PBS containing 0.1% Tween 20.

(e) *Second antibody* HRP labelled anti-mouse IgG, γ-chain specific (Sigma, Amersham, Dako or other company). In general, 1 ml of antiserum is supplied and recommended use is at a dilution of around 1 in 1000. For this, stock is diluted to 10 ml with PBS containing 0.5% BSA, and stored in 100 μl aliquots in polytubes at $-20°$C. Dilute 100 μl of this stock to 10 ml with PBS containing 0.5% BSA just before assay.

(f) *Substrate* Stock solution 3 mg/ml of 4-chloronaphthol in methanol, stored for up to 1 month in a dark bottle. Dilute with 5 volumes PBS and add H_2O_2 to 0.01%. It is important that the H_2O_2 be added *immediately* before use.

Procedure

(i) Wear gloves – nitrocellulose binds protein very readily. Rule off 5×5 mm squares on the sheet of nitrocellulose paper with a blunt graphite pencil while the paper is slightly damp, resting the nitrocellulose on clean filter paper. Square/cut off ten sections of this, each containing 12 across by 8 down squares and label all ten squares rows A–H (1–8) and columns (1–12) to give the equivalent of the ten ELISA plates in Protocol 2.2. Cut off the top left hand corners so that you know the orientation of the paper.

(ii) For each sheet, pipette 2 μl of the antigen solution. Pipette accurately and into the centre of the square. It is possible to allow the paper(s) to dry out to flexibility but not to the point of being brittle.

(iii) Wash the paper(s) for at least one hour by putting it (them) in a suitably sized very clean plastic container (the type of container which holds an ELISA paper is particularly useful) with sufficient PBS 0.05% Tween 20 to cover it (them) – 5 ml for a 15 cm/30 cm container – more for a larger one, covering this container with lid or clingfilm and rocking either by hand or on laboratory devices sold for this purpose.

Alternatively, one can obtain a commercial polythene bag sealer and a roll of polythene, and make a customised container, containing suitable volume for each set of squares.

(iv) Incubate the papers in blocking reagent for 2 hours with washing in the same containers and manner as that used for washing.

(v) In precisely the same central spot in the appropriate square of each paper, add 2 μl from each well of the tissue culture plates so that the papers precisely match each of the culture plates. Incubate for a minimum of 1 hour in humidified conditions, on no account allowing the paper to dry out. Wash as before.

(vi) Incubate the paper(s) in 2nd antibody (2 ml/cm^2) for 1 hour with rocking. Then wash as before.

(vii) Incubate the strip in 5–10 ml substrate solution. Positives are dark blue/ purple. Stop the reaction by washing the paper in distilled water.

(viii) Inspect by eye, photograph. Scan by reflectance densitometry if necessary.

Attend to the following points

(a) The control wells which contained only myeloma cells should give a low reading. More relevant are the wells which only contained spleen cells. These will often give quite a high reading at early stages as the spleen cells themselves will continue to secrete antibody for about 10 days. A well can only be scored as positive if it is above these controls.

(b) If there are too many positives to clone, wash the paper with 0.15–0.2% Tween in washing buffer and proceed as from step (vii). This will select only those Mabs which bind strongly to the antigen.

(c) The positive wells should be checked with the original tissue culture papers to examine the size of the clone producing the antibody. If there are enough cells, they should be cloned as soon as possible (Chapter 8).

(d) The tissue culture plates should be rescreened after 3–4 days.

2.7.5. Dot-blotting for particulate/cellular antigens

While there were many earlier reports that this technique was successful, particulate antigens may readily detach from paper and the technique seldom gives good duplication with such complex antigens.

2.8. Screening for cellular antigens by FACS

In the early days of Mab technology, ELISA was used to screen for cellular antigens. This proved largely unsuccessful in that antibodies which bound at low affinity to major intracellular structural proteins tended to dominate the results. Immunocytochemical assays in which the precise localisation of the antibody can be determined were more successfully employed but these are very labour intensive and also subjective. In addition, if the cell has a large nucleus and minimal cytoplasm, as do, for example, many tumour cells, it is quite difficult to differentiate staining in the cytoplasm from staining on the cell membrane.

If the final use of the antibody involves binding to the external surface of a cell, it is advisable to screen with live cells which are impermeable to antigen. One of the most efficient methods for this is a flow cytometry assay which will, in addition give information as to whether the antibody binds to all or only a subset of the cells under test. Flow cytometry can also be readily used to screen antibodies to bacterial populations.

2.8.1. Screening by flow cytometry

Flow cytometers or FACS (Fluorescent Activated Cell Sorting) instruments used to be cumbersome, expensive and difficult to operate. There have been many advances in technique and design and a flow cytometer is usually present in, or available to, most well found laboratories. Where a laboratory does not have one, it is usually possible to lease time on one owned by a nearby haematology, immunology or biochemistry laboratory. The two main firms marketing the instruments are Becton Dickinson and Coulter Electronics. Both companies market not only instruments which physically sort fluorescent cells, but also much less expensive but highly efficient instruments designed for analytical use only. The modern instrument is user friendly and can be operated by a junior technician.

The FACS great advantage is that the subjective element of immunocytochemistry is removed and data can be obtained from several thousand cells in 2–5 minutes. It can differentiate a weak positive from a control where an operator has difficulty as the cells bleach under microscopic examination. FACS is superior to live cell ELISA assays in that it indicates whether there is a *strong* signal from a *small* population or a weaker one from the entire population of cells under analysis. It is inferior to immunocytochemical assays in that it does not indicate the distribution of antigen on the cell surface and many cell types and epithelial cells in particular regularly show localised staining. This can only be seen by direct microscopy. The ideal protocol involves preliminary FACS screening followed by detailed immunocytochemical analysis.

FACS instruments are laser powered and the monochromatic emission of the laser does not excite all dyes. Table 2.4 gives a spectrum of the absorption and emission characteristics of various laser types. The commonest type, the argon ion laser, cannot be directly used with some of the red fluorescent stains used in immunofluorescence such as rhodamine and Texas Red, although it can be used in fluorescence transfer where an antibody labelled with biotin can be linked to an antibody labelled with 'duochrome', a streptavidin label which contains a fluorophor excitable at the wavelengths relevant to the argon ion laser such as phycoerythrin linked to a molecule such as Texas Red, emitting in the long red wavelength, where argon ion excitable fluorophors seldom emit. The end result is to extend the emission range of the laser to encompass a wide variety of fluorescent probes.

The minor problems of screening in this manner relate largely to Fc receptor binding, which can be checked by using a control with a Mab of the same isotype, and to antibody bivalence. For this reason screening with a fluorescent Fab rather than whole second antibody may be preferred for some uses, for example in the case of very high-density cell surface antigens. The flow cytometer will see an aggregate as a large single particle and only recognise this as one event so that an aggregate indicating a number of positive cells may only be registered as a single event. Large aggregates will, of course block the in-

TABLE 2.4
Fluorochromes and instrumentation used in Mab detection

Primary excitation wavelengths of hardware
Argon ion laser 488 nm
Helium Neon Laser 632 nm
Mercury line 545 nm
Krypton line 568 nm

Fluorochromes
(i) FLUORESCEIN (FITC)
Excitation range 400–530 nm. Max 490 nm.
Emission max 530 nm
Used extensively in immunofluorescence microscopy and FACS
Green on low-density staining, yellow on high density. Easily attached to proteins. 0.05 mg FITC/mg protein in total volume of 0.5 ml or less 0.25 M carbonate buffer, 0.15 M NaCl pH 9 at 4°C overnight. Separate bound from free on small Sephadex G-25 column (Johnson and Holborow, 1986)

(ii) R-PHYCOERYTHRIN
Excitation range 420–580 nm. Max 480, 545, 565 nm.
Emission max 580 nm
Protein (Mol wt 240,000). High fluorescence yield/molecule (30 × fluorescein yield)
Used extensively in two colour FACS analysis.
Orange/red. Has to be attached to protein by protein–protein cross-linking methods (Hardy, 1986). Activated R-PE for direct linking to thiol groups can be purchased (Molecular Probes, Oregon). Alternatively, biotinylated probes can be used with streptavidin R-PE.

(iii) B-PHYCOERYTHRIN
Excitation range 460–580 nm. Max 545, 565 nm.
Emission max 575 nm
Protein (Mol wt 240,000). High fluorescence yield/molecule (30 × fluorescein yield)
Suitable for mercury lamp. Used in immunofluorescence microscopy
Orange/red. Has to be attached to protein by protein-protein cross linking methods (Hardy, 1986). Activated B-PE for direct linking to thiol groups can be purchased. (Molecular Probes, Oregon). Alternatively, biotinylated probes can be used with streptavidin B-PE.

(iv) TEXAS RED
Excitation range 500–630 nm. Max 550 and 600 nm
Emission max 620 nm. Not compatible with primary wavelength of argon ion laser (488 nm) but can be used in conjunction with R-phycoerythrin to absorb at R-PE wavelengths and emit at TR wavelengths (Duochrome) thus making three colour FACS experiments possible.

TABLE 2.4 *(continued)*

The long emission wavelength means that, provided the correct filters are used Texas red can be used in immunofluorescence cytochemistry simultaneously with fluorescein to give lower background and stronger signal than rhodamine.

(v) RHODAMINE
Excitation max 522 nm. Not compatible with primary wavelength or argon ion laser.
Emission max 570 nm. Red.
Easily attached to proteins. 0.05 mg TRITC/mg protein in total volume of 0.5 ml or less 0.25 M carbonate buffer, 0.15 M NaCl, pH 9 at 4°C overnight. Separate bound from free on small Sephadex G-25 column.

(vi) PROPIDIUM IODIDE
Excitation max 493 nm. Compatible with primary wavelength of argon ion laser
Emission max 630 nm.
Red. Used to stain DNA, also stains RNA. Can be used with R-PE or B-PE but not Texas red on FACS.

(vii) 7-AAD (7-AMINO ACTINOMYCIN D)
Excitation max 523 nm
Emission max 647 nm. Red. Can be used with primary wavelength of argon ion laser.
Used to stain DNA (GC selective).

(viii) DAPI (4′,6-DIAMINO-2-PHENYLINDOLE HYDROCHLORIDE)
Excitation max 345 nm
Emission max 455 nm. Blue
Used to stain DNA (AT selective). Weak only with RNA. Ten fold more sensitive than PI.
More usually employed in microscopy than in FACS.

(ix) HOECHST 33258 AND 33342
Excitation max 345 nm
Emission max 480 nm. Blue
Used to stain DNA (AT selective). Weak only with RNA. More usually employed in microscopy than in FACS.

strument collecting systems but these are usually visible by eye. Aggregation is most likely to occur when both first antibody and second antibody are polyclonal (i.e., in the screening of the serum of the mouse to be used in fusion but not in screening of the Mabs themselves).

Flow cytometry is generally considered to be a technique only suitable for use with cells such as lymphocytes which grow in suspension but it can readily be used with adherent cells if they are removed from the plastic of the tissue culture vessel without extensive application of proteolytic enzymes such as trypsin. This can be achieved by the use of 0.25% (w/v) trypsin, 0.2% (w/v) versene (EDTA) in PBS, pH 7.5, for a short period of time (generally 1–2 minutes) which will 'round up' most epithelial cells on the plastic so that they can be shaken off with a vigorous slapping of the culture flask. The amount of trypsinisation required is variable among cell lines and must determined for each one. A check on whether the treatment has left the cell surface proteins intact can be made by using a Mab directed to MHC Class I antigens as these are vulnerable to proteolysis and present on most cell types with the exception of erythrocytes.

PROTOCOL 2.5: TESTING MOUSE SERUM TITRE BY FACS

Materials

(a) *Hardware* Scanning flow cytometer and centrifugable 5 ml capacity round bottomed tubes which can be attached directly to the flow cytometer (e.g., Falcon 2052 for FACScan). Low speed bench centrifuge.

(b) *Antigen* 3×10^6 antigen bearing cells, preferably fresh but may be used frozen. For frozen storage use 90% FCS, 10% DMSO and liquid nitrogen for freezing periods of more than 3 days.

(c) *First antibody*. 100 μl each of mouse serum diluted 1/100, 1/250, 1/500 and 1/1000 with PBS containing 0.5% BSA. Control mouse serum (pre-immune or same strain and age) diluted 1/100 in the same manner.

(d) *Second antibody* FITC labelled anti-mouse IgG, preferably γ-chain specific. Keep in the dark.

(e) *Propidium iodide* (PI) 1 μg/ml to stain dead cells (Caution–mutagenic – wear gloves)

Method

(i) Keep cells on ice at all times. Wash the antigen bearing cells twice in 3 ml PBS containing 0.5% BSA, centrifuging gently at 1000 rpm. Resuspend in 3 ml PBS/BSA.

(ii) Pipette 250 µl antigen bearing cells into 10 round bottomed tubes compatible with instrument as above, labelled 1–10. Avoid using any clumps of material from dead cells which may be present if the cells have been frozen. Centrifuge gently at 1000 rpm (150 × g). Pour off supernatant.

(iii) To tubes 1 and 2 add 25 µl PBS BSA. To tubes 3–6 respectively add 25 µl 1/100, 1/250, 1/500 and 1/1000 immune serum and to tubes 7–10 add 25 µl 1/100, 1/250, 1/500 and 1/1000 control serum, respectively. Mix by gently finger flicking at the bottom of the tube. Incubate on ice for 1 hour.

(iv) Add 3 ml PBS/0.5% BSA to each tube and centrifuge gently at 1000 rpm for 5 minutes.

(v) To tube 1 add 25 µl PBS/BSA. To all other tubes add 25 µl FITC labelled second antibody (1/100 in PBS/BSA). Incubate in the dark on ice for 1 hour.

(vi) Pour supernatant off gently and briefly vortex the pellet. Resuspend in 0.5 ml filtered PBS (no BSA), keeping in the dark (under tin foil) and on ice. Add 10 µl of propidium iodide (PI) to all tubes.

(vii) Scan on FACS collecting 2000–5000 events using a 'red for dead' collection 'gate' to exclude all dead/permeable cells which stain strongly with PI.

Interpretation of data

For each sample, examine firstly the scatter plot. If the cells have been significantly aggregated by the antibody then they will have been shifted to the right on the forward scatter plot with respect to the controls and this may increase the brightness but reduce the number of the positive signals obtained. In addition to this, any very small material on the scatter plot may represent debris from cells which have been damaged by handling. These can bind antibody non-specifically and it is wise to draw an analytical gate to exclude them from the assessment of the antiserum. Analysis with and without such a gate will give an indication of the extent to which they affect results.

Tube 1 gives autofluorescence of cells which can be quite high if the cells have been grown in a tissue culture medium containing a pH indicator dye such as phenol red.

Tube 2 shows the extent to which the cells bind second antibody alone, if this is high, then the amount of second antibody should be reduced.

Tubes 3–6 and 7–10 show the reaction of the immune and control serum with the cells. If the fluorescence intensity on the green (FITC) channel is clearly stronger in tube 3 than tube 7 then the antiserum is positive at 1/100, if it is stronger in tube 6 than tube 10, then the antiserum is positive at 1/1000. A fusion can be performed with an animal which gives a titre above 1/500.

The FACS will analyse cells according to cell volume or to the intensity of any fluorescence label according to programming and give a statistically relevant result. It is, however, a very good idea to check out your FACS technique by taking a small sample from all tubes, or at least tubes 3 and 7, once antibody staining is complete but before addition of PI. The cells are simply dried in the dark and examined under the fluorescent microscope. This gives a check on the FACS data and allows the investigator to check for uniformity of staining over the cell surface. What the FACS sees as a bright cell may be a single cell stained brightly in one patch on the membrane, a spotted stain, or an overall stain. It is always a good idea to view the stained antigen by eye where possible.

PROTOCOL 2.6: SCREENING A MOUSE FUSION BY FACS

Unlike ELISA screening, FACS screening is only performed on wells where there is a clearly visible emerging clone and is a continuing process with new clones being screened every day.

Materials

(a) *Hardware.* Scanning flow cytometer and centrifugable 5 ml capacity round bottomed tubes which can be attached directly to the flow cytometer (e.g., Falcon 2052 for FACScan). Low-speed bench centrifuge.

(b) *Antigen* For each clone to be assayed, 2×10^5 antigen bearing cells (it is possible to use fewer if cell numbers are at a premium), preferably fresh but may be used frozen. For frozen storage use 90% FCS, 10% DMSO and liquid nitrogen for freezing periods of more than 3 days.

(c) *First antibody.* Fusion plates. Micropipettes with sterile tips. 25 μl of culture supernatant from those wells which contain clones ready for assay (0.5–1 mm diameter – see Chapter 8)

(d) *Second antibody* FITC labelled anti-mouse IgG, preferably γ-chain specific. Keep in the dark.

(e) *Propidium iodide* (PI) 1 μg/ml to stain dead cells (Caution–mutagenic–wear gloves).

Method

(i) Keep cells on ice at all times. Wash the antigen bearing cells twice in PBS containing 0.5% BSA, centrifuging gently at 1000 rpm. Resuspend in 3 ml PBS/BSA.

(ii) Pipette 2×10^5 antigen bearing cells in PBS into each of as many flow cytometer tubes as there are clones to assay, adding two tubes (1 and 2) for the controls. Centrifuge gently at 1000 rpm (150 $\times$ g) and pour off supernatant.

(iii) To tubes 1 and 2 add 25 μl PBS/BSA. To each of the test samples add 25 μl supernatant from the tissue culture wells. It is better to do this directly in the sterile hood to avoid loss of antibody on transfer. Mix by gently finger flicking at the bottom of the tube. Incubate on ice for 1 hour.

(iv) Add 3 ml PBS/0.5% BSA to each tube and centrifuge gently at 1000 rpm for 5 minutes.

(v) To tube 1 add 25 μl PBS/BSA. To all other tubes add 25 μl FITC labelled second antibody (1/100 in PBS/BSA). Incubate in the dark on ice for 1 hour.

(vi) Pour supernatant off gently and briefly vortex the pellet. Resuspend in 0.5 ml filtered PBS (no BSA), keeping in the dark (under tinfoil) and on ice. Add 10 μl of propidium iodide (PI) to all tubes.

(vii) Scan on FACS collecting 2000–5000 events using a 'red for dead' collection 'gate' to exclude all dead/permeable cells which stain strongly with PI.

Interpretation of data

For each sample, examine firstly the scatter plot. If the cells have been significantly aggregated by the antibody then they will have been shifted to the right on the forward scatter plot with respect to the controls and this may increase the brightness but reduce the number of the positive signals obtained. In addition to this, any very small material on the scatter plot may represent debris from cells which have been damaged by handling. These can bind antibody non-specifically and it is wise to draw an analytical gate to exclude them from the assessment of the antiserum. Analysis with and without such a gate will give an indication of the extent to which they affect results.

Tube 1 gives autofluorescence of cells which can be quite high if the cells have been grown in a tissue culture medium containing a pH indicator dye.

Tube 2 shows the extent to which the cells bind second antibody alone.

The other tubes show the extent to which the culture supernatant carries an antibody which binds to the cells. These should be overlaid on data analysis against tube 2. Any supernatant which shows a shift to the right with respect to this tube is worth considering. A large shift to the right obviously indicates binding. A small shift to the right indicates (i) an antibody which is present in too low a concentration to give a bright signal or (ii) an antigen which is present at low density on the cell surface or (iii) an antibody binding with very low affinity

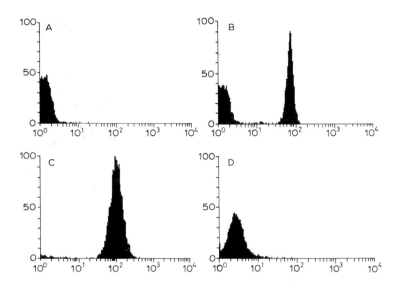

Fig. 2.6. Typical FACS screening profiles. (A) Control cells stained with second poly-clonal fluorescent antibody alone. (B) A Mab that reacts strongly with a proportion of the test cells. (C) A Mab that reacts strongly with all the test cells. (D) The common-est situation. A Mab that reacts slightly with the test cells. This could be a more valua-ble reagent than B or C. See text.

(Fig. 2.6). The first two are both potentially useful reagents. (i) can be distinguished by reassaying after 24–48 hours when more antibody has built up in the supernatant and (ii) by giving the cells an extra wash on reassay. A high-affinity Mab binding to a low-density cell surface protein should remain where a low-affinity one will be dis-lodged (Section 2.2.2). If the screening is with a γ-chain specific probe, most of the antibodies should have reasonably high affinity.

A common feature encountered in this type of assay is that only a certain proportion of the cells react with the antibody and some remain unstained. This suggests an antibody which reacts with a sub-set of cells due to the fact that the cell population is heterogeneous in some way (for example some antigens are only present at certain stages of the cell cycle). It is worth checking the positions of stained and unstained cells on the scatter plot to determine whether they can also be differentiated by size. It is wise to check the immunofluorescence pattern by microscope at this stage (see 2.8.1 above) but also to remember that a weak positive, which may be to a low-density antigen of great interest, may not be as readily detectable on this subjective assay as by FACS.

2.8.2. Preservation of cells for FACS assay after staining

After the cells are stained, they can be stored for up to 48 hours after fixation in 2% paraformaldehyde.

2.8.3. Preservation of cells for FACS assay before staining

Cell suspensions can be frozen in liquid nitrogen in a mixture of 10% DMSO, 90% foetal calf serum. Lymphocytes can be stored for some months in this manner as can established tissue culture lines. Primary cells other than lymphocytes store less well and a high percentage will be made permeable to antibody on freezing. It is not possible to obtain intact cells from frozen pieces of tissue and any solid tissue should be disaggregated into a cell suspension before freezing.

2.8.4. Detection of intracellular antigens by FACS

For fixed cells, or cells with leaking membranes (and these may look intact – check with PI or other dyes which stain DNA) this is not recommended. Antibodies to high-density structural proteins will be detected. Even an established Mab generated against a pure protein antigen with intracellular location may end up bound weakly to high-density proteins such as to actin, fibronectin etc.

2.8.5. Detection of bacterial antigens by FACS

The problems experienced with eukaryotic cells are reversed in this case as the most highly repetitive elements are generally on the outside of the bacterial cell. Mabs of varying quality directed to the external components of bacterial cells are readily produced and many have been described. These can be screened by ELISA (Section 2.7) and also by FACS. Many Mabs aggregate bacteria in which case FACS assay and screening is obviously inappropriate. However, the antigens most of interest in the 1990s are those inside bacterial cells. Most bacteria are rendered permeable by organic solvents and/or heat. However, a Mab to an intracellular bacterial protein tested on a whole cell, will tend to bind weakly and non-specifically to the protective outer coat. Unless a laboratory strain with no protective coat is used to express the required antigen, FACS has limited value.

2.9. Screening for cellular antigens by immunocytochemical methods

Immunocytochemical analysis is time consuming and labour intensive but rewarding. It is a classical technique which has had to be adapted from polyclonal to monoclonal analysis (see Polak and Van Noorden, 1986 for recent developments). Immunocytochemical methods have the potential to give the greatest amount of information about the antigen defined by a Mab. For any single cell it can give the intracellular location or, for a membrane antigen, the type of membrane staining involved (uniform, polar, patchy etc). Where tissue sections are used, immunohistochemistry can indicate the geographical location of positive cells with respect to other cells of the same and of different phenotype within the framework of the overall architecture of the tissue. It is a vital tool in characterising a Mab but a tedious and subjective system for screening, and a preliminary screen by ELISA or FACS can be invaluable in cutting down the number of wells for which further immunocytochemical screening is required.

2.9.1. Preparation of cells and tissues for immunocytochemistry

Adherent cells which can be grown in culture are generally grown on coverslips, in petri dishes, or in multiwell slide chambers. They generally attach within 1–2 hours but should be cultured at least overnight to allow them to be growing normally. To some extent the transfer may synchronise the cells and if a cell cycle dependent antigen is thought to be involved it is advisable to use cells which have been grown on the slide for different times.

Non adherent cells such as lymphocytes can be cytocentrifuged onto slides, or a drop of cell containing suspension in PBS/5% BSA may be smeared on a slide by spreading with the edge of a coverslip to give a film which is less than one cell deep. They can also be stained in suspension as for FACS as described above and then air dried on a slide.

In either case, the cells can be permeabilised by gently air drying (leave in sterile hood with fan running), by fixation by immersion in organic solvents such as acetone, methanol or a mixture of the two, or by fixation in 4% paraformaldehyde in PBS. The choice depends on the antigen. Organic solvents may disrupt membranes and alter membrane proteins, the aldehydes will alter all the amino groups on protein epitopes and may also alter hydroxyl groups. Air drying alone is preferable if the cells under study do not detach during the washing procedures involved in subsequent staining.

Tissue sections are prepared from two sources:

(a) Paraformaldehyde fixed paraffin embedded tissue sections   This has been the classical method for storing tissue samples and is the one which best preserves the overall architecture of the tissue. In consequence, most pathology departments have extensive banks of tissue samples from normal and diseased tissues of many types. Thus, for example, in a retrospective study of whether the expression of a particular antigen in a primary tumour is a prognostic indicator of its long-term metastatic capacity, it is usually possible to obtain paraffin embedded tissue from patients who first presented 20 years earlier.

Unfortunately paraffin sections have proved of slightly restricted value in Mab screening and characterisation since the procedures involved in preserving the samples involve processes such as heating to 60° and can destroy the antigen. The paraffin sample is cut to a 4–5 μm sample with a microtome, baked on a alcohol pre-cleaned slide at 60°for 30–60 minutes, 'dewaxed' by 2–3 immersions in xylene, and gradually rehydrated by washing twice each in absolute ethanol, 95% ethanol, 50% ethanol and water before immersion in the staining buffer. Having been fixed before storage, these sections need no further fixation and are ready for blocking and staining.

(b) Frozen tissue sections   These are more commonly used for Mab work. This tissue is frozen in liquid nitrogen where it will keep for over a year (it is convenient to cut the primary tissue in elongated sausage shaped chunks approximately $7 \times 3 \times 3$ mm before storage), and sliced while still frozen on a cryostat. Most pathology departments have such instruments and will lease time on them but it is a good idea to purchase your own blade since this is a critical factor in obtaining good sections. Sections should be as thin as possible, in practice 4–5 μm, and as evenly cut as possible since a thicker part of a section will show higher background staining and confuse interpretation. The section is placed on a slide which has been precoated with either 1% gelatin or 0.1% poly(L-lysine) and either air dried (preferable if the section will remain attached during subsequent staining), or alternatively fixed with acetone/methanol or formaldehyde/glutaraldehyde as described for attached cells above.

2.9.2. Blocking in immunohistochemical assays

These present a blocking problem in that the antibody is exposed to a wide variety of antigens, each of which have their own set of ideal blocking conditions. 1% goat, rabbit or other irrelevant serum is recommended but it should be remembered that these may have a low but detectable affinity for Fc receptors on the surface of haemopoietic cells.

2.9.3. Incubation with Mab (or test polyclonal serum)

This is similar to the other assays described in Protocols 2.2–2.4. Tissue culture supernatants are used neat, serum starting at dilutions of 1/100 and ascitic fluid at a generally higher dilution but titred over a wide range. The use of an IgG (γ-chain) specific second antibody is very strongly advised (Table 2.2). 100 μl or less will usually cover the cell mass on the slide. Incubation is for a mimimum of one hour. This is then washed in a multislide container which is gently immersed 2 to 3 fold in PBS for a defined period of time (3 min). Tween 20 or Triton X-100 may be added to the washing solution up to 0.02% if the background staining is too strong.

The main difference with other screening methods is the number of necessary controls. A first and second antibody system challenged with such a wide range of antigens will show extensive non-specific binding. For serum, these controls should include:-

(i) Pre-immune serum from the same animal plus second antibody plus substrate.

(ii) If there has been a long immunisation period, serum from a non-immunised animal of the same strain and age, kept under the same conditions.

(iii) PBS, 5%BSA in place of first antibody and otherwise treated identically (same washes and detection system).

(iv) PBS, 5% BSA in place of second antibody and otherwise treated identically (same washes and same detection system).

(v) PBS, 5%BSA in place of both first and second antibodies and otherwise treated identically (same washes and detection system).

2.9.4. Choice of staining method

The main staining methods are enzymes or fluorochromes. In addition, noble metals can be used. Second antibody is usually applied in a more concentrated form than for ELISA and a single aliquot is diluted in 1 ml PBS/3% BSA rather than the 10 ml used for ELISA.

(a)   Enzymes. The use of detecting enzymes has been discussed extensively in Section 2.6.7 and the relevant substrates and conditions of use are detailed in Table 2.3. In immunocytochemistry there is limited resolution as the insoluble enzyme product is deposited over a broad area, 10–50 μm beyond the precise attachment site of the first antibody. Thus for example, an antibody directed to cytoskeletal proteins at the outer rim of a cell is not readily differentiated from one directed to the cell surface proteins.

(b) Fluorescent labels. The main fluorochrome detecting systems are listed in Table 2.4. Fluorescein is used in both fluorescence microscopy and in FACS analysis and the suitability of probes depends on wavelengths available if a laser excitation system is used, or filters available if a mercury lamp is used for excitation, together with the filter and compensation systems used to detect emission. The most useful guide current to detection systems is the comprehensive and detailed handbook by Haughland (1989) produced for Molecular Probes Inc,Oregon.

Most Mab researchers use second antibody labelled with FITC (fluorescein) for staining cells at screening and then proceed to use this together with other antibodies labelled with rhodamine or texas red for immunocytochemical study or R-phycoerythrin for FACS analysis during further characterisation.

(c) Gold labelling. Gold labelling has been less common but has always had certain advantages. The resolution is much finer than that of enzyme immunohistochemistry since the gold is directly bound to the second antibody and there is not the same spread of enzyme product. Gold labelled antibodies are marketed by most major firms. Gold labelling can be greatly enhanced by the use of silver coating which yields a dark brown stain. Most major firms (e.g., Sigma) market solutions for silver enhancement which are mixed and applied to the slide for 2–3 minutes, washed, and then incubated in sodium thiosulphate fixative together with detailed instructions for their use. A dark room is not required.

2.9.5. Counterstaining

Counterstaining with haematoxylin makes it possible to view the enzyme or gold stain in relation to the major structural components of the cell more clearly. Harris's hematoxylin is used for alcohol insoluble products and Mayer's hematoxylin for alcohol soluble products.

These are not used with fluorescence microscopy where the same field is photographed in phase contrast and then under fluorescent illumination.

2.9.6. Mounting

Mounting media come in two basic types, aqueous and non-aqueous, the latter being required when the enzyme product is readily soluble (Table 2.3). Both types can be readily purchased from several suppliers. If fluorescein has been used, then it is important that the pH of the mounting medium is at the optimum (8.5) as fluorescein is readily quenched at lower pH values. Many manufacturers include chemicals to limit quenching in the mountant such as 2.5% (w/v) DABCO (1,4-diazobicyclooctane), 5% (w/v) n-propyl gallate, or p-phenylenediamine.

The aqueous mountants are the polyvinyl alcohol based Gelvatol, Mowiol, or Elvanol. These are made up by the method of Osborne and Weber (1982). 2.4 g of the mountant is stirred in 6 ml glycerol for an hour, 6 ml distilled water is added with further stirring for 2 hours, and then 12 ml 0.2 M Tris, pH 8.5, is added and the mixture is incubated at 50°C for 15 minutes. The solution is clarified by centrifugation at $5000 \times g$ for 15 minutes and stored at -20°C in the long term. In the short term, it can be stored at room temperature for up to two weeks.

For short-term mounting many people simply use 50% glycerol in PBS. Alcohol soluble reaction products can be mounted in glycerol/gelatin (Sigma). The main non-aqueous mounting medium is DPX (10 g distrene, 5 ml dibutyl phthalate, 35 ml xylene) which must be applied to a completely dry sample.

2.10. Screening for catalytic antibodies

Ideally, screening for catalytic monoclonal antibodies (Section 1.14) would involve direct assay of enzyme activity in the tissue culture supernatant. However, this would require an antibody with a high K_{cat} and a very sensitive assay. One type of assay which may be further developed for hydrolytic activity is the use of mutually quenching fluorescent probes on either side of the bond to be hydrolysed. Hydrolysis leads to an increase in fluorescence. For example if the 2-aminobenzyl group is used on the carboxyl side of a peptidyl group to be hydrolysed and the 4-nitrobenzylamide group on the amino side, the latter will quench the former until hydrolysis occurs (Nishino and Powers, 1980). Alternatively, a system can be used employing enzymes which act on one of the products but not the substrate to give a fluorescent or coloured product.

A major factor in such assays is that there must be no endogenous enzyme activity in the tissue culture supernatant as even a small contaminating activity is likely to give too strong a background against which the antibody activity has to be detected.

The most common method of screening for catalytic Mabs is simple binding on an ELISA plate or nitrocellulose filter using as antigen, the transition state analogue bound to a different protein from that used as carrier in the original immunisation. If KLH is used as carrier in the immunisation, BSA is generally used in the assay. These assay methods will lead to the production of antibodies which bind the transition state analogue. However, they may not actually catalyse the required reaction.

2.11. Screening recombinant libraries

Recombinant libraries (Section 9.6.4) can yield a very large number of clones so that, in principle, screening capacity can be the limiting factor. There is no point in having a library with 10^{12} possible clones if the screening system cannot accommodate it. The capacity of the average laboratory to screen very large numbers of clones on even the usually efficient ELISA system is clearly limited with the standard 96 well plates.

A further complication is that such libraries only tend to contain the variable regions or variable and first constant regions and will be poorly detected by a second antibody directed to the entire constant region. For this reason, peptide 'Tags' which can be detected by a previously established monoclonal antibody are usually incorporated into the vector. This Tag, can however be lost by proteolysis in cloning. An antibody to the V gene in question can be used to overcome this in a model system (Ward et al., 1989) but obviously not when screening is required to detect new variable region combinations.

Screening for a hapten or protein is most readily accomplished by using a radioactive labelled protein (or haptenated protein) to identify plaques actively secreting the relevant binding activity by the standard nitrocellulose overlay techniques used in recombinant DNA methodology. The filter is overlaid on the plaques to absorb the recombinant protein, blocked, treated with the radioactive antigen, and then developed and compared to the original plate. Positive plaques can be picked off and rescreened (Huse et al., 1989).

While this type of method makes it possible to screen a large number of recombinant clones, it is limited to nitrocellulose bound protein and is unlikely to be an ideal system for screening for, say, binding activity against membrane proteins and more sophisticated detection systems which can also cope with large numbers will need to be developed.

CHAPTER 3

Selection of animals, tissues and cell lines

3.1. Animals in which hybridomas may be generated

There are only three main systems used for classical monoclonal antibody production and these are mouse, rat and human. It is not possible to make hybridomas from rabbits as suitable myeloma lines are not readily generated in these animals. For the same reason, sheep, goat and bovine systems, which would yield extensive amounts at low cost in ascites, have been attempted but remain poorly developed. A system which has been of some use in generating Mabs for basic immunological research on mouse antigens is the Syrian or Armenian hamster system which is reported to yield stable hybdridomas on fusion with mouse cell lines (Sanchez-Madrid and Springer, 1986). Human hybridomas can be further subdivided into chimaeric ones reconstructed to humanise the immune responses of rodent Mabs by the use of recombinant DNA technology (Chapter 9) and 'genuine' human Mabs generated from humans themselves, both methodologies involving fairly complex manipulations (Section 3.6).

Both mouse and rat systems are widely used and the choice between the two remains fairly open. The mouse system is the original one developed by Kohler and Milstein (1975) and the better known. However, the rat system has been very successfully used by the Cambridge groups of Hale and Waldmann and has a highly committed advocate in Bazin (1990), from whose laboratory all the rat myeloma lines originate.

3.2. Whether to choose the rat or mouse system

My own laboratory has used both systems extensively and ended finally by using the mouse system. Our main reasons for choosing it were (ii) to (iv) below. Other laboratories may have different factors to consider.

The choice between the two can be affected by several factors:

(i) The antigen should be foreign and therefore mouse antigens will be more successful in rat hybridoma production and vice versa. Basic research immunology is usually performed on the mouse and hence rat hybridomas are convenient.

(ii) Most rat cell lines are under patent restrictions. The main mouse ones are not. For any projected commercial use, this gives mouse hybridomas a widely perceived advantage.

(iii) Rat systems are usually technically more difficult for the non-expert at tissue culture as the myeloma cell lines are less robust.

(iv) Rat fusion frequencies are generally lower. A good mouse fusion from a single spleen can yield several hundred colonies. A rat fusion yields a comparatively small number.

(v) Rat systems are, however, often more stable once fusion has been achieved and chromosome loss leading to lack of secretion is less common. This is true not only immediately after fusion, but also years after fusion. A rat hybridoma seldom needs recloning and is stable in industrial bulk culture (Section 3.2.5).

(vi) Rats are very much (approximately 10 fold) larger than mice and can yield up to 50 ml of ascitic fluid at a single draining where a mouse yields less than 5 ml. The Lou strain is also claimed to have larger litter sizes and these two factors combine to provide a more economical system for the bulk production of ascites fluid.

(vii) Rat antibodies are claimed to be able to fix human complement better than mouse ones. This confers limited advantage since all rodent antibodies are basically too foreign to man for extended in vivo use, antibodies from both mouse and rat eliciting equally toxic anti immunoglobulin responses.

(viii) Where a simple protein antigen is involved, it is possible that the Lou rat will have the ability to respond to that antigen where the Balb/c mouse cannot or vice versa. It is, however, possible to change strains within a single rodent species rather than to change species (Section 3.4).

(ix) While rat hybridomas are claimed to be easier to purify than mouse hybridomas (Bazin, 1990), this probably reflects the fact there are less of them available to compare. Most laboratories who have used both rat and mouse systems extensively find this too simple a generalisation since even two Mabs of the same isotype from the same species may require quite different purification procedures. If any generalisation can be employed, rat Mabs are less amenable to purification on Protein A which is one of the major purification systems (Chapter 10).

3.2.1. Choice of cell lines as myeloma partners

There are several desirable characteristics in a good myeloma line as the fusion partner and some of these occasionally conflict. The major mouse ones are discussed below and can be obtained from commercial companies such as Flow or Gibco (Life Technologies) or the ATCC (American Type Culture Collection) and its equivalent ECACC (European Collection of Animal Cell Cultures) at the Public Health Laboratory Service, Porton Down, U.K. (Appendix 2). Most of these suppliers will send cell lines certified as currently mycoplasma free and such a certificate of health is very strongly advised (Section 5.4.3). The major mouse lines are not under any patent restrictions.

3.2.2. Myeloma antibody synthesis

It is clearly preferable in a fusion experiment to use a myeloma partner which does not itself make antibody. If this is not the case then the resultant hybridomas can produce antibodies with a variety of specificities giving overall lower affinity and possible non-standard affinity and specificity. The ideal situation is shown in Fig. 3.1A. The situation for a myeloma line which makes light chain (whether or not

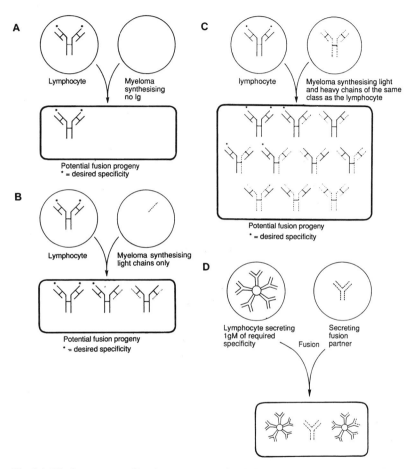

Fig. 3.1. The importance of having a non-secreting fusion partner. (A) Is the ideal situation which can be achieved in the mouse system. (B) Is an acceptable situation, common to most rat systems. C and D reflect the human system.

it originally secreted it) is shown in Fig. 3.1B and the situation for a fusion partner which makes/secretes both heavy and light chains in Fig. 3.1C. An IgM antibody is similarly 'diluted' in affinity by light chain, but not heavy chain association (Fig. 3.1D).

The consequences of this are considerable since commercial or therapeutic use requires that a completely pure and highly defined antibody preparation is employed.

3.2.3. Hybridoma antibody secretion

Despite the fact that it should not make antibody itself, the myeloma line employed for fusion should lead to the production of clones secreting large amounts of antibody. It is important here to understand the difference between a 'plasmacytoma/myeloma' cell line which is a tumour of highly differentiated antibody producing cells and a 'lymphoblastoid' line which is a tumour of a much earlier stage of B cell differentiation where the cell has antibody on its surface but secretes little. The two types are readily distinguished under the electron microscope since plasmacytoma/myeloma cells carry large amounts of endoplasmic reticulum and lymphoblastoid cells do not. Clearly a parent fusion line which has any defects in its ability to make or secrete all immunoglobulins rather than its own particular (and irrelevant) one would be an unsuitable fusion partner. The best fusion partner is therefore a plasmacytoma/myeloma line which has ceased to be able to make or secrete its own antibody, not because of a defect in genes encoding the general synthetic or secretion apparatus, but because of a defect in the precise gene encoding either synthesis or secretion of the irrelevant internal antibody. Statistically this is a rare event.

Figures for hybridoma secretion rates are difficult to quantify. Many papers quote values for 10^6 cells over 24 hours but do not specify the stage of growth, despite the fact that it is well known that cells in early growth at high percentages of serum divide but do not make much antibody while those at later stages of growth or in lower percentages of medium do not divide, but make a much increased level of antibody per cell. Most of these quoted secreted rates have very limited meaning.

3.2.4. Ability of myeloma partners to support effective fusion

Cell lines suitable for fusion are very rarely described. There is only a single mouse line (P3K) which has led to all the currently used mouse fusion partners and the same is true for the S210 progenitor of the three known rat fusion cell rat lines. Thus, in 15 years of hybridoma research only two cell lines with the ability to fuse and give clonable antibody producing progeny have been established. In such a context, it is not surprising that suitable human cell lines, which rely on the rare myeloma patient being available to a laboratory interested in human hybridoma technology, have not been established.

The precise requirements for a good myeloma fusion partner are unknown. However, they are more likely to relate to the stability of secretion of fused gene products rather than the membrane plasticity at the time of fusion.

Reports of this 'ability to fuse productively' parameter have varied widely among research groups and within particular schedules and is inevitably linked to factors such as operator skills. It is clearly important to have cells in active growth for fusion and it is assumed that S phase, G2 phase or metaphase cells must be responsible, but no published work has proved this. Experimentally however, a mouse cell line which originates from the original P3K cell line referred to above, can yield 1000+ clones when fused with a single mouse spleen.

3.2.5. Reversion frequency and stability

Reversion frequency relates to the phenomenon of a high yield hybridoma becoming non-secreting. At the early stages of hybridoma production this is anticipated and expected and early and frequent cloning (Chapter 8) can overcome it. However, it can occur at any time after the establishment of a clone, and while such a situation can be reversed by repeated recloning, it is obviously a major problem for procedures such as bulk culture where continuous secretion is an absolute requirement – if a single non-secreting cell outgrows the others in a 1000 litre culture then there is a considerable financial loss for the company involved. With established rat hybridomas reversion almost never happens, with established mouse ones it is slow, and with (non-recombinant) human ones, it happens all too often.

3.3. Selective drug markers

3.3.1. HAT medium

It is vital that the myeloma parent cell line can be selected against in tissue culture so that non-fused cells may be eliminated from the fusion mixture. The commonest method for carrying out this procedure is to use a parent myeloma which has been selected for its sensitivity to Hypoxanthine, Aminopterin and Thymidine (HAT) medium (Fig. 3.2). Figure 3.3 shows the manner in which the selection procedure

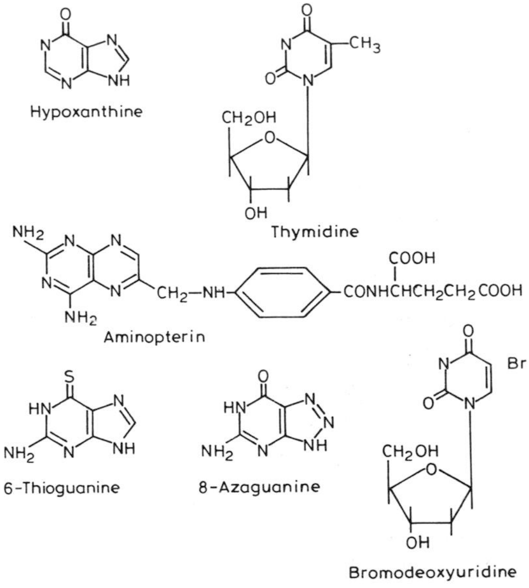

Fig. 3.2. The structure of some of the common chemicals involved in the selection of HAT sensitive cells.

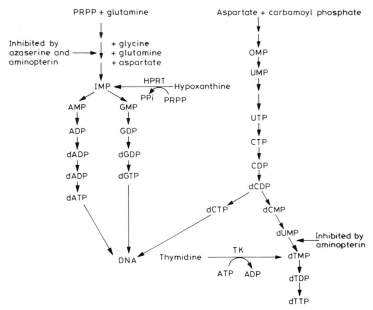

Fig. 3.3. The main pathways of purine and pyrimidine biosynthesis and major sites of aminopterin and azaserine blockage. Azaserine may also inhibit pyrimidine biosynthesis but at comparatively higher concentrations.

works. Aminopterin blocks the main biosynthetic pathways for purine and pyrimidine synthesis in animal cells principally by inhibition of the enzyme dihydrofolate reductase. There are, however, salvage pathways by which exogenous nucleosides may be utilised instead. The pyrimidine pathway involves the enzyme thymidine kinase (TK) and utilises exogenous thymidine. The purine pathway utilises the enzyme hypoxanthine (guanine) phosphoribosyl transferase (H(G)PRT) with exogenous hypoxanthine. Cell lines can be made deficient in either one of these enzymes by growth and selection in either bromodeoxyuridine (which selects TK negative cells) or azaguanine or thioguanine (which select HPRT negative cells). In normal cells these inhibitors are converted to the appropriate nucleotides which are cytotoxic and consequently only mutants deficient in the appropriate enzymes survive. Nearly all the rodent cell lines currently in use have been selected on azaguanine and are consequently HPRT negative. Commercial constraints are such that, particularly with the human system, it is sometimes expedient to select an HPRT or TK negative cell line in the laboratory rather than acquire one from other sources.

3.3.2. Selection for azaguanine, thioguanine and bromodeoxyuridine resistant mutants

In general it is easier to select for HPRT negative cells rather than for TK negative ones. In most mammals, the chromosomal locus is on the X chromosome and whatever the sex of the original tumour donor, only one X chromosome is generally transcriptionally active in established cell lines. Consequently only one mutation is required in theory for an HPRT negative mutant to be generated. 6-Thioguanine is probably better than 8-azaguanine for the selection of HPRT negative mutants (Evans and Vijayalaxmi, 1981). The latter is reported to be incorporated into RNA as well as DNA which effectively protects cells against its mutagenic effect (Nelson et al., 1975). More importantly, nearly all mutants selected in thioguanine are HPRT negative whereas selection in azaguanine can lead to the production of cell lines with normal levels of the enzyme (Littlefield, 1963; Cox and Masson, 1978). Cells are selected in gradually increasing concentrations starting at around 1 μg/ml (it is a good idea to vary this within a small range as different cell types may show different sensitivity) and leading up to levels from 30 to 300 μg/ml after 6–8 weeks. The cells may be mutagenised first with irradiation or treatment with ethyl methanesulphonate but this is not necessary. If there is extensive cell death, the surviving cells can be purified on Ficoll. The resistant cells are cloned several times and clones are chosen for high growth rate and low reversion frequency to growth in HAT medium. TK negative cell lines are selected in a similar way with bromodeoxyuridine as the selecting agent.

Human parent myeloma lines which have been selected in azaguanine or thioguanine are usually re-passaged regularly with the selecting drug to check for any reversion mutants. Again this is because new human cell lines are being speculatively developed and their stability for drug sensitivity is less assured than that of the small number of solidly established mouse lines.

3.3.3. Selection for ouabain resistant mutants

Ouabain resistance is a convenient additional property, particularly where human cell lines are involved. Rodent cell lines grow in levels of ouabain up to $10^{-3}M$ where human ones die at levels of $10^{-7}M$ so that in human rodent fusions ouabain can be used as a selective agent against the unfused human cells. To prepare a rodent or human ouabain-resistant mutant it is usual but not essential to mutagenise the cells with irradiation (100–200R) or with mutagens such as ethyl methanesulphonate (100 $\mu g/ml$). The cells are then selected with ouabain levels increasing from $10^{-7}M$ gradually over a period of several weeks.

3.3.4. Other methods of selection

The main alternative method of selection involves the use of selective medium containing hypoxanthine and azaserine (HAz) with HPRT negative cells. Azaserine blocks the pathways of purine biosynthesis but not that of pyrimidine biosynthesis (Fig. 3.3) and consequently thymidine need not be included in the medium. Thymidine inhibits DNA synthesis at millimolar concentrations in most mammalian cells and some cell types are susceptible at lower concentrations. Hypoxanthine and azaserine containing medium avoids this problem and the medium has therefore been used in T cell fusions (Foung et al., 1982) and human B cell fusions (Edwards et al., 1982).

3.3.5. Dominant selection systems

It should also be noted that since HAT systems were developed, techniques involved in selecting eukaryote cells which have acquired new genes have become much more sophisticated. HAT systems are essentially recessive since they require that recipient myeloma cell be made deficient in a gene function prior to use. New methods such neomycin (neo) resistance or the transfer of bacterial guanosine phosphoribosyl transferase (GPT) (Chapter 9) are dominant in that they employ drugs which will kill a normal cell which has failed to acquire the selecting DNA sequence. This is an important technical distinction as, while recessive selection systems can only be applied to established cell lines, dominant selection systems can, at least in principle, be applied to primary cells.

3.4. The mouse system

3.4.1. Mouse cell lines to use

All the available mouse fusion partners have their origins in the Balb/ c mouse which is susceptible to the induction of IgA producing plasmacytomas on intraperitoneal injection with mineral oils such as pristane. In consequence, most of the cell lines are prefixed with the letters MOPC for Mineral Oil Induced PlasmaCytoma, contain the letters Ag for azaguanine resistance and a multiplicity of other letters which simply relate to clone identification. Most of the commonly used ones originate from a single cell line, P3K (Horibata and Harris, 1970) and its subline P3-X63-Ag8, which secretes antibody but is HPRT negative (Kohler and Milstein, 1975). In the last edition of this book, a Table listing all possible lines was published. At the time, it was thought that a superior fusion partner might be developed. However, it is now clear that there are only three major lines used throughout the world, all developed from P3K, and all readily available without patent restrictions. These are:

(i) *P3 X63 Ag8 653*. This line was selected from P3-X63-Ag8 for non-expression of antibody but retention of HPRT negativity (Kearney et al., 1979). The cells have the normal mouse DNA content and shed extraneous chromosomes rapidly after fusion.

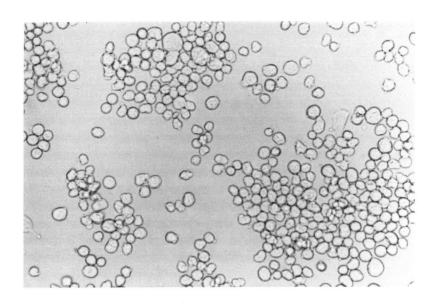

Fig. 3.4. Cells of the mouse myeloma SP2/0. Magnification × 300.

(ii) *SP2/0 Ag14* (Fig. 3.4). This line was selected from P3-X63-Ag-8 by fusion with non-immunised mouse spleen cells leading to a cell line which no longer made or secreted antibody (Shulman et al., 1978). SP2/0 cells have almost twice the normal amount of DNA of a normal mouse cell but have remained stable throughout the years. Immediately after fusion, they shed chromosomes and revert to a DNA content close to that of the original SP 2/0 line. SP 2/0 cells are slightly adherent and tend to stick slightly to plastic. They are readily dislodged by a sharp sideways slap on the flask.

(iii) *NS0/1* This line was independently established by Milstein's group from the original P3K line after selection for both HPRT loss and non-secretion. It yields clones at lower frequency than the SP2/0 or Ag153 in most laboratories but is a perfectly adequate fusion partner.

All of these lines work well in fusion and the choice of line is highly personal according to health of the line in the lab and the initiate is advised to obtain at least two lines or several samples from different sources, making sure that all are mycoplasma free (Section 5.4.3). The only other line that occurs sporadically in the modern literature is the FOX-NY line, also established from the original P3K line for double sensitivity to HAT and AAT (Taggart and Samloff, 1982). Other lines are referenced in older texts or the first edition of this book.

3.4.2. Strain of mouse to use

From the foregoing, the Balb/c mouse is the logical starting point for immunisation. However, where small protein antigens are involved and if the mouse serum titre is poor, it is well worth trying other strains if available. The understanding of this in molecular terms lies in the fact that the antigen must be presented to helper T cells in a 'groove' on the MHC Class 2 molecule (Fig. 4.3). With inbred strains of mice or rats, which have a limited and defined repertoire of MHC molecules, it is possible that a simple antigen does not contain a peptide segment able to fit the groove and perform this function efficiently, and without T cell help, the antibody response cannot mature to high affinity. In this case, it is worth trying all available strains of animal and testing serum IgG titre (Chapter 2). All the Balb/c myeloma

TABLE 3.1
Main mouse strains and Class 2 MHC antigens

Strain	Class II MHC haplotype[*]
Balb/c	d
NZB	d
DBA/2	d
A/J	k
CBA	k
AKR	k
C57 BL	b
SJL	s
I 29	b

[*] Note that Class II compatibility does not imply total histocompatibility but only identity at Class II loci.

lines recommended are totally compatible with splenic B cells from other strains of mice and the only technical complication comes at a later stage if ascites production is required in which case an F1 hybrid of the immunising strain and the Balb/c mouse is readily produced. Thus assuming that ascites expansion is not required (and this is generally the case), any mouse outwith those in Table 3.1 can be used and even an outbred strain might be an excellent choice. The full pedigree of most strains of laboratory mice is given in Festing (1979) and Class II haplotypes for inbred strains and given in Klein et al. (1983).

3.5. The rat system

Some of the advantages of the rat system have already been discussed in Section 3.1. The rat system was originally developed by Bazin (Bazin et al., 1972, 1973; see Bazin, 1990 for background). Rat myelomas rarely occur but two strains of rat were developed in Louvain by Bazin's group in the 1970s. Lou/C rats have a high incidence of ileocaecal tumours and Lou M strains a low incidence. The tumours showed characteristics of plasmacytomas but were not originally induced by mineral oils as are the mouse plasmacytomas. One of these myeloma lines which Bazin referred to as S210 was developed in the U.K. as the R210 line and clones which were azaguanine resistant and good fusion partners were isolated. There are two related lines from this source available in the U.K., both based on the R210.RCY3 cell line from Lou/C rats.

The Y3-Ag 1.2.3 (Known as Y3) cell line (Galfre et al., 1979) (Fig. 3.5) secretes a κ-chain. It is less easy to grow in culture than the mouse cell lines and yields fewer hybrids, but their antibody secretion remains stable.

The YB2/3 Ag 20 (known as Y/0) line is a myeloma line derived from a fusion between the original Y3 line and the spleen cells from an AO rat immunised with complement (Lachman et al., 1980). Y/0 makes no immunoglobulin and is in theory superior to Y3. In practice we have found the Y/0 line very much more difficult to handle than

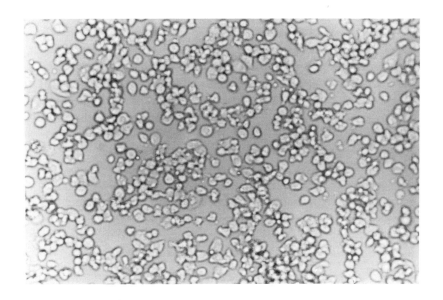

Fig. 3.5. Cells of the rat hybridoma Y3/Ag 1.2.3. Magnification × 300.

Y3 and clones derived from it less stable than those from Y3 but there is no doubt that it can yield successful hybridomas. The fact that it was obtained from a cross-strain fusion means that Y/0 cells can only be propagated in the ascites fluid of (Lou C × AO) f1 rats. These lines can be obtained from the European Cell Culture Collection (Appendix 2) and consent/patent forms must be signed.

The IR983F (known as 983) line was developed by Bazin's own group who have made large numbers of rat hybridomas (described in Bazin, 1990). It is a non-secreting line which can be obtained from Bazin himself at the University of Louvain or Zymed Laboratories, San Francisco. It is not specifically stated that hybrids from 983 are as stable as those from Y3 or not but inspection of the published cloning data would suggest that they are stable from the start.

As with the mouse system, a variety of strains of rat may be used in order to determine the optimal responding strain. The rat Class II MHC locus is much less well defined among strains than the mouse

locus but DA and AO rats have been shown to be particularly successful with antigens which are low responders in the Lou rat.

3.6. The human system

3.6.1. Background

The requirements for human hybridoma technology and some of the
difficulties have been discussed in Section 1.9. The technology has a
troubled history (Reviewed by James and Bell, 1987) but the prospects for the 1990s are more encouraging.

It was originally assumed that a human myeloma partner of equivalent fusion capacity and post fusion secretion stability to the original
mouse P3K or rat S210 lines could be established from myeloma patients. In theory, this could then be selected for HPRT negativity and
non-secretion in the same way in which the current rodent fusion
partners were developed from the parent lines. Many candidate lines
featured in patent applications in the early 1980s. While making lines
HPRT negative caused no problems, it proved very difficult to isolate
any which did not make their own antibody but were nonetheless able
to secrete the antibody coded by the relevant human B cell (Section
3.2.2). In addition, fusion frequencies were low in comparison to the
mouse system (Section 3.2.3), and the high secretion level myeloma
lines proved very difficult to establish in comparison to the low secretion level, less desirable lymphoblastoid ones (Section 3.2.2).

The realisation that the B95–8 Epstein Barr Virus (EBV) (Chapter 7)
secreting cell line was freely available without patent restrictions then
attracted interest. EBV was thought to immortalise comparatively immature CD21 + B cell populations to give lymphoblastoid cells which
are predominantly surface IgM positive (a few are IgG positive) and
which secreted very much less antibody than a myeloma. In addition,
EBV transformants lose the ability to make antibody after 2–3 weeks
in culture. Thus the technique was limited but seemed to have potential. It also became apparent that EBV was a polyclonal activator of

non-transformed B cells as well as a transforming virus so that culture wells which showed active cell division and good antibody secretion often derived the two properties from different populations of cells. Thus, productive EBV transformants came to be regarded as 'unclonable'.

In consequence of the general instability of EBV transformed lines, the idea of 'short term clonal expansion' by immortalising EBV susceptible (CD21 +) B cells followed by 'stabilising' fusion of transformants with human myeloma cells emerged. Such fusions generally proved unsatisfactory since the human myeloma cells had failed to prove good fusion partners in the first place and all made their own contaminating antibody which they tended to secrete preferentially (Fig. 3.6).

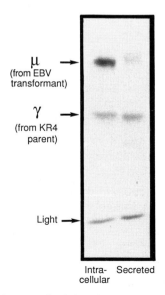

Fig. 3.6. Cells may make an antibody but do not necessarily secrete it. The autoradiograph is of a human IgM secreting unstable EB transformant fused with a stable human lymphoblastoid cell line. The resulting stable quadroma (double hybridoma) makes both the mu and gamma heavy chains but its secretion is heavily biassed towards the latter, which has the unwanted specificity.

The next development was the concept of fusion of EBV transformed cells with the well established mouse lines. These fusion lines made significant amounts of specific antibody but were chronically unstable, being interspecies fusions. Heteromyeloma lines which were hybrid mouse/human fusion partners to be fused with EBV transformants also frequently proved unstable. During this time, the fact that many of the IgM antibodies produced were polyreactive became clear.

In consequence, by the end of the 1980s, the prospects of immortalising the human B cell response looked little better than at the start. The extent of the current problem is summarised in Table 3.2. It

TABLE 3.2
Problems in human Mab production

Immunisation and tissue availability

(a) Humans cannot ethically be hyperimmunised with required, relevant, and often complex pathogens – more than half of the published human IgG Mabs have been selected using a well established purified bacterial secreted protein vaccine (tetanus toxin).

(b) Both practically and ethically, it is difficult to obtain tissue other than blood from pre-exposed/pre-immunised individuals. Blood does not, however, reflect relevant localised or mature B cell responses. In particular, blood B lymphocytes have very small numbers of IgG secreting B cells.

(c) A major problem in many potentially relevant cases has been that the patient has received previous therapy with generally cytotoxic or specifically immunosuppressive drugs.

Cell lines available for fusion

(d) Unlike the well known mouse myeloma lines, human fusion partners are almost all lymphoblastoid and therefore weak secretors (Section 3.2.2).

(e) Unlike mouse myeloma lines, human cell lines make their own antibody which dilutes any specific antibody on fusion (Section 3.2.1).

(f) Fusion to yield stable antibody secreting progeny is a rare property of B cell lines and most human fusion partners cannot do this.

(g) Human mouse fusion products are unstable in secretion.

Alternative transformation methods

(h) Epstein-Barr Virus transforms largely lymphoblastoid IgM secretors which are polyreactive with diverse antigens, and only rarely transforms IgG secreting cells. Secretion is unstable and most 'positive' results are due to polyclonal activation of non-transformed B cells.

should, however, be noted that several groups have had success in making a small number of good IgG Mabs to rhesus antigens for which immunisation and boosting are ethically permissible. This success has come from a variety of strategies, all involving EBV transformation (Chapter 7). Thus some groups have removed the T cells to avoid cytotoxic activity while others have retained and stimulated them to maximise helper T cell activity. Some have cloned EBV transformants alone and others have 'backfused' with mouse myeloma lines or human mouse heteromyeloma lines and then cloned the fused cells (Foung et al., 1987; Goosens et al., 1987; Melamed et al., 1987; Kumpel et al., 1989). Thus no clearly defined strategy has emerged, even for a single blood borne antigen in hyperimmune individuals.

3.6.2. New ways to approach the problems of human Mab production

3.6.2.1. Human rodent chimaeras
The production of these is outlined in Chapter 9. It is important to note that they reflect largely a rodent response to a human antigen and not an autologous human response (Fig. 1.7). The two undoubtedly detect different antigens and the genuine human response is preferable (Section 1.9)

3.6.2.2. Immunisation
The SCID mouse (see EMBO Workshop proceedings in Curr. Top. Microbiol. and Immunol.(1989) for a full description) is unable to produce either functional B cells or functional T cells. This is thought to be due to a deficiency in DNA repair enzymes which participate in the recombination process (Section 9.2) of antibody gene rearrangement (Fulop and Phillips, 1990). The SCID mouse therefore appears to have the potential to be repopulated by a functional human immune system without the normal processes of rejection. In consequence it appears to be the ideal candidate for hyperimmunisation of transplanted human immune cells. There is some indication that a human immune system transplanted into such mice does not function normally (Mosier et al., 1989) where only bone marrow or blood cells

are introduced, and it may be necessary to graft accessory human organs such as thymus and node (Kaneshime et al., 1990). Given the nature of the immune response to antigen and its requirement for T cell help (Section 4.1), this seems very likely.

3.6.2.3. Tissue availability

Tissue availability has largely been addressed by a shift to the study of relevant locally reactive tissues such as tumour draining lymph node or rheumatoid joints. However, many patients have undergone drug therapy of some sort (Table 3.2(c)) which reduces the effectiveness of the approach.

3.6.2.4. Polymerase chain reaction

The advent of Polymerase Chain Reaction (PCR – Section 9.6) makes it possible for libraries of potentially useful human clones from small numbers of cells to be immortalised, stabilised, and then screened extensively at leisure. This can be by two methods:

(a) By short term immortalisation and cloning of the relevant IgG producing cells (Chapter 7) followed by PCR of the matched relevant heavy and light chains from a single clone. This means that the cells must be expanded to form a large enough clone for genetic manipulation. While officially PCR can immortalise a single cell, in practice at least 1 μg of RNA is needed and this requires around 10^6 committed clonal cells plus experienced laboratory practice. Either of these requirements may be reduced by advances in the technology in the future.

(b) By immediate separate cloning of the heavy and light chain coding libraries of the diverse population of responding B cells followed by random joint re-expression in bacteria in the hope that an assay system can be devised to detect the relevant Fab fragments among the 10^{12} resultant bacterial clones (see Section 9.6 for more experimental detail).

3.7. T cell lines

The main thrust of Mab technology in this area has been towards establishing Mabs which react with the many possible T cell subsets such as the CD antigens and antibodies reactive with the variable region sequences in the T cell receptor.

T cells themselves are seldom immortalised by hybridoma technology and perhaps should be immortalised more by this method. Interleukin 2 (IL-2) can be used to prolong growth T cells in culture and is used in preference to fusion for studies on T cell biology. Like fusion, IL-2 selectively expands subpopulations but almost certainly different subpopulations from those obtained by fusion. Unlike fusion, most IL-2 uses are patented. For mouse T cell fusions the widely available, non-patented, BW 5147 line (Hyman and Stallings, 1974), derived from the AKR thymoma line is the most relevant, particularly for helper T cells. In the human system, original lines such as CEM referred to in previous editions have largely fallen out of use and it is presumed that they had the unacceptable characteristics of human B cell fusion partners.

3.8. Tissues used as sources of B cells

In the mouse and rat this is usually the spleen which has proved very suitable as source of tissue from mice boosted 4 days before fusion or mice with pathological conditions. Quantitatively, this is the best source and, while fusions with lymph nodes in the mouse (Appendix 1) yield successful hybridomas, they yield a much smaller number as the lymph nodes are small and the number of available B cells is therefore small.

It is, however, important to appreciate that more relevant tissue may be obtained in the case of localised infections or inflammations. This is obviously more widely studied in humans where the main source, peripheral blood lymphocytes, has often proved unsatisfactory. Table 3.3 shows the B cell composition of a variety of relevant

TABLE 3.3
Tissue sources of B cells

Tissue	% B Cells*
Tonsil	40–60
Spleen	30–40
Lymph node	20–40
Blood	10–20
Tumour infiltrating lymphocytes	1–10
Thymus	1–5

human tissues. In the case of more complex methods of immortalisation (Chapter 7) many protocols rely on T cell help in culture and this may also be a relevant factor. For example, lymph nodes are very rich in helper T cells (helper suppressor ratio 6/1) whereas tumour infiltrating lymphocytes are low (helper suppressor ratio 0.4/1). Blood averages a helper suppressor ratio of 2/1.

It should be noted that, while tonsillar tissue is often readily available, it is often heavily contaminated with mycoplasma and should be kept in isolation from all other cells.

CHAPTER 4

Immunisation

4.1. How the natural immune response operates

The natural B cell response is generated by regular challenge with diverse extracellular antigens in the environment. These invade non-sterile areas such as the gastrointestinal tract, and occasionally, by tissue damage, the bloodstream. Each alteration in the circumstances of mouse or man outside an enclosed environment generates a new challenge and mammals are equipped to respond to this with a local low-affinity IgM response which is only amplified to a high-affinity systemic response on precise signals from both T cells and antigen.

4.1.1. Early and immediate antibody responses

Stem cells in the blood are continuously differentiating into a variety of cells of the haemopoietic lineage (Fig. 4.1) including a very small percentage which become IgM secreting B lymphocytes. B lymphocyte precursors rearrange their antibody genes in a random process (see Section 9.2 for technical detail) to produce cells which make polyspecific IgM antibodies which can bind a variety of antigens at low affinity but high avidity (Sections 1.3 and 2.2). If these cell surface IgM positive B cells do not encounter antigen to stimulate them the cell which has offered a particular specificity is not selected. However, if the IgM producing cell encounters a 'foreign' antigen, even at low affinity, it is selected for clonal expansion, i.e., it proliferates until several daughter cells of the same clonotype are available to respond to the antigen (Fig. 4.1).

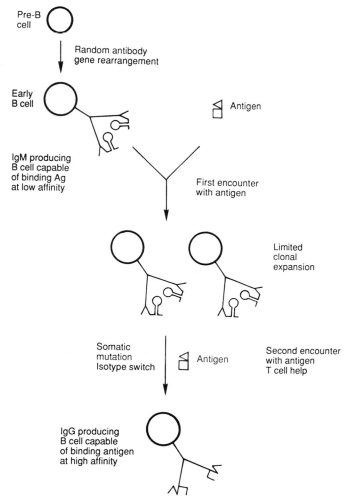

Fig. 4.1. Low-affinity antibodies are produced by first encounter with antigen. High-affinity antibodies generally only occur after somatic mutation during isotype switch.

4.1.2. After continued challenge with antigen

If the antigen persists, as in acute or chronic infection, these poly-specific, low-affinity clones must further selected. Only B cell clones with a high affinity for the antigen are required. In consequence, somatic mutation during replication is allowed to occur in the antigen binding regions of the original clone as it expands.

As in all selection systems, the second round is more exacting and many of the progeny of the original selected cell will not proceed to further growth and differentiation. In particular, T cells are required for B cell differentiation beyond (mouse) IgG3 production and the T cell can only accommodate peptides, not carbohydrate in their antigen binding groove (see below). The important factor about this somatic mutation is that it occurs during isotype switch (Fig. 4.2) where the antibody producing cell essentially changes its constant region function while increasing its affinity within the variable region (reviewed by Gritzmacher, 1989). The somatic mutation generates IgG,

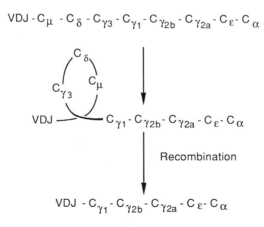

Fig. 4.2. Isotype switching at the gene level. The tightly coiled chromatin is opened up in response to a signal from the cell surface and the switch sequences in the intron in front of the constant chain gene are exposed and therefore able to recombine with those in front of the μ region. During this process, the VDJ sequence undergoes somatic mutation which increases its affinity for encountered antigen (Fig. 3.1).

IgA and IgE producing progeny of the original IgM-producing clone and increases their affinity for the original foreign antigen (Fig. 4.1). The selection process is thought to occur in the germinal centres of lymphoid tissue and is 'antigen driven' (Liu et al., 1989) so that only high-affinity cells are selected. The resultant high-affinity antibodies can be used as useful reagents. B cells immortalised earlier on in the differentiation process are of less value.

4.1.3. Ti or thymus independent antigens

These are generally high molecular weight polysaccharides in nature. In many respects they represent the natural B cell response since most Ti antigens are bacterial antigens bearing complex carbohydrate coats. In general the response is IgM and only in situations where the antigenic stimulus persists – acute or chronic, can this response switch, and then usually only to IgG3 in the mouse (IgG2b in rat). However, if the immune system also detects protein antigens then T cells also become involved. Activated T cells secrete lymphokines which provide the potential for further somatic mutation and further isotype switching.

4.2. Is it necessary to immunise?

The answer to this is emphatically positive, the only exceptions being in the study of an autoimmune response within the animal (see below). At the start of the hybridoma era, it was assumed that, since in theory the immune system is multipotent, it might be possible to make monoclonal antibodies from animals with low serum titres to antigen, or indeed with no immunisation at all. This is indeed possible but the monoclonal antibodies generated from animals with a low or zero serum titre are generally very poor reagents. The Mabs are usually of the polyreactive IgM isotype, with low intrinsic affinity for specific antigen and with the capacity to cross-react with molecules of totally unrelated structure. Even the new recombinant DNA methods for making antigen binding molecules from gene libraries, require prior immunisation of the animal from which the library is generated (Section 9.6). This is one of the main problems which remains in the generation of true human hybridomas where hyperimmunisation with the antigen of interest is not usually an available option. It is possible to take peripheral blood B cells from healthy individuals and generate EBV transformants secreting IgM to a variety of pathogens, autoantigens or lethal molecules such as ricin (Winger et al., 1983; Damato et al., 1988), and also possible to make IgM monoclonal antibodies from the spleen of an unimmunised rat or mouse which are reactive with a wide variety of non-encountered antigens. The logical conclusion is that these were produced in the host in response to some unknown environmental antigen and were sufficiently polyreactive to bind to the test antigen under assay conditions (Fig. 2.4). ELISA assays with large amounts of antigen on the plate are particularly prone to yielding such misleading data, whatever the antigen. Antigens with regularly repeating structures such as cytoskeletal proteins or DNA (Section 2.2) also tend to give spurious positive results in such systems, whatever the assay. This book recommends the use of screening systems which only detect IgG antibodies wherever possible, the only obvious exceptions being antibodies to molecules such as the ABO red blood cell determinants which are known to be natural IgM isohaemagglutinins.

In consequence, the only situation in which immunisation is not required is the study of an autoimmune response to an autoantigen or internally growing tumour antigen. In these cases, control syngeneic animals should be tested for IgM antibodies and, if these are also positive as is generally the case, care should be taken to select only IgG monoclonal antibodies by use of γ-chain specific probes (and not IgG reactive probes as these will detect IgM – Table 2.2).

4.3. Is it necessary to know precisely what the antigen is?

While it is not strictly necessary to know what the antigen is, it is preferable, forms a more logical scientific approach, and has generally been more successful. Many first generation monoclonal antibodies were generated to unknown antigens which were then characterised or partially characterised by use of the resultant hybridoma. The most common approach was with cell membrane antigens. Many of the Cluster Determinant (CD) markers (Table 1.3) on cells of the haemopoietic lineage have been obtained by immunising mice with whole cells or membrane preparations of a particular cell type and then screening the resulting fusion with panels of cells containing the immunising cell together with others of known or partially characterised phenotype in order to detect a new cell surface marker. The precise physicochemical nature of the marker was determined at a later stage. A key factor in making this approach successful has been the fact that haemopoietic cells tend to have a more straightforward membrane where the proteins are accessible. A similar approach with epithelial cells leads to Mabs generally directed to the high molecular weight mucins associated with their membranes rather than cell surface proteins.

4.4. Purity of antigen

Another assumption at the start of the hybridoma era was that it was possible to immunise an animal with a very impure mixture of antigens and isolate a monoclonal antibody which bound to molecules which constituted, say, 1% of the immunising antigen. This has been true in sporadic cases, for example with interferon as antigen and a bioassay for screening (Secher and Burke, 1980). However, in the great majority of cases it is advisable to have antigen as pure as possible for immunisation so that the spectrum of the response is focussed towards the correct target antigen. For example, if an antibody to a protein component of a gram negative bacterium is required, it is usually not possible to make it by immunising with the whole bacterial cells since the immune response will be totally dominated by the bacterial lipopolysaccharide. Another example is the previously quoted human ABO antigens which completely dominate the rhesus antigen when injected into a mouse (Fig. 1.7). Much depends on the nature of the contaminating material as well as the amount. In a mixture of

1% KLH, 99% histone, it is possible to make good Mabs to KLH but in the reverse mixture of 1% histone and 99% KLH it will not be possible to make good Mabs to histone.

4.5. The use of previously determined schedules

There is a tendency for protocols to group antigens according to physicochemical properties, i.e., protein, carbohydrate etc. and this is of limited value since any two within a group may be quite different in the extent to which the mouse or rat sees them as 'foreign'. For instance in the example above, KLH, keyhole limpet haemocyanin, is a protein which is a good antigen in most mammals since it is obviously foreign. Histones on the other hand, are very highly conserved throughout evolution and are very weak antigens. While both antigens are protein, the first injected in microgram amounts can elicit an immune response but the latter requires milligram amounts.

4.6. Strains of rodent

Most complex antigens should give a satisfactory serum titre with the standard strains used. However, simple antigens may elicit no response in one strain and a substantial response in another and this is particularly true of small peptide antigens and repeated peptide polymeric antigens. For example the peptide sequence NANP which is present on the malarial sporozoite fails to elicit any response in some strains of mouse. This is probably due to the need for T cell help which may not be available with antigens of restricted complexity.

T cell help is provided by CD4 positive T cells which recognise antigenic peptides 'presented' in the groove of a Class II MHC antigens on antigen presenting cells such as macrophages or B cells (Bjorkman et al., 1987; Brown et al., 1988) (Fig. 4.3). These T cells then release lymphokines which can promote and mature the response of antibody producing B cells. Where inbred strains of animals are used, lack of

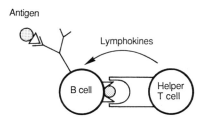

B cell recognising one epitope on antigen
internalises it and "presents" another epitope
to T cells in the groove of MHC class II
molecules

Fig. 4.3. Helper T cells do not recognise the same epitopes as antibody producing B
cells and both epitopes are necessary for the mature immune response.

appropriate Class II MHC molecules may result in failure to present
the desired peptide to T cells, giving rise to the 'low responder' phenotype. For this reason, it is often helpful to try an antigen to which
Balb/c (Haplotype H2 ^{d}) is a 'low responder' in mice of other H2 haplotypes, particularly those differing at Class II loci (Festing, 1979;
Klein et al., 1983) (Section 3.4). Any hybridomas produced will have
to be expanded in the f1 hybrid if ascites is required. This is not difficult as it is necessary to acquire only one male from the other strain
to mate with the Balb/c females to generate an f1 litter.

The fact that B cells can both present and recognise antigens does not
imply that both properties reside in the same sequence of the antigen
(Fig. 4.3). It is quite possible for a B cell to recognise one determinant
through its antibody receptor system and digest the antigen, presenting another determinant to the essential helper T cell on its Class II
MHC antigens.

4.7. Age and sex of rodent

Animals are not usually given their primary immunisation until they
are 4–6 weeks old and the nature of hybridoma production is such

that they are generally used while still under one year old. We have, however, had comparable results with animals which are considerably older at first immunisation and age does not appear to be an important factor.

Either sex of animal can be used and the main advantage of females which are recommended in some texts, is that they fight less in the cage. Fighting often results in wounds which can become infected and divert the immune response. Among the many factors involved in the generation of the immune response, steroid hormones undoubtedly play a part, but a good panel of Mabs to injected antigen can be as easily generated from a male as from a female mouse.

However, if autoimmunity is under study and animal models are being used, then the disease is frequently sex linked and the appropriate sex should be used.

4.8. Tolerance, overimmunisation and underimmunisation

The general area of tolerance is a complex one, still poorly understood, and dealt with in greater depth in the major immunological texts. Hybridoma production has never been sufficiently sophisticated to use mechanisms of tolerance to manipulate responses in a positive way and the main concern is to avoid B cell tolerance. Neonatal tolerance is obviously not a problem unless the newborn animal has been exposed to the antigen. Low zone tolerance is induced by repeated injection with subimmunogenic amounts of antigen and does not generally complicate hybridoma production schedules. However, repeated injections of large amounts of antigen can lead to functional deletion of B cells and /or blockade of antigen producing cells by antigen itself. If the general advice given below is used, then this problem should not be encountered, since an animal is not used for fusion unless it has a good mature serum response and the final boosting dose is small.

4.9. Adjuvants

4.9.1. Freund's adjuvant

The purpose of adjuvant is to maximise the immune response to the injected antigen and the major way in which adjuvants do this is by slowing the release of the antigen into the body so that the immune system is maximally exposed to antigen. A foreign protein injected in saline will be quickly removed but a foreign protein as an emulsion or solid complex will remain in the body for much longer, eliciting a greater immune response. There is no doubt that this is a useful function for stimulating the immune response. The addition of killed bacteria to such adjuvants was originally thought to enhance the response and this is a concept which is becoming increasingly less tenable. As knowledge of the nature of B cell development and maturation has progressed, no clear role for the bacteria in CFA has become apparent and it seems very possible that they only potentiate nonspecific local polyclonal response at the site of injection.

The best known adjuvant is Complete Freund's Adjuvant (CFA) which is a suspension of killed mycobacteria in mineral oil, first described over 50 years ago (Freund and McDermott, 1942; Freund, 1956). Incomplete Freund's Adjuvant (IFA) is mineral oil without the killed mycobacteria. Thus many people successfully use only IFA since the mineral oil emulsion is invaluable for slow release.

Both CFA and IFA, but especially the former can cause unpleasant local inflammation and care must be taken not to inject oneself while immunising the animal.

Mixing antigen in aqueous solution with either CFA or IFA is very similar to making mayonnaise which is also an oil-water emulsion. Equal volumes of oil and aqueous solution are used. While original methods involved injecting the aqueous solution from the barrel of one syringe across into the barrel of a second 'head-to-head' linked syringe containing the oil, glass syringes are comparatively rare in modern times and the standard polypropylene syringes are unsuitable. Thus many laboratories use repeated vortexing. 100 μl of aqueous solution containing enough antigen to immunise a single mouse is placed in a glass tube and the CFA or IFA is added in aliquots of 10–20 μl with vigorous vortexing between each addition. The final emulsion should be thick and creamy and should not separate after standing for some hours. While many texts suggest that it is essential to add the aqueous solution to the adjuvant rather than the other way round, in practice it makes very little difference and the immune system is able to see the antigen whether it is injected on the outside or inside of oil droplets.

A remarkably simple method of mixing the two is to give the mixture of antigen and oil a quick burst of sonication. However, this is only useful for robust antigens.

4.9.2. Aluminium hydroxide (alum)

This is less toxic than CFA or IFA. The antigen is either trapped onto the surface of the aluminium hydroxide as it is precipitated from solution or adsorbed onto the preformed aluminium hydroxide. The starting material in either case is 10 ml of a 10% (0.2 M) solution of aluminium potassium sulphate $(AlK(SO_4)_2 \cdot 12H_2O)$ which may contain antigen.

If it does contain antigen then the adsorbed alum is precipitated with 5 ml of $NaHCO_3$, with vigorous stirring, centrifuged at $500 \times g$ and resuspended for immunisation.

If it does not contain antigen, it may be precipitated with either 5 ml $NaHCO_3$ or 5 ml of the more rigorous NaOH. The particles are then washed in saline and the antigen is then adsorbed passively at a weight ratio of approximately 10/1 (Alum/Antigen).

Older protocols which involve the addition of killed *Bordetella pertussis* (whooping cough) organisms are both impractical because of lack of availability and, as with the myobacteria in complete Freund's adjuvant, probably irrelevant to the specific antigen under study.

4.10. In vitro immunisation

While the primary aim for in vitro immunisation has been to find methods of immunising human B cells, it has also been used in mouse systems where thymocyte conditioned medium from young mice is used to stimulate the B cells (Reading, 1986). The main claims for it have been that it requires very small (nanogram) amounts of antigen and that it has led to the production of antibodies suppressed in the in vivo immune response. There is now some scepticism about the process since it has become apparent that it is possible to produce a panel of polyspecific IgMs, and also the occasional IgG, from any unimmunised animal to almost any antigen. In addition, basic research has indicated that antibody maturation is essentially an in vivo process requiring many unknown factors present in germinal centres and there is some doubt as to whether this can be reproduced in vitro. In the rodent system, in vitro immunisation has therefore currently fallen out of use. The protocol is quite simple and involves the growth of thymocytes (Protocol 5.7) in medium containing 5×10^{-5} M mercaptoethanol for 2-4 days to provide thymocyte enriched medium and incubation of this together with sterile antigen with the spleen cells for a further 2–4 days before fusion.

In the human system, where hyperimmunisation is a major ethical and technical barrier, Borrebaeck (1989) has argued a fairly solitary case for the use of methylleucyl dipeptide to destroy lysosome rich suppressor cells and therefore make human B cells more susceptible to stimulation by antigen.

A variation on this has been intrasplenic immunisation which had a brief period of fashion in the mid 1980s (Spitz, 1986). This also yields largely IgM antibodies of poor specificity and is not advised. The animal manipulations are extensive and the antibodies produced do not justify the trauma caused.

4.11. Production of specific antibody isotypes

4.11.1. The requirement for specific isotypes

Different isotypes of IgG can have different functions. For example some fix complement better than others or bind to Protein A more readily. However, it is possible to alter the isotype of an established hybridoma by recombinant DNA methodology (Chapter 9) and so specific isotypes from a direct fusion are usually required primarily for research purposes. IgA Mabs are usually required in the study of mucosal immunity and IgE Mabs in the study of hypersensitivity. One obvious way of selecting a specific isotype is to use a probe specific to the appropriate heavy chain as described in Chapter 2 for the selection of IgG producing cells. IgA or IgE producing cells can be selected by the use of α- or ε-specific second antibodies respectively.

4.11.2. Route of immunisation and tissue used for fusion

IgA producers can be selected by immunising the animal by gastric intubation (Colwell, 1986) followed by standard fusion with spleen cells. Other methods involve fusion with gut associated lymphoid tissue (Komisar et al., 1982; Dean et al., 1986).

4.11.3. Lymphokines and other biological response modifiers

Lymphokines normally act in a highly local manner and used systemically act as traumatic polyclonal stimulants. Lymphokines differ from other local stimulants such as bacterial LPS in that specific lymphokines can cause defined class switches (Table 4.1) both in vivo and in vitro. There are two ways in which they can do this. The first is 'directed' switching where all the cells in the culture are induced to rearrange their genes (Fig. 4.2) to produce the directed isotype. The other is selective expansion of cells which have previously switched in response to an earlier unknown stimulus. Thus the promotion of IgA production by TGFβ is thought to be a directed switch while the promotion

TABLE 4.1
Biological response modifiers selecting mouse isotypes

Protein	Favoured isotype
Bacterial LPS	IgG3
Interleukin 4	IgG1, IgE
Interleukin 5	IgA
TGF-β	IgA
Interferon-γ	IgG2a

of IgA production by interleukin 5 is thought to be selective expansion of IgA producers.

There is no evidence as to whether or not this lymphokine induced isotype switch is accompanied by the affinity enhancing somatic mutation characteristic of the natural in vivo process but in the absence of the accessory factors supplied by the environment of the germinal centre, it seems unlikely.

Human lymphokines can also cause class switching but there is no direct parallel between the effects of any human interleukin and its mouse counterpart (reviewed by Finkelman et al., 1990). Human Interleukin 4, is, however, definitely implicated in IgE production.

4.12. Routes of immunisation

The usual routes of injection are subcutaneous (s.c.), intraperitoneal (i.p.) and intravenous (Appendix 1). The intravenous route is used only for the final boost via the mouse tail vein 4 days before fusion and obviously must not contain toxic material such as adjuvant or pieces of polyacrylamide gel and is replaced by intraperitoneal injection in such cases. Some groups use an intraperitoneal final boost for all antigens and appear to have success.

Most soluble antigens emulsified with CFA or IFA are injected subcutaneously. On the other hand whole cells are usually injected intraperitoneally.

Other methods of injection such as intradermal or footpad are more suited to larger animals and generally not employed with mouse. In the U.K. the licence obtained under the Animals (Scientific Procedures) Act 1986 specifies procedures to be used and a detailed justification for using these comparatively traumatic procedures would have to be made.

4.13. Schedules

Immunisation schedules have three main injections. The first stimulates only a primary immune response and will yield IgM Mabs. The second stimulates isotype switching and the production of high-affinity antigen committed memory cells. If a good serum titre is not obtained at this point, then the second injection can be repeated. Once the animal has a satisfactory serum titre it can be rested for a short period of time. The final and critical immunisation is an intravenous boost 4 days before the fusion to activate the memory B cells in the spleen. Where the intravenous route is unsuitable, it can be replaced by intraperitoneal injection. It is important that this be a small boost (Fig. 4.4) as this will only expand the highest affinity clones of memory cells.

Schedule 1
(i) Primary immunisation. Four or more weeks before fusion, subcutaneously in CCFA
(ii) Secondary immunisation. Two-three weeks after the primary, subcutaneously in IFA
(iii) Serum test 10–14 days after secondary (e.g., Protocol 2.2, 2.4 or 2.6). If the IgG level rather than the IgM level in the serum is to be tested, then a second antibody specific to the γ-chain of IgG should be used. At this point, the animal can be rested if the serum titre is high (positive with an IgG specific probe with respect to control serum at a dilution of 1/500 or greater). If not, the secondary immunisation should be repeated until the titre is high. There is little point in doing a fusion without this.
(iv) Final boost 4 days before fusion one tenth of the original dose, intravenously in saline (intraperitoneally if toxic).

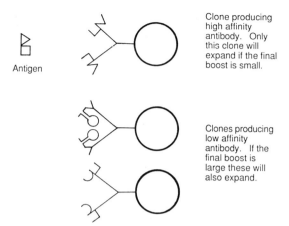

Fig. 4.4. Why the final booster immunisation should be a small amount. A larger amount will stimulate clones producing low-affinity antibody.

Schedule 2
(i) Primary immunisation. Four or more weeks before fusion, intraperitoneally
(ii) Secondary immunisation. Two-three weeks after the primary intraperitoneally
(iii) Serum test 10–14 days after secondary (e.g., Protocol 2.6). If the IgG level rather than the IgM level in the serum is to be tested, then a second antibody specific to the γ-chain of IgG should be used. At this point, the animal can be rested if the serum titre is high (positive with an IgG specific probe with respect to control serum at a dilution of 1/500 or greater). If not, the secondary immunisation should be repeated until the titre is high. There is little point in doing a fusion without this.
(iv) Final boost 4 days before fusion one tenth of the original dose, intravenously in saline (intraperitoneally if toxic).

4.14. Specific examples – proteins

4.14.1. Proteins from eukaryote sources

(i) Pure soluble proteins. The usual range is 10–500 μg for primary and secondary immunisation with Schedule 1 above. The amount used depends on how foreign the protein is to the mouse. A highly conserved protein will require that quantities at the upper end of the range are injected.

(ii) Insoluble proteins. These are generally more antigenic and so the range is smaller. 10–50 μg. Schedule 1.

(iii) Cell membrane proteins of haemopoietic/ lymphoid cells. Ideally membrane proteins should be presented to the immune system within the context of the membrane and outer membrane proteins can often be successful antigens injected as whole cell (10^6–10^7, Schedule 2) or whole cell membrane preparations from the same number of cells. However, if the protein is very low abundance and/or of limited antigenicity, some pre-purification will be necessary as the response will be dominated by the other proteins in the membrane. Ideally, for a low abundance protein, an overexpressing cell line should be sought or indeed generated by transfection of the gene coding for it. However, purified protein isolated from a gel by electroelution can be reconstituted.

Reconstitution within membrane lipids is a common procedure for mitochondrial proteins (Wohlrab et al., 1986; Kaplan et al., 1986). Selection should be by FACS (Protocol 2.6), or immunofluorescence of live cells.

Inner cell membrane proteins are generally less antigenic and if a membrane preparation is to be used for immunisation, the outer membrane proteins should be stripped by treatment of the whole cell for 2–5 min with trypsin prior to isolation of the membrane.

(iv) Cell membrane proteins of adherent cells. There is generally a lot of carbohydrate associated with such cells and in particular with epithelial cells. Immunisation with whole cells or membrane preparations will lead to a response dominated by this. In addition, the cytoskeletal proteins of such cells elicit a strong immune response so that if whole cells are used, the response to the membrane protein will be further diminished. Preliminary purification is nearly always required.

(v) Membrane proteins of intracellular organelles (Mitochondria, chloroplasts). The organelles should be purified first and it is important that they be free of cytoskeletal proteins. The procedure is then as for free floating haemopoietic cells in (iii) above.

(vi) Proteins from SDS-PAGE.

A band from an SDS gel can be lyophilised, ground up with a mortar and pestle and injected subcutaneously into the animal. There is no need for adjuvant as the gel itself acts as adjuvant. However, the local inflammation at the site of injection is considerable and this is not a suitable technique for a mouse. It is slightly less traumatic to the larger rat. A better strategy is to electroelute the protein from the gel through a porous membrane into a chamber where it is trapped by dialysis tubing. Apparatus for this can be purchased from most major protein separation firms (Bio-Rad, Pharmacia). The position of the protein in the gel can be determined either by light staining without fixation or by the staining of strips at each side of the gel to locate the antigen. The latter is the better procedure but less easy to line up if the band required is close to other contaminating bands since the staining procedure can alter the size of the strips. The standard Coomassie blue stain takes rather a long time to destain and brief staining in 0.3 M $CuCl_2$ (Lee et al., 1987) is equally sensitive and more suitable. This gives an overall white background with clear bands where the protein is located. The relevant band is excised and equilibrated with electroelution buffer. The electroeluted protein is then used as in Schedule 1.

4.14.2. Proteins from prokaryote sources

(i) Genuine prokaryote proteins
While in general the procedures described in 4.14.1 can all be applied, bacterial proteins can be dominated by even very small amounts of some of the highly antigenic bacterial polysaccharides – for example the gram negative bacterial lipopolysaccharides. While many rough laboratory strains of say, E. coli lack this LPS, wild type gram negative bacteria are generally of the smooth LPS expressing type. LPS can also be present, undetected, on SDS PAGE unless silver staining is used. The exosporium coat on the spores of some bacilli presents similar problems. Thus for Mabs to the protein components of antigens such a Salmonella or V. cholerae, it is usually necessary to use LPS negative strains. Bacterial proteins are good antigens and 10–50 μg, Schedule 1 should give a satisfactory titre in most cases.

(ii) Expressed proteins. These must be expressed in an LPS negative strain of bacterium. They can be either secreted into the periplasmic space (Section 9.5) or sequestered in insoluble inclusion bodies. Since insoluble material is highly antigenic, the latter are perfectly suitable for immunisation. However, the bacterial proteins will also be highly antigenic and compete for the immune response and in general, expressed proteins are better eluted from gels before immunisation. Schedule 1 is used with intraperitoneal rather than subcutaneous final boosting.

4.14.3. Peptides

Mabs to peptides are neither generally necessary nor advisable. Immunisation with a peptide defines the epitope for polyclonal serum. Selection of a single clone which binds to the epitope generally means that the additive affinity of the antibodies in the polyclonal serum is lost and most anti-peptide Mabs are of low affinity. If a Mab is required because of its standard nature, then it is more likely to be successful if the peptide is reasonably long. Under 12 amino acids should be avoided and 20 or more is preferable.

4.15. Specific examples – carbohydrates

4.15.1. Small carbohydrates

For many known small carbohydrate sequences there is no need to make a Mab since there are a wide variety of lectins which have sugar specificities. Outwith this range, small carbohydrates should be attached to antigenic proteins as haptens (see below).

4.15.2. Large carbohydrates

These are generally highly antigenic and tolerance (Section 4.8) can occur on over-immunisation. 1–10 μg is usually sufficient and IFA rather than CFA should be used. They also tend to elicit antibodies of low intrinsic affinity and high cross-reactive potential. IgM Mabs should, as usual, be avoided but in addition the IgG3 class in the mouse (IgG2b in the rat) which is the dominant IgG response can be cross-reactive. It is possible to encourage clones to switch to the other higher affinity IgG classes by attaching them covalently to protein antigens which can elicit the required T cell help (Fig. 4.3).

4.16. Specific examples – lipids and nucleic acids

These are poor antigens and not recommended. While Mabs to lipids have occasionally been reported, they have been largely polyreactive IgMs of little diagnostic or clinical value. While some texts suggest that immunisation with nucleic acid attached to protein may be antigenic, no useful reagents have been produced and the level of nuclease activity in most body fluids would suggest that injected antigen is unlikely to survive long enough to be seen by the immune system. It is, however, possible to obtain high-affinity anti-DNA IgG Mabs with some sequence specificity, from autoimmune animals such as the NZB × NZW f1 or MRL lpr/lpr mouse (Stollar et al., 1986). In this case, there is no need for immunisation and the animal is used when the disease is advanced enough to show a high serum IgG titre but before the animals become clearly unwell.

4.17. Specific examples – haptens

4.17.1. Size of hapten

The nature of antibody-antigen interactions (Section 1.3.1) and particularly the realisation of the extent of the number and range of contact points between antibody and protein antigens means that a small molecule which offers limited opportunity for antibody binding will not yield a high-affinity Mab. With polyclonal serum this is less important because of the additive effects of the different antibodies. In consequence, it is probably not sensible to expect to obtain high-affinity Mabs to small haptens such as acetylcholine, tyrosine phosphate etc. More substantial haptens such as steroids can elicit antibodies of useful affinity. However, a hapten has to be of considerable size before it can be detected in a double sandwich assay (Fig. 1.8) which depends on two Mabs, each binding at high affinity to different sites on the detecting antigen.

4.17.2. Conjugation

The precise method of conjugation of the hapten obviously depends on its structural groups and for example, amino groups can be conjugated to amino groups on the carrier with glutaraldehyde while carboxyl groups can be conjugated by amide bond formation. Higher affinity antibodies will be obtained if the linkage of hapten to protein is spaced at 6 angstroms or greater so that the antibody does not recognise the carrier as part of its epitope but T cell help from the carrier is still available. The interest in catalytic antibodies has led to the design of a wide variety of new heterobifunctional cross-linking agents (Reviewed by Shokat and Schultz, 1990; Tramontano and Schloeder, 1989) which perform this function.

The carrier protein is most commonly KLH or BSA and the main part of the antibody response is, of course, to the carrier. Typical conjugation levels of 20–40 haptens/protein are required for an efficient immune response and this puts the haptens into the category of polymeric antigens which are vulnerable to low-affinity antibody binding (Sections 1.3 and 2.2). A fairly rigorous immunisation schedule is required (Schedule 1, $100 + \mu$g of protein and it is likely that the secondary immunisation will have to be repeated several times).

4.18. Specific examples – whole cells and organisms

In general, it is now more usual not to immunise with complex antigens as a subset of material will tend to dominate the immune response. Individual proteins of interest are best used as separate antigens purified from overexpressed genes and/or SDS-PAGE in separate fusions. However, particulate antigens are good antigens and if the Mabs required are to the dominant antigen, it is possible to use the entire particle.

4.18.1. Viruses

Viruses are generally inactivated before injection but this is not strictly necessary if the mouse strain used is not susceptible and the virus is not one which will put the local animal or human population at risk. Most methods of inactivation involve formaldehyde or glutaraldehyde at 0.1–0.25% (v/v). These are not ideal as they can alter the chemical nature of the antigenic groups. Inactivation can also be achieved by placing the preparation close to a source of UV light for 5–10 minutes to cross-link the DNA. The exact conditions depend on the source used and it is best to do a test experiment to check that the inactivation has been effective.

If the whole inactivated virus particle is used as antigen then the cell surface glycoproteins will dominate the response. 10–20 μg of total virus protein, Schedule 1 will give a good response to these antigens. Virus preparations can be contaminated with host cell antigens and the screening system should select for Mabs specific to the virus.

Soluble viral proteins produced in infected cells will obviously be heavily contaminated with host cell material and these are best purified or partially purified first by the methods for proteins described above.

4.18.2. Bacteria

Bacteria must be killed before injection. The commonest methods are heating to 60–80°C with or without 0.1% phenol. The exact conditions depend on the bacterium used. Alternatively, they may be fixed with 0.1–0.25% (v/v) formaldehyde or glutaraldehyde but this will alter the structures of some epitopes.

If antibodies to LPS or bacterial capsular polysaccharides are required then immunisation with the whole organism is generally the most suitable method. The problem is that these (particularly LPS) tend to dominate the response to other bacterial antigens even when present in very small amounts and the best solution to date has been to use mutant bacteria which are deficient in their ability to generate carbohydrate coats, e.g., an LPS negative strain of gram negative bacteria. Gram positive bacteria carrying Protein A or G on their surface, will obviously bind a wide range of B lymphocytes non-specifically and elicit a polyclonal response.

Bacterial membranes can be prepared by digestion of the bacterial peptidoglycan with 10 mg/ml lysosyme. In the case of gram negative bacteria which only have a cytoplasmic membrane, this will produce protoplasts which can be lysed by 10 mg/ml lysosyme followed by lysis of the spheroplasts by osmotic shock to give membrane vesicles. Gram positive bacteria require that the lysosyme digestion be in the presence of 3 mM EDTA to permeabilise the outer membrane. The outer and inner membrane proteins can be purified from the resultant spheroplast lysate by density gradient centrifugation. Bacterial appendages such as flagella, fimbriae and pili can be partially purified by mechanical shearing of the cell followed by centrifugation.

4.18.3. Whole cells

Whole cells are excellent antigens and, particularly when antibodies to membrane proteins are required, are probably one of the best methods of immunising with cells of the haemopoietic system, the other being to use purified membranes. The approach is less successful with other cell types (Section 4.14.1) as it can be dominated by carbohydrate material associated with the membrane and highly antigenic intracellular cytoskeletal proteins. Screening should be by FACS where possible. The dosage is 10^6 to 10^7 cells on Schedule 2.

One particularly successful approach with whole cells has been to use cells which have been transfected with the DNA coding for a membrane protein so that they hyperexpress the protein.

4.19. Immunisation of human subjects

4.19.1. Non-toxic antigens and infected individuals

While even with non-toxic antigens, there is an obvious limit to which any individual can be hyperimmunised (for example CFA cannot be used), there are a variety of antigens, notably inactivated bacterial toxins, which give good serum titres. In addition, samples can be obtained from patients carrying infections. An important point to note with respect to immunisation is that the source of lymphocytes is generally peripheral blood and the method is not fusion but transformation. In the most successful cases of human hybridoma production, most of which involve the rhesus antigens, the optimum blood B cell transformable response is obtained longer than 4 days after the final boost and is closer to 2–4 weeks, possibly reflecting the production of EBV transformable memory B cells (Kozbor and Roder, 1981; Melamed et al., 1987; Kumpel et al., 1989).

4.19.2. Toxic antigens

The main problem with humans is obviously an ethical and practical one and is discussed in Section 3.6. While primates can be used (Van Meel et al., 1985; Van Meurs et al., 1986; Erlich et al., 1988), their availability is very limited, their cost is excessive, and the system is still foeign to man. The only current prospect for addressing this problem would therefore appear to be the use of the SCID mouse and this remains to be demonstrated as a suitable host for any simple working human immune system such as that generated by the injection of human peripheral blood lymphocytes into the mouse (Mosier et al., 1989). It is likely that, to obtain a high-affinity isotype switched response, akin to that which would occur in man, the Scid mouse will require grafting not only with human blood but also with organs important to the maturation of the immune response such as human thymus and lymph nodes (Kaneshima et al., 1990).

CHAPTER 5

Cell culture requirements for hybridomas

5.1. Introduction

Cell culture techniques cover a wide range of complex processes and many major aspects are dealt with in a recent edition of another book in this series (Adams, 1990). This chapter is addressed to cell culture requirements specifically for hybridomas.

5.1.1. Safety

Human tissue can be a source of a wide range of contaminating materials including mycoplasma and most Mab labs keep any material of human origin in hoods and incubators used solely for human work. Known or suspected HIV or hepatitis A or B infected material is obviously handled in separate hoods and incubators. All human material, from whatever source, should be treated as dangerous, handled in surgical gloves and both unused fractions and wash supernatants from cells should be autoclaved. Hoods should be serviced annually and filters changed. There is no evidence to date that hybridoma technologists working with human material have been contaminated by the material with which they work (and in comparison to surgeons the risk is very small) but the safety rules in most countries require such practices and the cost of a legal action against an individual or organisation is such that it is wise to have very rigorous observation of these rules.

5.2. Basic cell culture requirements

These are listed in Table 5.1 together with typical costs. In principle, it is quite possible to produce Mabs in any general research laboratory equipped with a sterile hood and a carbon dioxide incubator. In practice, however, it is very useful to have an area of the laboratory set aside for hybridoma work and it is particularly advisable not to share sterile hoods with a large number of people whose technique is not of the quality required.

It is essential to have an inverted microscope of the highest affordable quality to monitor the cells and, in particular, to monitor emerging clones. These are 'inverted' in the sense that the objective is below the stage holding the culture vessel and the light source is above. A vertical laminar flow cabinet which protects operator and sample from each other is also essential, although it does not replace good sterile handling techniques. Bunsen burners should not be used in such cabinets as the air is recycled and ethanol or methanol used to swab the working surfaces can build up to explosive levels. A jacketed carbon dioxide incubator capable of maintaining the cells at 5% CO_2 and high humidity is also required together with the appropriate replaceable gas cylinders, regulators and inlet valves. The other piece of major equipment is a liquid nitrogen storage vat. This will require topping up twice weekly and so regular arrangements with a liquid nitrogen

TABLE 5.1
Essential hardware for hybridoma production

Item	Typical cost (1990 U.K.)
Vertical laminar air flow cabinet with UV light	£3000
Water jacketed carbon dioxide incubator	£4000–£7000
Inverted microscope	£2500
Automatic carbon dioxide regulators and valves	£200
Liquid nitrogen storage vat (20 l)	£400
Autoclave and/or pressure cooker	£5000 and/or £35
Automatic pipetter for 10 ml volumes (rechargeable)	£200
Eight channel variable volume multipipettes for μl volumes	£300

supplier are necessary. Access to an autoclave is invaluable for all hybridoma work and essential for human hybridoma work. However, routine sterilisation of small items such as pipette tips is generally carried out in a domestic pressure cooker. An automatic pipetter for measurements of large (ml) amounts of media is invaluable and the most convenient are those with rechargeable batteries. While numerous device for sampling or feeding cells in 96 well plates were brought onto the market during the 1980s, most hybridoma labs feed and sample using 8 channel multipipettes and these are also listed since their cost is not small. Table 5.1 lists only major suppliers and approximate costs and a better local supplier may be available at lower rates. Anyone starting hybridoma work for the first time is advised to consult those local research and hospital laboratories which undertake a lot of tissue culture to find the lowest cost local system. It is assumed that other items such as refrigerators and freezers and a haemocytometer for counting cells are already available. In all these cases, it is, however, preferable to have one set aside for hybridoma work.

Suppliers (Appendix 2) are now many and most of the above items can be obtained from Bibby, Flow Laboratories, Gallenkamp, Scotlab etc. In the U.K. Olympus supply microscopes.

5.2.1. Plasticware

Table 5.2 gives a list of plasticware with typical costs. Tissue culture plates should have an independent rim to each well to minimise the possibility of transfer of material between wells by means of droplets of evaporation. The other requirements are petri dishes, tissue culture flasks of all sizes, pipettes and tips and large numbers of sterile 20 ml universal containers. Protective gloves and autoclave bags are not included but often required. Glass reusable pipettes with plugged cotton wool tips may also be used and these are undoubtedly of lower cost.

Again, there are a wide range of suppliers the main U.K. ones including Flow Laboratories, Gibco, Sterilin, Costar and Bibby.

TABLE 5.2
Essential plasticware for hybridoma production

Item	Typical number for one fusion with ten selected subclones (highly variable)	Typical cost (1991, U.K.)
98 well plates	24	£42/50
24 well plates*	4–10	£43/50
1 ml sterile pipettes	50	£60/500
5 ml sterile pipettes	50	£35/200
10 ml sterile pipettes	50	£93/500
Petri dishes (60 mm)	20	£63/500
Universal containers (20 ml)	50	£43/400
25 cm^2 tissue culture flasks	20	£190/500
80 cm^2 tissue culture flasks	20	£72/100
175 cm^2 tissue culture flasks	12	£61/50
Ampoules for liquid nitrogen storage	50	£7/50

*See Section 6.5.

5.2.2. Media

Two main types of medium are used for hybridoma production. These are Dulbecco's Modification of Eagles Medium (DMEM) and Rosewell Park Memorial Institute (RPMI) medium, formulation 1640. Both contain the amino acids, vitamins, salts and nutrients in varying proportions. Throughout this book RPMI 1640 is the medium specified. However, in all cases DMEM will perform equally well. There are differences in the media, for example basis DMEM has pyruvate where RPMI does not and DMEM has more bicarbonate buffer so that it may be more useful if for some reason it has to spend long periods of time in the absence of carbon dioxide. Media formulations are given in the suppliers catalogues (Appendix 2). Liquid medium is frequently supplied without glutamine because of its comparative instability in aqueous solution and it should be added to a level of 2 mM. Powdered medium is usually purchased with glutamine already added on the assumption that it will be made up immediately before use. Various protocols recommend further additions, notably pyruvate at 1 mM, oxaloacetate at 10 mM, mercaptoethanol at 50 μM, glycine at 100 mM and insulin at 1 unit/ml. None of these are essential for successful classical hybridoma production although none do any harm. In specialised cases where cells are being grown at low density (e.g., cloning of EBV transformants – Chapter 7), pyruvate and insulin in particular may be helpful. Media are made up in double distilled water, sterilised by filtration through 0.2 μm filters and stored in 500 ml aliquots for up to 6 weeks. Both the main recommended media are bicarbonate buffered with phenol red indicator. The correct colour for medium is bright orange indicating a pH of 7.2. Yellow medium is acid indicating strong growth of cells (or bacteria).

5.2.3. Sera

Foetal calf serum (FCS) is used in nearly all hybridoma work. This can be obtained from most suppliers of tissue culture equipment and media. Most reputable suppliers are prepared to send several samples from different batches for the laboratory to test and a bulk order can then be placed for the most suitable. Ideally, serum should be tested on a cell line which is comparatively difficult to grow and closely related to the work to be undertaken using the serum. This can be a poor growing but established hybridoma but also any slow growing myeloma lines. Our own laboratory uses a variety of such lines including the rat Y3 line (Section 3.5) which has always been a slow growing line in our hands. Serum is not only tested for its ability to support fast growth of bulk cultures but also for its cloning efficiency of these more difficult lines, i.e., its ability to support one cell/well growth on feeders and 100 cell/well growth without feeders. These two types of test do not measure the same qualities of the serum and the second one, for cloning efficiency can sometimes be quite poor for a serum which promotes good growth of bulk cultures.

FCS is usually obtained in sterile 100 ml aliquots which are kept frozen at $-20°C$. These are heated at 56°C for 30 min to inactivate complement and other serum proteolytic activities before use. FCS is always assumed to be particularly useful for hybridoma work because of its low level of contaminating immunoglobulin, although different batches can have up to 1.3 mg/ml bovine IgG (Underwood et al., 1983). However, it is also preferable for culture of many other cell types and it is likely that it contains additional nutrients not available in normal serum. Newborn calf serum is significantly less efficient than foetal at supporting growth. FCS is, however, one of the major costs incurred in hybridoma production, being £26/100 ml or greater at 1990 U.K. prices.

ECACC will supply fully tested FCS of American origin to the European market at negotiable prices. This may prove of particular value to individuals or firms who regularly ship hybridomas or their supernatants to America where regulations about imported material containing animal sera are very strict.

5.2.5. Serum free media

Serum free medium is not recommended for fusions and subclonings in general. The suppliers have tended to publish growth curves of a hybridoma in their serum free medium in comparison to growth curves in 10%FCS but since the quality of FCS used can be so variable, this can be a rather artificial comparison. In particular, few if any, serum free media give the same cloning efficiency as good FCS and FCS remains the choice for emerging clones. Most serum free media are also still quite expensive and represent little saving in comparison to FCS. They can be supplied as a complete medium or as a supplement to be added to RPMI 1640 which will abolish or reduce the requirement for FCS.

The advantages of serum free media lie in their standard nature and the consequent fact that it is possible to detect cell products which clearly come from the cells and not the serum. Thus, if a hybridoma or myeloma line, or primary splenocyte culture is being tested for the secretion of, or response to, lymphokines, serum free medium is obviously essential. A further advantage lies in bulk culture of hybridomas where serum can lead to frothing and poor aeration in oxygenated vats, where the minimal number of steps for purifying the product antibodies is a major factor in cost calculations, or where therapy is to be the final use of the Mab and it is necessary to demonstrate purity. This last is obviously a much simpler task when the components of the medium in which the hybridoma was grown are known but even then the cells themselves may supply further contaminants.

Nearly all serum free media or serum free supplements have albumin, pyruvate, transferrin and insulin and they may in addition include selenium, steroids,unsaturated fatty acids and ethanolamine. Serum free medium requirements are different for each cell type and even within cell types, can be different for different cell lines. Obviously a medium formulated for hybridomas only should be used. Two complex media for hybridomas were described in 1986 (Kawamoto et al., 1986; Kovar and Franek, 1986) but neither has been extensively used. All major firms market such media, notably American BioOrganics, Boehringer Manneheim, Collaborative Research, and Sigma (Appendix 2) and their content has been reviewed by Samoilovich et al. (1987). One of the better ones appears to be SF-1 marketed by Costar (Adams, 1990). For normal Mab production their expense does not justify their use.

5.2.5. Antibiotics

The basic antibiotics used for hybridoma production are penicillin and streptomycin (P/S). The former inhibits the growth of most gram positive bacteria and the latter the growth of gram negative bacteria. They are usually made up in $\times 100$ stock solutions containing 10^7 units of sodium benzyl penicillin and 10 g of streptomycin sulphate per litre. This is filter sterilised through 0.2 μm membranes and stored in 20 ml aliquots at $-20°C$. Prepared stock solutions may be purchased from all major tissue culture suppliers. It is *not* advisable to propagate stock myeloma lines in P/S in case resistant strains arise. P/S is permissible in fusions or transformations but is not otherwise a replacement for good laboratory technique.

P/S lasts only for a few days in culture solutions but this is unimportant since contamination with bacteria is largely introduced by manipulation and will be evident after 24 hours.

5.3. Basic cell culture techniques

5.3.1. General sterile technique

While all tissue culture requires good sterile technique, hybridoma production requires a particularly high standard because of the number of manipulations involved in feeding and sampling. The personnel involved should have a high standard of personal hygiene with clean hair, beards, clothes and fingernails. They should not drink beer, draught cider or especially real ale and not bake bread in the 24 h before fusion or cloning are carried out. (Pure spirits such as whisky are permissible provided they do not affect the competence of the operator.) Hands and forearms should be scrubbed clean and swabbed with 70% ethanol before they enter the hood (surgical gloves are also necessary for human material). The hood should be kept scrupulously clean and swabbed with 70% ethanol. Bunsen burners are not used in vertical flow hoods for safety considerations and in any case flaming is not a suitable technique for plastic material as it can release toxic substances. All bottles of medium etc. should be wiped and swabbed at the stoppers with 70% ethanol before being put into the hood. A 37°C water bath for warming medium is not recommended for routine use as it can be a major source of contamination and most laboratories use a separate 37°C oven in which to thaw serum and medium.

The CO_2 incubator is particularly important. As with the hood, all samples should be handled in the incubator with clean swabbed hands. Old cultures should be discarded and not left in the hope that they may grow better. The incubator should be cleaned weekly with disinfectant and the water in the bottom tray which keeps it humidified should be sterile double distilled water. If the incubator is too humid, contamination, particularly with fungal spores, spreads more readily and samples on the top shelf are particularly vulnerable to droplets with accumulated contaminating material. If the incubator is not humid enough, the outer wells of a 96 well plate tend to dry out. Some groups do not use these wells but fill them with sterile distilled water to give a plate its own internal humidity without having to rely on the incubator. It is possible to further insulate 96 well plates by wrapping them in clingfilm but this fogs the plastic and is only advised where contamination has been diagnosed.

The experimental material itself may be a source of contamination. Animals should not be handled in the sterile hood, even if they have been maintained under sterile conditions and working areas swabbed with ethanol. Every cell line received from elsewhere should be certified as mycoplasma free. Human tissues (Section 5.1.) should be treated as a potential source of bacterial or mycoplasma contamination and handled in separate facilities.

It will be evident from the above that shared equipment can present problems. The standard of sterility is effectively as high as that of the least hygienic operator. In a large group, it is sensible to have very firm cleaning and inspection rotas. Every new member of the group should be trained with extreme care, preferably on equipment outside the hybridoma hood and incubator.

5.3.2. Complete medium

Basic medium is usually made up in 100–500 ml aliquots. For a 100 ml batch containing 10% FCS, 90 ml of RPMI with glutamine are combined with 10 ml FCS and 1 ml stock solution of P/S. This medium can be used for propagation of the parent line and is also adequate for the growth of established hybridomas. However, in situations where a small number of clones are present in a well (after fusion and during cloning), some laboratories prefer to use 20% FCS (80 ml RPMI, 20 ml FCS and 1 ml stock P/S). It is important to emphasise to students what 'medium' is in any protocol so that they use either RPMI alone and RPMI + FCS where appropriate.

5.3.3. Freezing and thawing of cells

5.3.3.1. Liquid nitrogen stocks

This procedure is obviously important in hybridoma work. Unless recombinant DNA technology is used to immortalise the genes, the liquid nitrogen bank containing valuable hybridomas is a bank in more than one sense.

Liquid nitrogen is at $-186°C$ and cells maintained at that temperature remain viable for months and sometimes years. However, liquid nitrogen vats require regular topping up. There are two types of vat. The small laboratory one and the large automatic one. The small laboratory one is topped up twice a week from a storage vat by the laboratory involved. The large automatic ones are topped up directly by the supplier. Both systems can fail totally or, more frequently, be topped up less often than is ideal. In the latter case, the samples at the top of the vat are most vulnerable.

It is therefore important to store a valuable hybridoma
(i) In several vats
(ii) At several levels of the vat
(iii) Preferably also in a totally independent geographical location.
In respect of this third requirement ECACC (Appendix 2) will store hybridomas and myelomas for a small charge and guarantee not to release them to other users without consent/patent acknowledgements being signed. However, most people use exchange agreements with other laboratories in their home town with neither laboratory knowing the precise specificity of the clone it is storing for its neighbour.

5.3.3.2. Preparation of cells for freezing

With all hybridomas of value, at least 10 vials should be kept in liquid nitrogen at any one time. All cells should be frozen slowly to avoid damage by intracellular ice crystals. They are also best protected by medium which has a reduced freezing point. The best freezing medium for hybridomas or myelomas is 90% FCS, 10% DMSO (dimethyl sulphoxide). Other freezing media containing less FCS or glycerol as a replacement for DMSO may work but do not work as well. There is usually no need to autoclave the DMSO but it should be handled under sterile conditions. Cells should be frozen in logarithmic growth and quality (i.e., viability) is better than quantity.

PROTOCOL 5.1: FREEZING OF HYBRIDOMAS AND MYELOMAS

(i) Grow the cells to logarithmic stage (around 10^6 cells/ml). Harvest by centrifugation at $400 \times g$. There is no need to wash.
(ii) Resuspend the pellet in 1 ml 90% FCS, 10% DMSO for every 5×10^6 cells.
(iii) Pipette 1 ml aliquots into into sterile freezing ampoules and screw the top down tightly.
(iv) Wrap in bubble plastic or place in a polystyrene container and place in a $-70°C$ freezer for 24–48 hours. For short- term storage (a few weeks) $-70°C$ is adequate. For long-term storage, transfer to liquid nitrogen within 3–4 days wearing gloves and facemask.

Programmed freezing devices which reduce the temperature of the cells in a controlled manner and avoid local freezing and thawing eddies in the ampoule can be obtained from Cryoson.

It is possible to freeze cells in whole 96 well tissue culture plates (Wells et al., 1983) but recovery is generally less good. It can be optimised by adding 100 μl of FCS to each well, centrifuging the plate for 5 min at $800 \times g$, removing the supernatant, and resuspending the cells in each well in medium containing 20% FCS (de Leij et al., 1987).

5.3.3.3. Thawing of cells
In contrast to freezing, thawing of cells is done speedily. Recovery is never 100% and is very dependent on the health of the cells when they were frozen down.

PROTOCOL 5.2: THAWING OF HYBRIDOMAS AND MYELOMAS

(i) For each ampoule to be thawed, prepare a small (25 cm^2) plastic flask containing 5 ml complete medium (10% FCS) at 37°C.
(ii) Wearing a facemask and gloves, remove the ampoule from liquid nitrogen. Very occasionally, they can explode at this point.
(iii) Thaw the ampoule in a (clean) 37°C water bath by swirling it around until the material is almost liquid. Swab the outside with ethanol and transfer to the sterile hood. Draw the contents of the

ampoule into a pasteur pipette or 5 ml sterile pipette and then draw up some of the medium from the flask.

(iv) Return the cells and medium to the flask and incubate for 24 hours before subculturing.

If the cells do not recover well in this procedure. Lay down 100 μl spleen feeders in two rows (24 wells) of a 96 well tissue culture plate in medium containing 20% FCS supplemented with 5 mM sodium pyruvate. Thaw the ampoule into 5 ml medium containing 20% FCS, harvest the cells by centrifugation and resuspend in 2.4 ml medium containing 20% FCS and plate out on the two rows of feeder cells.

5.3.4. Cell counting and viability checks

Cell counting is generally by means of the Neubauer haemocytometer or counting chamber. These vary slightly but each one is supplied with exact specifications and amplification factors. In order to check viability, the cells are stained with a dye which differentiates dead from live cells. Typical dyes are trypan blue (0.2 g/l in 0.15 M NaCl) and eosin (0.05 g/l in 0.15 M NaCl) both of which stain dead cells. Nigrosine (0.2%) is also used. If a FACS is available the dead cells can be estimated using low concentrations of propidium iodide (final concentration 0.1 μg/ml), and the proportion of live cells in S phase can be estimated by the method of Vindelov et al. (1987). These checks are particularly important before fusion where high viability is required (Chapter 6).

5.4. Contamination

Contamination is best avoided by the precautions given in Section 5.3. If it occurs, whatever the source, the culture is best removed and autoclaved immediately without opening. Any attempt to rescue a contaminated culture may put all the other cultures in the laboratory at risk and if any attempt is to be made to save a culture, it should be strictly quarantined. In multi-operator situations it is vital to encourage an open attitude over contamination so that those sharing the same equipment are warned when it occurs.

There is no doubt that the failure of most hybridoma experiments is due to contamination and of the possible sources of contamination, the commonest and most serious is mycoplasma. Bacterial and fungal contamination do also occur but they are more readily detected, avoided, and dealt with should they occur.

5.4.1. Bacterial contamination

Bacterial contamination is very readily detected by microscopic examination. In addition both an overnight change to a yellow acid colour and turbidity in the medium are usually evident by inspection of the plate without the need for a microscope. The use of penicillin and streptomycin usually minimises bacterial contamination but resistant strains can develop. It is for this reason, in addition to the avoidance of changes in phenotype, that cells should not be routinely grown in culture without a clear end aim but should be kept as frozen stock when not in use.

Should bacterial contamination develop the following order of priorities should be adopted.

If the contamination is in a stock culture of which there are ample frozen supplies it should be disposed of immediately by autoclaving without opening of the flask or plate. Fresh cells can then be brought up from liquid nitrogen. The incubator should be resterilised.

If the contamination is in a vital cell line in a flask and there are no backup supplies, it is possible to use a third antibiotic such as gentamycin (200 μg/ml), and/or tetracycline (50 μg/ml) which affect a wide spectrum of gram positive and gram negative bacteria. The cell suspension should be centrifuged over 10 ml Ficoll at $500 \times g$ with the myeloma/hybridoma layer being carefully pipetted from the interface, replaced in fresh medium containing the new antibiotic and placed in an incubator wrapped in clingfilm or in a sealed gassed box.

Cells passaged through the ascites fluid of histocompatible pristane primed mice can sometimes be cleared of bacterial contamination

(Section 10.4). They should be washed free of medium and preferably purified on Ficoll as described above before injection to minimise the number of bacteria injected into the mouse. Since the bacteria are physically distinct from the cells, it is possible for the murine immune system to fight the bacterial infection, if not too many bacteria are injected, while allowing the hybridoma or myeloma to grow.

If the contamination is in only one or two wells of a vital tissue culture plate it is possible to aspirate the contents of the affected wells and replace them with sterile 5 N NaOH.

5.4.2. Fungal and yeast contamination

These are handled in much the same manner as described for bacterial contamination above. The antibiotics used for these are fungizone (Amphotericin B, 2.5 μg/ml) and/or nystatin (50 μg/ml). Fungal contaminants grow fast and are often not detected until they form a fluffy ball on the top of the culture. At this stage the fungal spores will be very infectious, and immediate autoclaving is advised. Again, if the contamination is not too far advanced, it is possible to isolate the myeloma hybridoma cells on Ficoll and put them into ascites growth in a pristane primed mouse.

5.4.3. Contamination with mycoplasma

This is the contamination that all hybridoma technologists dread. Mycoplasma contamination can lead to laboratories having no successful fusions for months. In addition, infected long established hybridomas can give greatly reduced or totally negative antibody secretion. The best thing to do is avoid it by adopting the procedures outlined in Section 5.3. Scrupulously clean working practice, separate handling of human material and in particular human tonsils or lungs, and quarantining of all incoming cell lines until they have been mycoplasma tested. However, it is likely that any reader addressing this otherwise apparently tedious section already suspects his or her laboratory to have the problem. In this case, even before diagnosis, they should take the remedial action advised in Section 5.4.3.3 below for any vital cell line.

Mycoplasma are small prokaryotes without a cell wall which can pass through 0.2 μ filter as can viruses. Mycoplasma can grow independently of eukaryote cells in rich medium, but, more relevantly, also grow in the cytoplasm of the mammalian cells which they have infected. Their biology is reviewed by Smith (1971) and much greater detail than below is given by Adams (1990). Mycoplasma are also known as PPLO (plueropneumonia like organisms). The family is broad ranging over a variety of eukaryote systems and there are many types with precise fastidious nutritional requirements, so that, in consequence, they can selectively deplete the culture medium of vital nutrients.

The main sources are

(a) Humans – the names of the human derived mycoplasma, *M. hominis*, but also *M. orale, M. pharyngis, M. salivarium* speak for themselves. While these will obviously be introduced by human samples of tonsil or lung, the most likely cause is primary transfer from breath or secondary transfer from skin or material which has been exposed to breathing. Internal organs of mouse or man never test positive for mycoplasma and any contamination comes through their extraction and handling.

(b) Cell lines which originally became infected by serum samples. These are mycoplasma such as the bovine *M. arginini* or *A.* (for a mycoplasma subset known as *Acholeplasma*) *laidlawii*. Many well established cell lines are mycoplasma positive and these must not be allowed to transfer into a hybridoma lab.

Their undoubtedly disastrous effect on fusions has been attributed to the fact that many mycoplasma, notably *A. laidlawii* cleave thymidine to its component sugar and base thus making selective HAT medium ineffective. However, the true situation is undoubtedly more complex.

Mycoplasma co-exist within the cell as intracellular parasites. They usually do not kill the cell but retard its growth rate and mycoplasma infected cells can sometimes look remarkably healthy down the microscope. They will, however, clone poorly if at all at 1 cell/well, whatever the feeder system, and tend to lose specialised functions such as antibody secretion. Above all they will not give antibody producing fusions.

5.4.3.1. Detection of mycoplasma

Mycoplasma are most conveniently detected as uncharacteristic deposits of cytoplasmic DNA and the simplest method of seeing this is to use a fluorescent dye which intercalates and stains double stranded DNA such as Hoechst 33258 (Hilwig and Gropp, 1972) or 4,6-diamidino-2-phenylindole (DAPI) at 0.1 μg/ml (Russel et al., 1975). The Hoechst stain is generally used on fixed cells but DAPI can be used with unfixed cells. Commercial kits using either stain and giving detailed instructions can be purchased. In addition, ECACC will undertake the entire screening process for any laboratory for a comparatively small sum.

Most of the classic methods for mycoplasma detection have been developed for adherent cells and in order to detect them in free floating cells such as myelomas or hybridomas, it is necessary to co-culture the suspect myeloma cell line with adherent cells which have been shown to be mycoplasma negative. These can be mouse 3T3 cells or any standard laboratory line. The two cell types should be grown together for 4–5 days so that the mycoplasma may transfer to the adherent line. An alternative is to cytocentrifuge the myeloma or hybridoma cells directly onto a glass slide and fix them.

PROTOCOL 5.3: DETECTION OF MYCOPLASMA BY HOECHST 33258

(i) Co-culture the myeloma/hybridoma cells with mouse 3T3 cells in medium containing 10% FCS (no antibiotics) for 4–5 days. Transfer to a cover slip grown in a petri dish or culture chamber slides (Labtek). Culture also 3T3 cells alone as negative control. Grow to 60–70% confluence. Positive, mycoplasma containing controls are desirable for detection but not for introduction into the laboratory. Some firms will supply slides of these with the mycoplasma securely fixed and not presenting any danger.

(ii) Remove the medium, wash the cells gently with PBS and fix them in 3/1 ethanol/acetic acid with two changes over 10 minutes. Wash the cells with PBS to remove the fixative.

(iii) Make up a stock of 5 mg/100 ml Hoechst 33258 in PBS, filter through a 0.2 μ membrane and store on the dark. Dilute 1/1000 with PBS before use.

(iv) Add the Hoechst solution to the cover slips or slide chambers so that all the cells are immersed and incubate in the dark for 30 min at room temperature.

(v) Wash the cells three times with distilled water and mount with aqueous glycerol mountant (Section 2.9.6). If coverslips have been used, these are placed face (cells) downwards on the slides. If slide chambers have been used, these are overlaid with coverslips.

(vi) Inspect under the fluorescence microscope exciting at 360 nm. The positive control cells are essential to give a background reading. Mycoplasma infected cells have grainy spots of fluorescence in the cytoplasm.

There are a wide variety of other ways of detecting mycoplasma, covered in greater detail by Adams (1990) but many are less sensitive and some are more complex or more expensive. They include the conventional orcein staining method of Fogh and Fogh (1968), autoradiography of incorporated thymidine (Nardone et al., 1965), the use of 6-methylpurine deoxyriboside (6-MPDR) in a mycoplasma induced cell toxicity test (McGarrity and Carlson, 1982), genetic probe tests for mycoplasmal rRNA (Johanssan and Bolske, 1989), and, perhaps inevitably, Mabs to mycoplasma supplied by various firms. Most labs still use the Hoechst system. It is, however, worth noting that methods utilising cytoplasmic staining for DNA are not always suitable for all cell types. For example, the cell line B95–8 used to produce Epstein-Barr Virus (Chapter 8) for human B cell transformation, secretes large amounts of double stranded DNA containing virus and will always therefore tend to have a certain level of cytoplasmic DNA staining.

5.4.3.2. Getting rid of mycoplasma – decontamination of equipment
The immediate response to the discovery of mycoplasma infected cells must be to test all the other cells which have been growing over the

period of time since mycoplasma is suspected to have come into the lab. All non-essential lines which have mycoplasma should be autoclaved. Hoods and incubators should be fumigated with formaldehyde in a manner suitable for the ventilation systems involved. Formaldehyde is a potential mutagen and this procedure must involve the laboratory safety officer. If he or she is unfamiliar with the problem, best advice as to how to decontaminate is obtained from laboratory safety officers of labs which routinely handle pathogens such as HIV. Hoods and incubators which ventilate to a safe external location are treated with the fans on with a beaker of formaldehyde placed in a heated container while the hood, incubator and/or room is sealed off from personnel involved.

5.4.3.3. Getting rid of mycoplasma – strategies for saving a vital hybridoma

The main advice here is not to try. If a hybridoma has been made once, it can be made again and continuing to grow mycoplasma infected cells puts the whole laboratory at risk. It is probably worth trying to save only very rare hybridomas – for example human ones which have come from individuals with rare diseases and which have already been extensively cloned.

However, for people who insist on trying, the following strategy is suggested.

PROTOCOL 5.4: STRATEGIES FOR ELIMINATING MYCOPLASMA FROM VITAL CELL LINES

(i) Antibiotics. The classical ones are kanomycin (100 μg/ml) (Fogh and Hacker, 1960), and tylosin or tylocine (6 μg/ml – see Gibco, Appendix 2). Others are lincomycin and vanomycin. Most laboratories have found these unsatisfactory. The newer ones are the quinolones such as ciprofloxacin (Schmidtt et al., 1988) and MRA (Flow laboratories). Ciprofloxacin at concentrations of 10 μg/ml is very effective – it kills many of the mycoplasma producing cells and so the first impressions are alarming but emerging mycoplasma free cells do grow out of the culture, much as in a fusion.

(ii) Cloning at 1 cell/well on feeders. This idea came from a procedure described by Schimmelpfeng et al. (1980) which used activated macrophage feeders together with some of the less effective antibiotics in an attempt to purify non-infected cells free by cloning. However, any method which acknowledges that other cells in a 96 well plate may be infected is probably doomed because of the ease with which mycoplasma move between and within plates. It is a perfectly sensible strategy to clone after antibiotic treatment with the modern drugs such as ciprofloxacin, although probably not with activated macrophages but rather with spleen feeders.

(iii) Passage through the ascites fluid of a primed histocompatible mouse or rat. This can work well for parent myeloma lines. For hybridomas, it is, as is all ascites work, dependent on the health of the cells injected. If the mycoplasma infection has been well advanced so that the majority of the injected hybridomas have ceased to secrete, then the yield may have many cells, but they will be non-secreting revertents.

In consequence, any laboratory which suspects it may have mycoplasma infiltration should put vital cultures into cyprofloxacin, and also inject them into ascites fluid. Then it can proceed with diagnosis and fumigation.

5.4.4. Contamination with viruses

Viral contamination is not usually a problem in rodent hybridoma work and relates largely to human cells. If human lymphocytes are used there is a high probability that they will be infected with Epstein-Barr Virus (EBV) and will become spontaneously transformed in culture, especially if T cells have been removed (Chapter 8). It is very difficult to perform a human fusion without spontaneous transformation overtaking the procedure. Lymphocyte donors can be tested for antibody to the EBV viral capsid antigen (VCA) by use of the cell line P3 HR1 which secretes non-transforming EBV. The P3 HR1 cells are suspended in 2×10^6 cells/ml, dried or cytocentrifuged onto a slide, and acetone fixed for 10 minutes at 4°C. Large batches of slides may be prepared and stored at $-70°C$. Serum samples are then tested in doubling dilutions of PBS and one drop is added to each slide. The slide is incubated in a humidified atmosphere (i.e., a plastic box with wet tissues on the bottom) for 1 hour, washed, and reacted with anti-human IgG (γ- specific – Table 2.2), washed again, and covered with aqueous mountant. Most human B cells will be positive in this test but the titre (lowest dilution to give a positive result) is highly variable from 1/100 to 1/10,000.

This test is particularly useful for laboratories which routinely use EBV to transform cells as it can indicate which workers (the majority) were seropositive before working with EBV infected cells, clarifying any rare but expensive legal action from a worker claiming this to be a source of infection. To the author's knowledge, there is no recorded case of seroconversion among laboratory workers to date in 1991.

5.5. Feeder cells

5.5.1. Feeders for mouse fusions

Feeder cells, or conditioned medium of very high quality, are quite essential for cloning of hybridomas. They can be provided in almost all cases by mouse spleen feeders at low cost. Naturally, companies which sell specific medium additives would prefer that this were not the case. Cells are not used to growing alone at high dilutions and must be provided with nutrients in addition to those supplied by the RPMI medium and FCS. Most of these nutrients are unknown growth factors and the reported metabolic feeding agents (glycine, oxaloacetate, pyruvate), rely on weak evidence and occupy such central positions in metabolism that it is impossible to guess where the main requirements are focussed. They are, in any case, superfluous and inadequate in the presence of feeder cells. Insulin is often reported as essential but again the experimental evidence is weak and there is a suspicion that almost any newly marketed growth factor will be advertised as capable of improving fusion or cloning. Interleukin 6 (IL-

6) was first marketed as 'hybridoma growth factor' with very limited experimental proof of superiority to good FCS. There is a general assumption that the requisite growth factors will be known ones. Given the rate of discovery of new growth factors, this would appear to be an over-optimistic assumption.

Feeder cells provide a wide variety of largely unknown ingredients and at critical stages of fusion, cloning, or recovering sick cells, far outstrip any media supplements in effectiveness. It will take some years before the range of material they provide is known but it may well involve close cell to cell contact. In the meantime, they cost little and provide the best support system.

Conditioned medium from feeder cells has largely gone out of fashion for hybridoma work. Its advantage was that it was more defined. However, cells fare best with direct contact with other cells and not their products. Similarly, irradiated feeder cells are now seldom used in the context of human or murine hybridoma production.

Mouse thymocytes are an excellent source of feeder cells but require several thymuses from very young mice. The thymus is assumed to provide T cell derived lymphokines. Mouse blood is very rarely used but can be employed at 1% (v/v). It has the advantage that the emerging clones are readily viewed against the erythrocyte background.

In the 1980s, several papers suggested that macrophages provided the best feeder systems. In particular, there was an idea that 'activated' macrophages secreted a wider range of growth factors than normal macrophages or other cell populations. In addition, macrophages can remove debris from dying cells as part of their natural function. Experience has shown that these are usually no more effective than mouse spleen feeders for any hybridoma cloning procedure.

With human cells, there is a considerable theoretical validity in the idea of using human rather than mouse primary cells as feeders since the relevant lymphokines are highly species specific (Section 4.11.3). However, at least for EBV transformed cells, mouse spleen feeders have proved to be as effective as any human cell and this suggests that the feeders supply non-species specific factors.

Feeders are not necessary immediately after the fusion step but may be helpful where low cell densities are involved. As fusion frequencies increase there has been an increasing trend to attempt to clone cells from the start (although initial positives will still cease to secrete in the mouse and human systems) and fusions can now be plated out in as many as 40×96 well plates. While a fusion plated out in $8–10 \times 96$ well plates (Chapter 6) has sufficient unfused mouse spleen cells to feed it, fusions plated out at very high dilutions should be supplemented with additional feeder cells.

In the case of cloning, or nursing of weak cultures, feeders are essential and invaluable. To a considerable extent mouse spleen feeders can also fill this role.

In consequence, mouse spleen feeders are recommended as the first feeder system to try. If this proves unsatisfactory, then it is possible to move on to thymocytes or macrophages.

PROTOCOL 5.5: MOUSE SPLEEN FEEDER CELL PREPARATION

(i) Use 100 ml complete medium with 10% FCS – for very delicate clones this may be raised to 20% FCS.

Lay out sterile dissecting instruments, 100 ml RPMI, 100 ml complete medium, 2×6 cm petri dishes, 3×21G and 3×25G disposable needles, 2×10 ml disposable syringes, 6 of sterile conical based 20 ml universal containers, a stock of 10 each of 5 and 10 ml sterile pipettes, a haemocytometer, two eppendorf (1 ml polytubes) tubes containing 0.3 ml 0.9% ammonium chloride, and the PEG solution. It is unrealistic to give precise quantities of small pieces of plasticware as minor alterations in technique change requirements. Pipette some sterile RPMI into a sterile universal container.

(ii) Kill an 8–10 week old non-immunised mouse histocompatible with the cells to be fed. Do this outwith the tissue culture lab and not in the sterile hood. Contamination scarcely ever results from an animal dissected on an ordinary laboratory bench. Soak the area of abdominal skin to be dissected in 70% ethanol and dissect out the spleen with sterile instruments, placing it in the sterile universal containing the RPMI.

(iii) Move the spleen to the sterile hood. Wash twice with serum free

RPMI and dissect off any fatty tissue. Put the spleen into a 6 cm petri dish containing 5 ml RPMI. Gently tease the spleen cells from the capsule using two 21G needles to break up clumps. Draw the spleen cell suspension into a 10 ml pipette through a 21G needle and pipette it out again. Repeat once with a 21G needle and then twice with a 25G needle. Use moderate pressure only (no frothing). Discard clumps which may jam the finer needle. Pipette the cells gently through the 25G needle into a universal. Centrifuge for 5 minutes at $500 \times g$, pour off the supernatant, tap the pellet to resuspend it in the dregs and then wash again a further two times in RPMI.

(iv) Count the spleen cells. This is not essential and you may, if you prefer, simply assume that there are 10^8 of them. Pipette a 0.05 ml aliquot into one of the eppendorf (1 ml polytubes) tubes containing the 0.3 ml ammonium chloride. This will lyse any red blood cells and swell the spleen cells. Leave for 3 minutes before counting and remember the additional 1 in 7 dilution factor in your calculations. If the number of spleen cells departs significantly from 10^8, adjust the number of myeloma cells accordingly.

(v) Resuspend spleen cells to 10^6 cells/ml (for 10^8 cells this is in 100 ml complete medium) and plate out in 96 well plates at 10^5 cells/well, i.e., 100 μl/well. For a normal size spleen this should give 10 plates of feeder cells.

PROTOCOL 5.6: MOUSE MACROPHAGE FEEDER CELL PREPARATION

(i) Make up 100 ml complete medium + 10% FCS. Lay out 100 ml sterile PBS, 2×10 ml syringes, 2×21G needles, several 20 ml universal containers, several 5 and 10 ml pipettes.

(ii) Kill an 8–12 week old mouse histocompatible with the cells to be fed. Prepare the macrophages according to Appendix 1 (Section A.1.6.2.4). Keep the cells cool to avoid the tendency of macrophages to clump. Centrifuge at $400 \times g$ for 5 min, wash with PBS twice and count. Each mouse should yield 4×10^6 macrophages.

(iii) Resuspend in 40 ml complete medium and plate out at 100 μl (10^4) cells/well in 96 well tissue culture plates.

Note. Activated macrophages may be obtained by intraperitoneal injection of 1 ml 10% sodium thioglycollate four days before sacrificing the animal. Activated macrophages are also common in older animals. Some groups do not recommend these as they are thought to be too active and liable to damage the injected hybridomas.

PROTOCOL 5.7: MOUSE THYMOCYTE FEEDER CELL PREPARATION

(i) Make up 100 ml complete medium + 10% FCS. Lay out 100 ml sterile PBS, 2×10 ml syringes, a sterile wire mesh or domestic tea strainer, 2×21G needles, several 20 ml universal containers, several 5 and 10 ml pipettes.

(ii) Kill two 12–14 day old mice histocompatible with the cells to be fed. It is important to use young animals as the thymus is smaller and less active in older ones. The thymus is above the heart as shown in Appendix 1. Rinse the animals with ethanol before dissection and do not rupture the oesophagus or the trachea as this will increase the chances of contamination. Rinse the organs well in serum free RPMI.

(iii) Press the organs through a sterile stainless steel wire mesh into a 6 cm petri dish containing 5 ml serum free RPMI. A domestic tea strainer is very suitable for this purpose. Alternatively, the organs may be teased apart with two 21G needles. Discard the capsule and further disperse the clumps by sucking them twice up and down into a 10 ml sterile disposable syringe with a 21G needle and then twice with a 25 G needle with moderate pressure.

(iv) Wash the cells twice in sterile serum free RPMI by centrifugation at $500 \times g$ in a sterile universal. Count the cells. Two mice should yield in the order of 10^7 cells. Resuspend at 2.5×10^5 cells/ml (this should be approximately 40 ml) in complete medium and aliquot at 100 μl/ well. Cells may be plated at a five fold lower density in round bottomed plates but clones are less readily viewed in such plates.

5.5.2. Feeders for human fusions/transformations

A substantial proportion of human transformants or hybridomas will clone well on mouse spleen (Ghosh et al., 1987) macrophage, (Edwards et al, 1982; Cote et al., 1983) or thymocyte feeders and there is no need to use human feeders. However, human hybridomas or transformants tend to have their own specialised growth requirements and may respond better to one feeder system than another. The general advice is to start with simple feeder systems and only move to more complex ones if these clearly fail to do the job.

Where human cells are used as feeders, irradiated fibroblasts (Kozbor and Roder, 1981), enriched monocytes (Brodin et al., 1983) or cord blood have all been used. However, the majority of human feeder systems are almost all from peripheral blood for obvious reasons. Most laboratories use an 'in house' donor but it is also possible to obtain buffycoats from the local blood transfusion service. In choosing a donor, it may be relevant to know whether the individual is Epstein-Barr Virus positive or not (Section 5.4.4).

Human PBL feeder cells are generally irradiated, largely to stop spontaneous transformation with EBV permitting the cells from the feeder donor rather than those from the test individual from growing.

PROTOCOL 5.8: PREPARATION OF HUMAN PBL FEEDERS

(i) Prepare 100 ml complete medium (10% FCS). Lay out Ficoll, 20 ml universal containers, RPMI, and 10 ml pipettes. Obtain access to a radiation source.

(ii) Withdraw 20 ml fresh blood from a donor into a heparinised tube. Dilute the blood 1 in 2 with RPMI. Layer over Ficoll in sterile 20 ml universal containers. Centrifuge at $500 \times g$ for 15 min.

(iii) The peripheral blood mononuclear cells including B and T lymphocytes and some monocytes will be at the interface. Remove the interfacial layer and dilute with an equal volume of RPMI. Centrifuge at $500 \times g$ for 5 min.

(iv) Resuspend the cell pellet in complete medium, count, and adjust to 3×10^6 cells/ml (for 20 ml blood this should be in the order of 10 ml).

(v) Irradiate at 2000R. Dilute in complete medium to 5×10^5 cells/ml and plate out in 100 μl aliquots (5×10^4 cells/well) in flat bottomed 96 well plates. Round bottomed 96 well plates may be used at the lower concentration of 10^4 cells/well. Clones are, however, less easy to view in round bottomed plates.

CHAPTER 6

Fusion procedures

6.1. The use of polyethylene glycol

6.1.1. Introduction

While early experiments in cell fusion were performed with enveloped viruses such as Sendai virus (Harris and Watkins, 1965), nearly all fusions designed to produce hybridomas are now performed with chemical fusogens and polyethylene glycol (PEG), which has the structure

$$HO(CH_2CH_2O)_nCH_2CH_2OH$$

is the major chemical used. Early fusions also involved mammalian cells which grow adhering to the tissue culture vessel and fusions of cells grown in suspension require slightly different conditions (Gefter et al., 1977). The mechanism of fusion is complex, involving cell agglutination, membrane fusion and cell swelling, the optimal environmental conditions for the three processes being frequently at variance (Knutton and Pasternak, 1979). It is interesting to note the wide variation in concentration, in molecular weight, and in the medium in which the PEG is dissolved, all having apparently led to successful hybridoma production. In addition, there are a large number of other chemicals which will also promote cell fusion (Klebe and Mancuso, 1981).

6.1.2. Molecular weight

PEG may be obtained in the molecular weight range 200–20,000. It is toxic to cells and low molecular weight PEG is more toxic than high molecular weight PEG. Furthermore, the toxicity varies for each particular cell type. High molecular weight PEG is viscous and difficult to work with. Most successful fusions are performed with PEG in the molecular weight range 600–6000 (Davidson et al,, 1976; Klebe and Mancuso, 1981). The supplier of the PEG may also be an important factor and it may be relevant to note that the number stated on the supplier's bottle does not always refer to the exact molecular weight of the PEG. There is always a range of molecular weights rather than a single species in each preparation. In view of the toxicity of the low molecular weight material, it is obviously important to obtain an undegraded preparation. Many laboratories use Merck 4000 as a result of an early and very limited study by Fazekas de St Groth and Scheidegger (1980) suggesting that this was the best, but most main suppliers now make an effort to supply PEG which has been specially tested for fusion with full specifications.

6.1.3. Temperature and pH

Many published protocols suggest the use of PEG at 37°C. This is not necessary and is often inconvenient in a sterile hood although suitable heating blocks may be obtained. Most people simply keep the PEG solution in the 37°C incubator until immediately before use. There is, however, little evidence that 37°C is superior to room temperature and some studies indicate the reverse (Klebe and Mancuso, 1981). 4°C is very much less effective and the PEG must be well thawed (Fazekas de St Groth and Scheidegger, 1981). The range of optimum pH is also wide, peaking at around pH 8.0 (Sharon et al., 1980).

6.1.4. Concentration

While the exact mechanisms of fusion are not fully understood, it is thought that the main function of the hydrophilic PEG solution is to occupy the 'physical free water' space leading to the agglutination of the cells. This occurs at concentrations of PEG in the region of 40–50% and most fusions are performed within this range with short exposure time. There is, however, some variation of the optimum concentration with cell line (Gefter et al., 1977) and successful fusions can be performed at lower PEG concentrations such as 35% with a longer exposure time.

6.1.5. Cell lines

Different cell lines can have very different membrane properties and this has only fully been appreciated since electroporation became a standard technique for introducing DNA into cells and it became apparent that quite different conditions were required for different types of cell. This includes cells of apparently very similar source and phenotype. If one is performing a large number of fusions with the same pair of cells, it may be worth playing with the system once it is established. While it would be rather difficult to prove, it is more than possible that fusion conditions could be adjusted to favour hybridomas producing, for example, IgGs from mature B cells rather than IgMs from immature ones.

6.1.6. Other components of the PEG solution

Many fusion protocols used to recommend the use of PEG in 10–15% DMSO, largely due to an initial report from Norwood et al. (1976) who reported greatly enhanced fusion frequencies for attached fibroblasts by addition of this reagent. DMSO does disrupt cellular aggregates and may facilitate the mixing of the two cell types. However, most myeloma lines and B cells do not aggregate and the value of it for hybridoma production is very doubtful. It is certainly not necessary for a good result.

A wide variety of buffers can be used to dissolve the PEG. The most common is serum free medium of the type employed in the fusion e.g. RPMI or DMEM. However, phosphate or Tris buffers have also been used successfully. While calcium ions have been reported to be both essential to fusion (Ahkong et al., 1973) and inhibitory to fusion (Klebe and Mancuso, 1981), common practical experience suggests that they are neither of these. As no systematic studies are published and most buffers work, the use of serum free medium is recommended here. The refinement of adding 2 × medium to the autoclaved PEG is unnecessary.

6.2. The components of HAT medium

There is happily less variability in the components of HAT medium and most fusion protocols utilise similar concentration ranges. Variation of these concentrations is only applied under specific experimental conditions. Hypoxanthine is generally not toxic to cells and concentrations of 0.1 mM are used. Thymidine on the other hand can cause cessation of DNA synthesis at millimolar levels due to a feedback inhibition leading to a reduced pool size of dCTP. For this reason the concentration of thymidine is maintained at 0.016 mM. Thymidine inhibition is reversed by the use of deoxycytidine which allows the blockage to be bypassed and some protocols incorporate deoxycytidine for this reason. T cell hybridomas are exceptionally sensitive to thymidine by two orders of magnitude lower than most mammalian cultured cells and selection in the presence of deoxycytidine (Fox et al., 1980) or in 0.1 mM hypoxanthine with azaserine at 1 μg/ml is sometimes used under these conditions (Foung et al., 1982). Azaserine blocks the pathway of purine biosynthesis but not of pyrimidine biosynthesis. Thymidine deficiency is often responsible for the difficulties encountered in attempts to fuse mycoplasma contaminated cells as many species of mycoplasma carry an enzyme which cleaves the base-sugar bond (Section 5.4.3). Aminopterin inhibits metabolic pathways distinct from those involved in nucleotide biosynthesis, notably the synthesis of some amino acids such as glycine and is therefore used at minimal effective dosage which is in the region of 0.4 μM. Some protocols incorporate additional glycine for this reason but it is not necessary as there are substantial quantities in RPMI or DMEM.

6.3. Selection of hybridomas by fluorescent activated cell sorting (FACS)

This is the one method which can be employed without the use of drug selection techniques and, in consequence, the FACS was originally thought to be a very powerful tool for the isolation of single hybridomas. However, a FACS with full sorting ability is less frequently encountered than a FACScan which can analyse but not sort cells and access to a full FACS can be expensive because such instruments involve high powered, usually water cooled, lasers and committed highly trained operators. The antigen is coupled to a fluorescent label and the hybridomas expressing an antibody capable of binding this label can then be separated from other cells in the fusion mixture (Parks et al., 1979). The subject was reviewed by Dangl and Herzenberg (1982) and is now best approached by technical instructions supplied with the instruments. Since most FACS instruments have an accessory device which allows the appropriately stained cells to be aliquoted into a feeder containing 96-well tissue culture plates at 1 cell/well (or more if required) it is theoretically possible to select and clone shortly after fusion. There are, however, various technical problems associated with the process. Shortly after fusion there will be many splenic B cells which are unfused but still viable and expressing antibody on their surface and these must be 'gated out' by virtue of their smaller size which gives them different light scattering properties from fused cells. The technique is also only applicable to hybridomas which express antibody on their surface and immediately after fusion while the cells are concentrating on growth, there is comparatively little surface immunoglobulin. It is however, an excellent method for obtaining stable clones at a later stage where there is overgrowth from non-secretors as it effectively assays and selects only positive clones all at the one time. The technique has also been used for T cell hybridomas (Taniguchi and Miller, 1978; Arnold et al., 1979).

6.4. Preparation of stock solutions

6.4.1. Preparation of PEG

Weigh out 20 g PEG 1500 (Boehringer, Merck or Serva) in a glass 20 ml universal container. Autoclave at 15 lb/square inch for 10 minutes. The PEG will now be liquid. When it is still liquid but cool enough to handle, add 20 ml RPMI in a sterile hood to obtain 50% PEG (or, for alternative protocols, 37 ml RPMI for 35% PEG, or 30 ml RPMI for 40% PEG). Aliquot in 2 ml samples and store at $-20°C$. The solution should keep for several months.

6.4.2. Preparation of HT and HAT

Dissolve 136 mg of hypoxanthine and 39 mg thymidine in 100 ml distilled water (HT). Hypoxanthine is not very soluble but will dissolve if heated to 50–60°C. Sterilise the solution by filtration. Store at $-70°C$ in small aliquots. If the hypoxanthine comes out of solution on thawing, heat to redissolve. Use 1 ml HT for every 100 ml culture medium.

Although it is quite possible to make up complete HAT medium, it is usually more convenient to make up the aminopterin (A) component separately. This is for two reasons. After the control myeloma cells in a fusion have died and aminopterin is no longer necessary, hypoxanthine and thymidine (HT) should still be added for a few days to allow for medium dilution and cell adaptation. Also, aminopterin is the most labile of the three chemicals and has be to checked separately. The simplest method is therefore either to buy aminopterin already in solution (Flow laboratories) or to make up and aliquot a 0.04 mM solution. This may be done by dissolving 1.8 mg aminopterin in 50 ml of 5 M NaOH, neutralising with HCl, and making up to 100 ml with distilled water. However, since 1.8 mg is not readily weighed, it is more common to dissolve 18 mg of aminopterin in 50 ml 5 M NaOH, neutralise by titrating with HCl, and make up to 100 ml with distilled water. Of this solution, 10 ml are then diluted to 100 ml with distilled water to make a 0.1 mM solution which is sterilised by filtration and stored in aliquots. 1 ml of this solution is usually added to each 100 ml of culture medium but 0.5 ml is equally effective if the cells are very sensitive. Aminopterin is light sensitive and should be kept in the dark at all times. It is stored at $-70°C$.

6.4.3. Other selective media

HAz (hypoxanthine azaserine) is made up by dissolving 136 mg hypoxanthine and 10 mg azaserine in 100 ml distilled water, sterilising by filtration, storing in aliquots and using 1 ml per 100 ml medium. When the azaserine is removed, the cells should be maintained on hypoxanthine alone for 7–10 days while they adapt.

HMT medium uses methotrexate (49 mg/100 ml stock, use 1 ml per 100 ml medium) instead of aminopterin.

6.5. Fusion frequencies and plating densities

Fusion frequencies are discussed in greater detail in Section 3.2.3. In general these range between 10 and 100 per 10^7 lymphocytes for the rodent system and somewhat lower for the human system (unless EBV transformed cells are involved – Sections 6.6. and 7.5). In a typical mouse fusion 800–1000 clones may be expected. Good fusions with experienced operators are better handled in 96 well tissue culture plates at densities in the region of 10^5 cells/well. This means that there statistically is not likely to be more than one clone in each well (although in practice they tend to occur in bunches, having disaggregated slowly from each other after PEG treatment). Provided that the chosen assay system can handle 800–1000 assays in a short period of time (Chapter 2), this is the most efficient way of operating. However, the capacity of 96 well plates is only 0.2 ml medium/well and in some makes of plate there is extensive evaporation at the outer edge. In addition, if the assay system cannot cope at that level, there is no point in having such a large number of wells. Thus in certain circumstances experienced operators use 24 well plates at 10^6 cells/well and 24 well plates are also advised for beginners. The clones are easier to see in the larger wells, evaporation from outer wells is less dramatic, and it is possible to put the fusion down in 1 ml and feed after a few days with a further 1 ml without disturbing the emerging clones. If there are clearly two or more emerging clones in a 24 well plate it is quite possible to aspirate the clones from a mouse fusion (but much harder with a rat one) independently with a sterile pasteur pipette or plastic tip and propagate them separately. Most beginners start with 24 well plates, move on to splitting a fusion between 24 and 96 well plates and finally use 96 well plates. If fusions are going badly with low frequency, it is obviously useful to move back to 24 well plates until the cause of the low frequency has been detected and removed.

6.6. Fusion protocols for mouse experiments

There are a large number of fusion protocols in general circulation and most of them work. The basic differences relate to whether one prefers to expose the cells to a high concentration of PEG for a short period of time or a low concentration for a longer time.

PROTOCOL 6.1: GENERAL FUSION PLAN FOR MOUSE HYBRIDOMAS

(i) 3–4 weeks before fusion. Start immunisation schedule (Chapter 4).
(ii) 7 or more days before fusion. Make up stock solutions of HT (Section 6.4.2), A (Section 6.4.2), P/S (Section 5.2.5), freeze and check equipment.
(iii) 7 days before fusion. Bring up the myeloma line (SP2/0) from liquid nitrogen. This is much better than keeping a continuous stock growing and vulnerable to mutation (Chapter 3). *The parent myeloma line should be in active logarithmic growth at the time of fusion.* Grow the cells in RPMI + 10% FCS + P/S and monitor the growth rate keeping the cell density in the region of 3–5 $\times 10^5$ cells/ml. Do standard mycoplasma and viability checks. You will need around 3×10^7 cells at greater than 95% viability on fusion day. Laboratories with a FACS

can do a quick check to see how well the myeloma cells are cycling on the morning of the fusion (Vindelov et al., 1987). At least 35% should be in S or G2 phase.

(iv) Boost the animal intravenously with a small dose in PBS or saline.

(v) One day before fusion. Lay down feeder cells if you have decided to use them (Section 5.5). Check sterile equipment. Split myeloma cells to ensure logarithmic growth. Remember that the key to successful fusion is healthy dividing myeloma cells.

(vi) Fusion day. See Protocol 6.2.

(vii) Emerging clones should be visible 5 days after fusion and earlier to the experienced operator (Fig. 6.1). Cells should be fed at this time. If the fusion is in 24 well plates, 1 ml HAT medium is added. If it is in 96 well plates, 0.1 ml medium should be replaced with 0.1 ml HAT medium with minimum disturbance to the emerging clones.

(viii) Assay is between 7 and 14 days after fusion depending on the rate of growth and also on the detection limits of the assay (Chapter 2). Subclone positives immediately (Chapter 8).

PROTOCOL 6.2: FUSION

(i) Prepare the materials, all sterile. Thaw the FCS, HT and A and make up the HAT medium ($2 \times$ HAT if feeders have been used) containing 20% FCS, P/S and 1 ml each of HT and A. Keep in the 37°C incubator. Put an aliquot of 50% PEG solution in the 37°C incubator. You will also need 500 ml of (preferably) warm serum free RPMI for washing.

Lay out at least two 6 cm petri dishes, 3×21G and 3×25G disposable needles, 2×10 ml disposable syringes, a large number (around 10) of sterile conical based 20 ml universal containers, a stock of 10 each of 2, 5 and 10 ml sterile pipettes, a haemocytometer, two eppendorf tubes containing 0.3 ml 0.9% ammonium chloride, and the PEG solution. It is unrealistic to give precise quantities of small pieces of plasticware as minor alterations in technique change requirements. Pipette some sterile RPMI into a sterile universal container.

(ii) Count a small sample of the myeloma cells. Check their viability

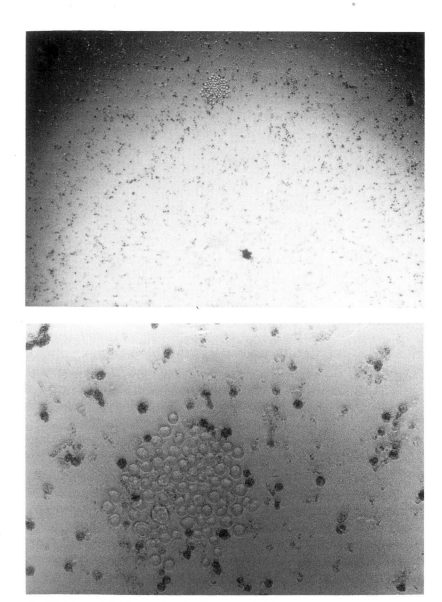

Fig. 6.1. Mouse hybridoma at low ($\times 60$ – top) and high ($\times 300$ – bottom) magnification one week after fusion. Note the number of surrounding dead myeloma and spleen cells.

and/or cell cycle (see Protocol 6.1). If this is below 90% postpone the fusion. It should be above 95%.

(iii) Kill the animal (Appendix 1), taking a sample of blood for positive assay control if required. Do this outwith the tissue culture lab and not in the sterile hood. Contamination scarcely ever results from an animal dissected on an ordinary laboratory bench. Soak the area of abdominal skin to be dissected in 70% ethanol and dissect out the spleen with sterile instruments, placing it in the sterile universal containing the RPMI.

(iv) Move the spleen to the sterile hood. Wash twice with serum free RPMI and dissect off any fatty tissue. Put the spleen into a 6 cm petri dish containing 5 ml RPMI. Gently tease the spleen cells from the capsule using two 21G needles to break up clumps. Draw the spleen cell suspension into a 10 ml pipette through a 21G needle and pipette it out again. Repeat once with a 21G needle and then twice with a 25G needle. Use moderate pressure only (no frothing). Discard clumps which may jam the finer needle. Pipette the cells gently through the 25G needle into a universal and top this up with RPMI. Centrifuge for 5 minutes at $500 \times g$, pour off the supernatant, tap the pellet to resuspend it in the dregs and then wash again a further two times in RPMI.

(v) Harvest 2×10^7 myeloma cells in sterile universal containers and wash twice by tapping and resuspending in RPMI and centrifuging at $500 \times g$. This can be done at the same time as washing of the spleen cells. It is important however that you do not harvest the myeloma cells too early, since they must be washed free of serum but will quickly respond to the lack of nutrient in their surroundings by becoming less viable.

(vi) Count the spleen cells. This is not essential and you may, if you prefer, simply assume that there are 10^8 of them. However, some antigens alter the spleen considerably (for example many parasitised animals have greatly enlarged spleens). Pipette a 0.05 ml aliquot into one of the eppendorf tubes containing the 0.3 ml ammonium chloride. This will lyse any red blood cells and swell the spleen cells. Leave for 3 minutes before counting and remember the additional 1 in 7 dilution factor in your calculations. If the number of spleen cells departs significantly from 10^8, adjust the number of myeloma cells accordingly.

(vii) Resuspend spleen and myeloma cells separately in 10 ml RPMI and from each universal remove a separate aliquot of 0.5 ml for controls. Then mix the spleen and myeloma cells together and spin at $500 \times g$ for 5 minutes. The ratio should be around 5/1 spleen/myeloma. Pour off the supernatant gently but completely and tap the pellet to loosen it.

(viii) Using a 5 ml pipette, add 2 ml PEG solution evenly over a period of 30 s shaking the cells by gently flicking of the tube and stirring the pellet with the pipette tip as you add the PEG. Over the next 30 s, gently pipette the PEG + cell suspension up and down the pipette. allow the cells to stand while you change to a fresh 5 ml pipette and fill it with 5 ml RPMI. Add this dropwise to the PEG + cell suspension over a period of 90–120 s shaking very gently to dilute out the PEG slowly. Then add another 5 ml RPMI all at once. Leave to stand for 3 minutes and then centrifuge for 5 minutes at $500 \times g$.

(a) For a 4×24 well plate 'beginner's fusion' which has not used feeder cells resuspend in 100 ml HAT medium. Aliquot 1 ml into each well with the exception of A1 and A2 on each plate. Centrifuge both control samples at $500 \times g$ for 5 minutes and resuspend in 5 ml HAT medium. Aliquot 1 ml myeloma cells into well A1 of each plate and 1 ml spleen cells into well A2 on each plate. If feeders have been used, resuspend in 50 ml $2 \times$ HAT (and controls in 2.5 ml $2 \times$ HAT) and aliquot 0.5 ml.

(b) For a 8×96 well normal fusion which has not used feeder cells resuspend in 160 ml HAT medium. Aliquot 0.2 ml into each well with the exception of A1 and A2 on each plate. Centrifuge both control samples at $500 \times g$ for 5 minutes and resuspend in 8 ml HAT medium. Aliquot 0.2 ml myeloma cells into well A1 of each plate and 0.2 ml spleen cells into well A2 on each plate. If feeders have been used, resuspend in 80 ml $2 \times$ HAT (and controls in 4 ml $2 \times$ HAT) and aliquot 0.1 ml.

6.6.1. Protocol variations for mouse fusions

It has been emphasised throughout this book that the number of variations in procedure is very large and most variations work. However, some major variations in technique together with their rationalisations are outlined below.

Step (i) Fusions can be quite successful and less expensive in 10% FCS and if there are strong financial considerations, it is possible to use this or the median of 15%.

Step (iv) The spleen has many cells other than B lymphocytes which comprise only about 30% of the total. If the whole spleen is put through a sieve or tea strainer then more cells will be obtained but these will include cells such as fibroblasts which grow very well for some weeks in primary culture and can dominate the fusion, taking all the nutrients in the medium. On the other hand, the rapidly dividing cells which are most likely to participate in a good fusion are mobile and a predominance of these is obtained by 'flushing out' the spleen with a combination of syringing and teasing with needles. In teasing the spleen cells apart, most of the mobile cells are obtained. This is therefore a median position and very easy to perform. It may, however, leave clumps and some people like to remove these by a gentle preliminary centrifugation. This requires very low speeds which are difficult to judge and maintain on most laboratory centrifuges. The needle technique described is the simplest and it works well.

Step (vii) The controls are quite important and only very experienced operators can afford to dispense with them. Basically they monitor cell death and in the case of the myeloma control, the effectiveness of the aminopterin which tends to be unstable. The spleen control also monitors the point at which the spleen cells themselves cease to secrete. This is important in early assay to establish a spleen background against which to assess positives. With a strong antigen, the spleen background can be quite high for periods of time up to two weeks.

The ratio of spleen cells to myeloma cells in protocols varies from 10/1 to 2/1. Only actively growing cells fuse. In the case of the myeloma cells this should be all of them while in the case of the spleen cells the fact that only 30% are B cells (Table 3.3) and not all of these are actively growing has to be taken into account. Fusion is not cell specific and splenic T cells, which will also be stimulated by the final boost, will also fuse with B myeloma lines to yield cross-phenotype hybridomas. These may grow quite well but they will not make antibody.

Step (viii) The procedure described here derives from the method of Oi and Herzenberg (1980). A common and successful variation is to expose the cells for longer (5–8 minutes) to a lower percentage of PEG (30–35%) while centrifuging them gently down together through the PEG at $200–300 \times g$. These 'spinning techniques' derive from the protocol of Gefter et al. (1977) and and Claflin and Williams (1978) which rely heavily on the early techniques established for adherent cells such as fibroblasts and epithelial cells. Fazekas de St Groth and Scheidegger (1980) compared three completely different protocols for PEG fusion and found all to be comparable in terms of number of clones produced. If the myeloma cells are healthy, almost any method works and the variations all relate to balancing out the toxicity of PEG against its fusogenic role.

Many protocols recommend that the fused cells are incubated for an hour before the post fusion centrifugation. This is claimed to improve the number of clones. However, it is possible to obtain a very large number without this.

Step (ix) For plating densities, see Section 6.4.

HAT is conveniently added at this stage. Several protocols suggest that it is better to add HAT 24 hours after fusion when the cells have settled. As ever, there is no detailed evidence for this and it is logical to suppose that the unfused myeloma cells will meantime have started to outgrow the hybridomas in the culture wells. Indeed it is quite common to lay feeders down in HAT 24 hours in advance and add the fused cells to established feeders. This also works and may suit those who want to minimise the (albeit already small) workload on the day of fusion.

The general experimental approach to a fusion is probably best if the fusion itself is not regarded as critical. With a well prepared expe-

riment only a single fusion should be necessary but with difficult antigens several fusions may be required and most laboratories regard a
fusion not as a major event, but as an established procedure which
can be fitted into a short session of laboratory work.

6.6.2. Variations in fusion protocols for the rat system

Rat fusions are carried out in a manner similar to mouse fusions. The
rat myeloma lines are particularly sensitive to their growth conditions
and need good serum (Section 5.2.3). It is quite common for a lab to
have successful mouse fusions simultaneously with poor rat ones but
seldom the reverse. A ratio of 2:1 spleen/myeloma cells is recommended (Galfre et al., 1979) and the emerging clones are diffuse and more
difficult to detect. A rat spleen usually gives about double the number
of cells of a mouse one, i.e., around 2×10^8.

6.6.3. Variations in fusion protocol for human systems

It should be emphasised that these are not recommended until better
human fusion systems can be developed. The recommended procedure for making a human monoclonal antibody from a human subject
(as opposed to 'humanising' one from a rodent – Section 1.9 and
Chapter 9) is to put the cells into short term culture (e.g., by EBV
transformation as described in Chapter 7) and then to use Polymerase
Chain Reaction (Chapter 9) to amplify the message in cells with the
chosen specificity.

    As with all matters relating to human fusions, there is a very wide
range of technique and this is not surprising since both the myeloma/
lymphoblastoid partners and the source of the human lymphocytes
are so variable. An extensive range of protocols has been published
but each has been usually to promote a particular cell line and there
have been no good comparative studies with a single parameter being
varied at any one time (see James and Bell, 1987 for a review). If primary human lymphocytes are used then fusion ratios are usually between 2/1 and 5/1 primary cells/fusion partner and frequencies are

generally lower than the mouse since the necessary boosting procedure is less well established. Much depends on the tissue source, tonsils, for example, being high in B cells (Chapter 3). However, where the antibody secreting lines are, for example, EBV transformed B lymphocytes, it is quite usual to fuse at 1:1 ratios and since both partners in the fusion can be put into logarithmic growth, fusion frequencies can be excellent.

Possibly because of the difficulties which are encountered with human fusions, extra ingredients are often incorporated into the medium and, in particular 2×10^{-5} M mercaptoethanol is frequently used. HAz (hypoxanthine azaserine) selection is also used more frequently, particularly in the case of human T cell hybridomas.

6.7. Electrofusion

Electrofusion is a technique which allows a high fusion frequency to be obtained with a comparatively small number of cells (Bischoff et al, 1982). Its perceived use has always been with small numbers of specialised B cells in the human system, for example within a rheumatoid joint. However, since the main problem in the human system is not lack of fusion per se but lack of post fusion stability due to the absence of any good human fusion partner (Section 3.6), it has not found a major role in Mab production to date. If a situation in rodent system which requires fusion of small numbers of B cells should occur, it would be a very suitable method. It is covered in a recent volume edited by Borrebaeck (1990).

CHAPTER 7

Alternative strategies for the immortalisation of antibody producing cells

7.1. Introduction

These alternative strategies fall into two groups.

The first is transformation of the B lymphocyte population with a virus or oncogene. Viral transformation generally yields a continuous line of transformed cells whereas transfected oncogenes often only confer transient stability to the recipient cells. Both viruses and oncogenes generally only immortalise a subset of the exposed B lymphocyte population which is presumed to be those expressing the appropriate virus receptor or having developmentally specific oncogene product vulnerability (Nussenzweig et al., 1988). This heterogeneous transformed subset of the original population has very limited cloning capacity at the level of a single cell specificity although it can be grown for longer (indefinitely in the case of some viruses) at higher cell density. The transformed subset may or may not include B cells which have the relevant specificity for the antigen of interest. In general, genetic techniques have the disadvantage of transforming mainly low-affinity IgM producing, immature B cells.

The second strategy is growth in lymphokine enriched medium which permits most primary B lymphocytes to expand clonally from single cell culture but only to the level of a few hundred fully differentiated antibody producing cells. This can yield sufficient mature, isotype switched clones originating from each B cell in the culture to permit analysis of antibody isotype and specificity but not sufficient for the encoding genomic or cDNA to be cloned. It is likely that PCR techniques will overcome this problem in the near future (Section 9.6). Both viral and lymphokine approaches yield different populations of B cells and both may be required to generate any panel of Mabs with a suitable specificity range.

7.1.1. Purification of lymphocytes from complex tissues

Before either of these strategies is used, it is frequently necessary to purify the relevant B cells free from the complex control mechanisms exerted by T cells. If a complex tissue with many irrelevant cells is used (and this generally applies to most human tissue samples) then it is necessary first to purify the entire lymphocyte population. If the sample is blood, then this is achieved by density gradient centrifugation on Ficoll Hypaque. The blood is gently layered over an equal volume of Ficoll and centrifuged at $600 \times g$ for 15 minutes. The population at the interface will contain lymphocytes together a few monocytes. This is harvested and washed before being subjected to the next stage of selection. 10 ml blood will yield over 10^7 lymphocytes of which 20% will be B cells.

The same procedure is also applied to lymphocytes extracted from solid tissue samples as these generally contain fibroblasts which can very quickly dominate other cells in tissue culture. In the case of solid tissue (e.g., infiltrated transplants or tumours) even if the lymphocytes 'spill' very readily by chopping of the tissue with a sterile scalpel, collagenase digestion (200 units/ml/g tissue dissolved in 5 ml RPMI + 10% FCS for 2–4 hours) is used to free any lymphocytes which may be trapped in the tissue since those lymphocytes which are least resistant to 'spilling' may possess adhesion molecules which attach them to the primary tissue (Springer, 1990). The released lymphocytes are then purified on Ficoll as above.

7.2. Pre-selection of lymphocytes with defined cell surface markers or antigen binding capacity

B lymphocytes, or a subset of antigen specific B lymphocytes are not generally selected for conventional mouse Mab production. With simple antigens, selection is not necessary. With weak antigens or unknown antigens pre-selection can reveal new specificity ranges. Pre-selection does not remove the need for assay and cloning after a conventional fusion since the relevant clone may lose the antibody coding genes, but does mean that every initial clonal growth is of interest. This means that the cells can be seeded at a low-density (on feeders) from the immediate post fusion stage. A more practical reason to avoid pre-selection of B cells is that the process is generally expensive as, with the exception of AET rosetting for purification of human B cells, it involves the purchase use of established phenotype specific Mabs.

However, for all human systems and for any rodent system involving the stimulation/immortalisation of B lymphocytes, B cells are usually first selected from other contaminating cells such as T cells, monocytes, neutrophils etc. In addition, they may be selected for antigen binding capability which gives a useful affinity 'sieve' to yield the subset of B cells which bind antigen at high affinity. It should be noted that the number of antigen specific B cells obtained from the blood of a non-immunised animal or human is very small.

Selection techniques fall into the main categories listed in Table 7.1 and the main choices are whether to use positive or negative selection. In positive selection the desired population is captured on a matrix coated with an antibody reactive to all B cells, or, more specifically with antigen itself. While at first this may seem to be the obvious choice, it is less frequently used. The reasons are that (i) it is often difficult subsequently to extract the B cells from the selecting matrix without damage, (ii) that if the captured antibody is either anti-immunoglobulin or antigen, the homogeneous population of B cells will then 'cap', i.e., internalise their surface antibody for a variable period of time and (iii) for many subsequent manipulations, B cells which

TABLE 7.1
Methods for selecting relevant B cell populations

Positive selection
(i) Mouse
Rosetting on anti CD45R (LyB5) or anti-Ig coated sheep red blood cells or antigen coated sheep red blood cells
Panning on anti CD45R (LyB5) or anti-Ig coated petri dishes or antigen coated petri dishes
Separation with beads coated with anti CD45R (LyB5) or anti-Ig coated beads or antigen coated beads
FACS selection of anti CD45R (LyB5) or anti Ig +ve cells or antigen +ve B cells (fluorescent antigen required for latter)

(ii) Human
Rosetting on anti CD19/anti CD20 coated sheep red blood cells or antigen coated sheep red blood cells
Panning on anti CD19 or CD20 coated petri dished or antigen coated petri dishes
Separation with beads coated with anti CD19 or CD20
FACS selection of CD19 and/or CD20 +ve cells or antigen +ve cells (fluorescent antigen required for latter)

Negative selection*
(i) Mouse
Rosetting on anti Thy-1-coated sheep red blood cells
Panning on anti-Thy 1 coated petri dishes
Separation with beads coated with anti Thy-1
FACS selection of Thy-1 −ve T cells
Complement mediated killing of Thy-1 +ve cells.

(ii) Human
Rosetting on AET coated coated sheep red blood cells+
Panning on anti CD3 coated petri dishes
Separation with beads coated with anti CD3
FACS selection of CD3 −ve cells
Complement mediated killing of CD3 +ve cells

* Recommended
+ Specific to human cells but inexpensive
(See table 1.3 for CD classification)

have 'seen' antigen outwith the context the normal in vivo situation may be downregulated rather than upregulated and become more difficult to work with. However, if antigen is to be used to select B cells, the positive selection system must be used.

In the generally preferred negative selection systems, the 'contaminating' cells are captured and removed and the required cell population remains.

7.2.1. Pre-selection of B lymphocytes from T lymphocytes

Once a comparatively pure population of lymphocytes has been purified from other cells in the primary tissue, the T cells can be separated from the B cells.

7.2.1.1. Rosetting

T lymphocytes are readily removed from a human (but not mouse) mixed lymphocyte sample by E rosetting with sheep red blood cells to leave a cell population enriched in B cells and monocytes. The most frequent application of this technique is in the transformation of human B lymphocytes with EBV but it is also used for the subsequent growth of B cells in short term culture. Over 90% of the human population carry latent EBV infection which is kept in control by cytotoxic T cells directed against the virus infected cells. Thus, it is widely believed that B cells cannot efficiently be transformed in culture when these T cells are present. The corollary of this is that when they are removed, the remaining B cells may occasionally appear to be spontaneously transformed if they have a high level of endogenous virus which is released from T cell constraint.

While lymphokines from helper T cells may be advantageous to the development of the B cell population, most groups believe that they are better added back in a more controlled and defined manner. It is, however, worth noting that some groups deliberately leave T cells present and stimulate them with PHA to aid EBV transformation for human hybridoma production (Doyle et al., 1985; Melamed et al., 1987; Kumpel et al., 1989).

The basis of the rosetting technique is that human and swine but not mouse or rabbit T cells bind to the CD2 antigen on Sheep Red Blood

Cells (SRBCs) and can consequently be separated from the rest of the peripheral blood mononuclear cells on the basis of the greater density of the erythrocytes. SRBCs alone are not an ideal reagent as the ability to bind T cells is widely variable and protocols usually involve SRBCs which have been pretreated with enzymes such as papain or neuraminidase or with sulphydryl reagents. The protocol below is derived from Kaplan and Clark (1974) and is economical and reproducible.

PROTOCOL 7.1: ROSETTING METHODS FOR SEPARATION OF HUMAN T LYMPHOCYTES FROM B LYMPHOCYTES

This is a negative selection process removing T lymphocytes from a preparation of cells from spleen, blood, node etc. All preparations should be undertaken under sterile conditions.

(i) Weigh out 102 mg of 2-aminoethylisothiouronium bromide (AET Aldrich chemicals) and dissolve in 10 ml distilled water. Adjust to exactly pH 9, with NaOH. Filter through a 0.2 μm filter to sterilise.

(ii) Wash 2 ml of fresh packed sheep red blood cells (SRBCs) three times with serum free RPMI. Add 8 ml of the AET solution and incubate at 37°C for 20 min with occasional shaking. Add RPMI and centrifuge at $500 \times g$ for 5 min. Wash the cells at least five times in RPMI and resuspend in RPMI to a concentration of 10% (v/v).

(iii) Dilute the stored AET treated SRBCs to 2%. Prepare the lymphocytes from the primary tissue by centrifugation on Ficoll as described in Section 7.1. Wash the lymphocytes to be separated in serum free RPMI and then, in precise order, add equal volumes of the 2% AET treated SRBCs, RPMI and FCS. The cells tend to clump with FCS which is added last. Centrifuge at $200 \times g$ for 10 min. Do not remove the supernatant but incubate the tube for 90 min in an ice bath.

(iv) Resuspend by gently rocking the tube. Count the rosettes on the haemocytometer. About 60% of the PBLs should have formed rosettes.

(v) Layer the cells very gently onto an equal volume of Ficoll-Hypaque in a 20 ml universal container and centrifuge at $600 \times g$ for 15 min. The rosetted T cells centrifuge to the bottom of the tube and the

B lymphocytes remain at the interface. Harvest the interface and wash the cells twice with RPMI.

(vi) If the T lymphocytes are required from the pellet, the SRBCs can be quickly lysed by a 5 second exposure to 17 mM Tris-HCl, 0.15 M ammonium chloride, pH 7.2, followed by immediate addition of medium. Instead of the AET treatment, some laboratories use neuraminidase made up to 1 mg/ml in PBS and filter sterilised. 1 ml of this is incubated with 10 ml 10% (v/v) SRBCs at 30°C for 1 hour. The cells are washed and stored in medium containing 10% FCS until use as above from step (iii).

If the SRBCs are to be coated with antibody or antigen for more precise selection requirements, then a separate second rosetting step is carried out. A typical use of this would be negative selection to remove IgM positive B cells prior to transformation of only the unbound IgG secretors. It is sometimes used as a positive selection step to purify antigen binding B cells.

PROTOCOL 7.2: ROSETTING ON ANTIBODY OR ANTIGEN COATED SRBCs

(i) Make up a solution of 1% (w/v) hydrated chromic chloride in 0.15 M NaCl. Adjust pH to 5 and 'age' the solution for a few weeks. adjusting the pH to 5 regularly.

(ii) Prepare 0.5 ml of a 0.1–1 mg/ml solution of the soluble antigen or antibody.

(iii) Use a preparation of SRBCs not more than two weeks old. Wash by centrifugation at $500 \times g$ in sterile 0.15 M saline at least three times and more if the supernatant remains red. Take 0.5 ml packed cell volume and dilute to 4.5 ml in 0.15 M saline.

(iv) Add the 0.5 ml antigen solution.

(v) Dilute the stock chromic chloride solution 1 in 100 in 0.15 M saline and add 5 ml of this dropwise to the antigen-SRBC mixture with constant stirring. Continue to mix for a further 15 minutes. Then add 10 ml PBS, mix, and centrifuge at $500 \times g$ for 5 minutes. Wash the pellet twice with phosphate-buffered saline. This preparation will keep for up to one week.

(vi) Prepare the B lymphocytes by rosetting out the T lymphocytes as in Protocol 7.1.

(vii) React the B lymphocytes with the coated SRBCs as in protocol 7.1 steps (iii) to (vi). Positively selected B cells will be in the SRBC pellet and negatively selected B cells at the interface.

7.2.1.2. Panning

Panning has the advantage that it is a more standard technique than rosetting as SRBCs can vary in quality. It is also very simple to perform. However, it requires well defined antibodies to the cell population to be panned. The extent to which cells stick to the dish depends on the quality of antibody used and on the cell surface density of the molecule it detects. With a primary cell population, expression of the antigen will also depend on their position in the cell cycle.

Monocytes in any cell preparation will tend to adhere without any antibody coating and may contaminate the resulting bound population. These are often removed by pre-panning for 1 hour at 37°C (since adherence is an active process) on a sterile non-coated petri dish, or by filtration through sterile Sephadex G-10 columns. There are generally few monocytes after the preliminary Ficoll step (Section 7.1) and this additional step is usually not necessary if the object is simply to remove T cells.

The actual panning is done at 4°C and this is important if the selection is positive since antibody binding is a more passive process which can occur at 4°C. At higher temperatures, B cells can 'cap' surface antibody bound to antigen or anti immunoglobulin, and downregulate some surface antigens.

PROTOCOL 7.3: PANNING TO SEPARATE CELL POPULATIONS BEARING SURFACE ANTIGENS REACTIVE WITH KNOWN MABS

All operations should be performed under sterile conditions.

(i) Coat a sterile 10 cm petri dish with 10 ml 10–50 μg/ml antibody containing tissue culture supernatant in sterile filtered 130 mM NaCl,

0.05 M Tris-HCl, pH 9. If the antibody is pure, less may be used (1–5 μg). Leave this in an incubator for 1 hour at 37°C and then overnight at 4°C. It is important to use a sterile petri dish but not one specially prepared for tissue culture (i.e., coated with collagen or other material to help cells adhere).

(ii) Pour off and wash with 5% BSA containing 1 μg/ml of the same antibody. Wash five times with PBS.

(iii) Prepare the lymphocytes from the primary tissue by Ficoll $\pm$ collagenase as described in Section 7.1. Pre-pan the monocytes at 37°C if necessary. Adjust the final cell suspension to 10^7 cells/ml.

(iv) Add 5 ml cell suspension to the plate and leave for 1 hour at 4°C, gently rotating the plate after 30 minutes to allow cells to coat more evenly.

(v) Gently tilt the plate and remove unbound cells and medium from one curve. If the selection process is negative, these can then be used directly, or repanned on another plate to remove any residual bound cells.

(vi) If the selection is positive and the bound cells are required, wash very gently twice by slowly adding RPMI at the side of the plate gently agitating the plate, and removing the RPMI. It is useful to inspect the plate under the microscope at the start of, and during these washes. Then detach the bound cells by a vigorous jet of RPMI across the plate followed by rapid removal of the dislodged cells before they reattach. If the cells remain difficult to dislodge, mechanical methods may be used. A sharp slap on the side of the petri dish is often effective.

7.2.1.3. Negative selection using complement

Complement mediated lysis is a standard way to remove unwanted cells in the mouse system, more used by scientists with an immunological background. It is obviously irreversible and it is not possible to recover the lysed cells to find whether they were contaminated by the sub-population of the cells to be selected. The basis of the process is that complement, which is a complex series of serum proteins, can recognise antibody bound to antigen and if the antigen is on a cell surface, will kill the cell bearing that antigen. The defect of the complement system is that it is so complex. Certain components are exceedingly heat sensitive and one does not buy a defined reagent but rather a complex and generally irreproducible mixture. As an assay with numerous controls, it can yield new information. As a purification system, it is unreliable.

For those who wish to use it, 10–50 μg of antibody containing tissue culture supernatant (1–5 μg of pure antibody), are mixed with 5×10^7 purified lymphocytes and incubated on ice (to minimise capping) in serum free RPMI. The cells are then washed by centrifugation and incubated with 5% (v/v) complement from rabbit or guinea pig sources for 45 minutes at 37°C. The antibody bound cell population is lysed and the remaining cell population is therefore depleted of them.

7.2.1.4. FACS selection

The FACS (Fluorescent Activated Cell Sorter) can identify and select cell populations bound to any appropriate fluorescent marker. The old FACS instruments sorted very slowly so that it took several hours for a workable population to be obtained. The modern ones can sort 10^6 cells positive for the appropriate fluorescent label within a few minutes. FACS instruments have only two major and highly competitive sources – Becton-Dickinson and Coulter (Appendix 2). The initial instrument is often obtained at surprisingly low cost. However, service costs are very high and the sales agreement usually involves the purchase of 'in house' Mabs from the same firm as opposed to the less expensive Mabs offered by other companies. In addition, a cell sorter usually requires a committed operator. FACS instruments are capable of cloning required cells directly at 1 cell/well into a 96 well plate which is an extremely useful facility but replaceable at low cost by panning and conventional cloning. The use of FACS systems to isolate a large number of B cells is therefore clearly highly uneconomic in comparison to simple techniques. This should not in any way detract from the fact that such instruments are exceptionally good at analysis (Section 2.8.1).

As in all techniques, the effective use is dependent on the quality of the reagent (selecting Mab) and the technical expertise of the operator.

7.2.1.5. Magnetic beads

Magnetic beads are an exceptionally good method for negative selection if a small number of lymphocytes are involved. The beads can be obtained pre-coated with a range of possible antibodies and reacted with the lymphocyte population. They can also be reacted with chosen soluble antigens. The beads are mixed with the cells and the container is then put into a small laboratory magnet which fits readily into a sterile hood. The bead bound lymphocytes are attached to the magnetised side of the tube and the other cells can be removed. While the technique was developed for positive selection, it can only be recommended for negative selection because it is sometimes very difficult to remove bead bound lymphocytes. It is also only recommended for a situation where a small number of lymphocytes are involved as it is very expensive to use in comparison to rosetting or panning.

7.3. Pre-selection of T lymphocytes

Either pre-selection or enrichment of T lymphocytes before a T cell fusion is a common procedure. This is particularly relevant where selection or assay procedures after fusion relate to cell surface antigens as a B-T fusion may be confused with a T-T fusion (Taussig et al., 1980). Enrichment is usually by the use of nylon fibre which binds B but not T cells (Greaves and Brown, 1974) or by panning on anti-immunoglobulin coated petri dishes. T cells purified in this way may be expanded in lymphokine enriched medium before or instead of fusion (Beezley and Ruddle, 1982; Haas and Von Boehmer, 1982).

7.4. Transformation of B lymphocytes

Transformation is a method for the immortalisation of lymphocytes which may be used either prior to fusion to boost a suitable subpopulation for subsequent stabilisation, or as a replacement for fusion if the subsequent transformed population expresses the appropriate characteristics of lymphocytes. It is usually effected by viruses. In the case of human B lymphocytes, the virus is generally Epstein-Barr Virus (EBV). However, Murine pre-B lymphocytes can be immortalised by the use of Abelson Murine Leukemia virus (Alt et al., 1986) and such transformations have given much information as to the nature of the sequence of rearrangement of antibody genes.

Transformation can also be effected by electroporation or fusion of cells with the relevant transforming DNA molecules rather than whole virus but the process is comparatively inefficient and, since the DNA only enters a small percentage of the cells, it can only immortalise a small proportion of a mixed cell population, which may not include cells with the relevant characteristics. It should be re-emphasised that transformation will immortalise a different population of cells than the population immortalised by fusion. For viral transformation it is necessary for cells to carry the relevant receptor molecule (e.g., the CD21 receptor for EBV) and this will only occur at a specific developmental stage. Fusion, on the other hand, will tend to immortalise rapidly expanding B cell populations at all developmental stages (Burrows et al., 1983) but only a small proportion of these.

7.4.1. Transformation by Epstein-Barr Virus (EBV)

EBV has as its target human (but not mouse) B lymphocytes bearing the CD21 (also called Complement Receptor 2 – CR2) molecule on their surface. CD21 is generally present only on comparatively early B cells – most before commitment to isotype switch and memory cell production. As a result, EBV transformed cells are generally poly-specific IgM secretors. However, a small population of EBV transformed cells are IgG or IgA secretors and can be expanded into potentially useful reagents. The precise proportion of IgG or IgA transformable cells is always small but tissue dependent (Miyawaki et al, 1988). EBV immortalises some B cells and has the additional ability also to temporarily activate secretion by, but not immortalise, many others. The result is that, after exposure of a group of B cells to EBV, many Ab positive culture wells containing growing cells are obtained but the growing cells are often not those which secrete the relevant antibody. Consequently further cloning gives many cultures with good growth but negative antibody secretion. The precise population immortalised by EBV remains poorly characterised (Azim et al., 1990) and varies under different conditions. It is the general experience that the resultant stable clones which produce useful Mab are IgG secreting cells but the methods for obtaining these vary. Two strategies are fairly firmly established and both use peripheral blood or (occasionally) spleen from patients boosted 7–28 days or longer before the blood is withdrawn.

(i) The first is to remove the T cells by rosetting and transform the resultant B cell population, often with positive selection to obtain antigen specific B cells (Kozbor and Roder, 1981; Foung et al., 1987; Goosens et al., 1987).

(ii) The second is to retain the T cells and either treat with cyclosporin A (0.5–1 μg/ml) or with phytohaemagglutinin (PHA) (1%, v/v) (Doyle et al., 1985; Melamed et al., 1987; Kumpel et al., 1989). This will allow T cell derived lymphokines to be released into the culture and these may well encourage switching and/or CD21 expression. In consequence, the two methods may yield different populations of transformed cells. Most active groups use both methods. Mabs to HIV may be different in this case since the helper T cell population will be low and infective and is probably best removed.

After transformation there is an initial surge of antibody production, mostly of the IgM isotype and then a fall-off with slow growth in some wells. The cells are deceptive in that they clump to give the impression of a clone (Fig. 7.1). At this point occasional success has been obtained by groups who concentrate mainly on stabilising the transformants, frequently using repeated cycles of positive selection in the emerging clones to retain those which still secrete antibody. However, occasional success has also been obtained by those who 'backfuse' the emerging clones of transformants with either mouse myeloma cells or heterohybridoma cells (Section 3.6).

The word 'occasional' is used to emphasise the contrast with the

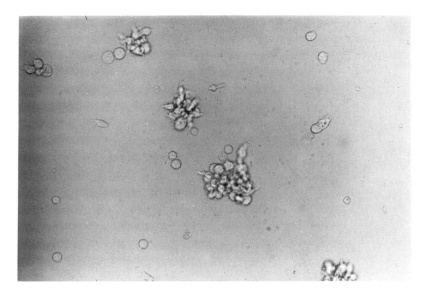

Fig. 7.1. A human EBV transformant clone. Magnification: ×300. Note that after transformation the cells tend to look like this in any case since EBV transformants clump. Thus all clumps are not clones. (Courtesy of Dr. Moira MacCann.)

mouse fusion system which can yield a large number of stable clones in a single fusion. In contrast, a large number of transformation experiments may have to be performed to yield a single stable transformant clone which is, even then, a significant achievement. For example Gorny et al. (1989) started with 14,329 culture wells from 58 patients and ended with 7 human Mabs. While their antigen was HIV which might be a special case, their statistics largely mirror those of groups with standard antigens.

The basic protocols are given below.

7.4.2. Source of EBV

The usual source is the B95–8 line of Miller and Lippman (1973) which is a marmoset line and the basic transformation method is not patented. The B95–8 line is very widely used to produce EBV for routine transformation for purposes such as karyotyping which only require temporary transformation of a few cells. Many sources of B95-8 are mycoplasma contaminated and it should be obtained from a good source.

While over 90% of the human population is EBV positive and have been exposed to the virus at some point, the stock concentrate of EBV is obviously rich in virus and should be handled with great care by all individuals. EBV causes infectious mononucleosis (glandular fever) which can be a lengthy and serious condition in certain individuals. While EBV is technically only a Category C pathogen (To be handled with routine good microbiological practice), an organisation that allows an employee to handle EBV without proper instruction can be vulnerable to legal action.

PROTOCOL 7.4: PRODUCTION OF EBV STOCKS

Work with care (see above)

(i) Obtain mycoplasma free B95–8 cells from a reliable source (readily available – ECACC, ATCC).

(ii) Grow the B95-8 cell line at a density of 10^6 cells/ml in good medium (i.e., 5% FCS in RPMI) and establish a good stock in liquid nitrogen.

(iii) Once you have established a stock, take a subculture and expand it under the conditions above. Then transfer it to poor conditions in which the dormant virus will emerge and make the B95–8 cells succumb and secrete. This means growing at the lower density of 2×10^5 cells/ml in 1–2% FCS at 30°C for about 2 weeks.

(iv) Allow the cells to settle at 4°C and collect the virus rich supernatant by centrifugation at $400 \times g$. Sterilise through 0.45 μ filters, and aliquot in 1 ml ampoules for storage in liquid nitrogen. Virus can be stored for several months. Use one ampoule/10^6 lymphocytes.

7.4.3. Transformation procedures

It is not possible to transform B cells efficiently unless the suppressive T cells are removed. There is also no point in transforming IgM producing B lymphocytes unless you are studying B cell developmental processes as they will not yield useful antibody. They will only confuse the assay and take up time and money. In consequence, on the day of transformation, it is possible to have to do three Ficoll separations, the first to purify lymphocytes from other cells in the primary tissue (Section 7.1), the second to remove T cells, (Section 7.2, Protocol 7.1) and the third to remove the low-affinity IgM secreting B cells (Protocols 7.2 or 7.3).

EBV transformants do not grow well in small numbers and feeder cells have limited effect. They were originally (Campbell, 1984) plated on human feeder cells from EBV negative donors but human donors are too variable and mouse spleen feeders provide a more reliable support system. The ideal support system for EBV transformants is fellow transformants or EBV stimulated cells (see above) and this requirement is obviously not compatible with cloning. Thus EBV transformants are plated at comparatively high density with a decreasing range on feeders. It is possible to achieve growth at lower density using U or V shaped 96 well plates which concentrate the cells but the resultant growths are difficult to view under the microscope.

Human cells are very variable in response and it is sensible to plate them at a variety of dilutions and undertake any further procedures with cells which respond to antigen best at the highest dilution.

PROTOCOL 7.5: TRANSFORMATION OF HUMAN B CELLS WITH EBV

(i) If the human subject is to be given a boosting immunisation and blood is to be the source of the B lymphocytes, boost at least 8 days and preferably 14 days before transformation.
(ii) Lay down mouse spleen feeder cells on 96 well plates (Protocol 5.5).
(iii) Purify the lymphocyte population from the human tissue (Section 7.1). Wash twice in RPMI.
(iv) Purify the B lymphocytes from the T lymphocytes (Section 7.2). Wash twice in RPMI.
(v) Purify the IgG producing B cells from the IgM producing ones by

negative selection utilising either rosetting (Protocol 7.2) or panning
(Protocol 7.3) with a human IgM (mu specific) polyclonal antibody.
Wash twice in RPMI.
(If the antigen involved is soluble, then purify antigen specific B cells
by positive selection using protocols 7.2 or 7.3. – but you may end
up with a very small number of cells)
(vi) Resuspend the finally selected B cell population in B95–8 supernatant at a concentration of around 10^6 cells/ml. Incubate at 37°C for
one hour. Wash three times in RPMI.
(vii) Resuspend the B cells in complete medium containing 10% FCS.
Count and adjust to 10^6 cells/ ml. Then plate half the cells on the feeder
cell plates at 10^5/well (depending on the source, this will be only 1–20
wells). To the remainder add an equal volume of complete medium and
plate the next half at 5×10^4/ well. To this second remainder, add an
equal volume of complete medium at 2.5×10^4/well. Continue the process through two further cell dilutions if there are enough cells to do so.
(viii) Assay after 7–10 days and be extremely careful to check whether
antibody positive cells also have cell growth.
(ix) Keep the positive wells growing but also clone on mouse spleen
feeders through the range of 1–10 cells / well.

7.5. Post-transformation strategies

7.5.1. Continuous cloning

This involves repeated selection of the clones secreting the highest level of antibody and immediate recloning. Some groups help this procedure along by positively selecting those cells which have the greatest
amount of surface antibody using any of the positive selection strategies outlined in Table 7.1 (i.e., to select for antigen or surface IgG).
As the transformed cell is no longer a primary cell, it is thought to
be less likely to downregulate its surface immunoglobulin when it encounters antigen and so positive selection, which is not advised for
primary cells, is acceptable in this situation.

7.5.2. Transformation followed by fusion

While the protocols given above for transformation may yield small clones of human B cells making an antibody of interest, it is very rare indeed to be able to establish a stable cell line from EBV transformation alone. Consequently techniques involving 'rescue' by backfusion have been developed. A brief flurry of activity generated by Kozbor and Roder (1981), who advocated 'backfusion' with human lymphoblastoid cells (KR4) or human lymphoblastoid/myeloma hybrids (KR12) was unproductive for the reasons outlined in Section 3.6 (see also Figs. 3.1 and 3.6). In almost all cases, the occasional successful results have been obtained by backfusion with one of the three standard mouse lines (Section 3.4). While mouse cell lines are naturally resistant to 10^{-5} M ouabain, they can be made even more resistant (Section 3.3) by sequential selection in gradually increasing amounts of ouabain if this property is considered critical.

Human mouse fusions are far from ideal since human chromosomes are preferentially and rapidly lost. In consequence, the operator is dependent on the rare stable fusion clone which is able to grow in culture expressing the relevant human antibody producing capacity at the same high frequency of the mouse fusion partner. Selection and cloning of such cells is very rigorous but possible. Heterohybridomas, which are themselves hybrids of human and mouse myeloma lines may also be used for backfusion but they are no better than mouse lines in most people's experience.

PROTOCOL 7.4: 'BACKFUSION' OF TRANSFORMED HUMAN LYMPHOCYTES WITH MOUSE MYELOMA CELLS

(i) Make up a stock solution of 10^{-3}M ouabain. This will be used at a dilution of 1 in 100. Add 1 ml of this to the culture medium of the intended mouse myeloma fusion partner and check that growth is normal. In any case, grow the myeloma cells in this medium for 2–3 weeks to ensure that they are adapted to ouabain.
(ii) Transfer the clones from the plate of transformed cells which ap-

pear to secrete the most specific antibody at the lowest initial cell seed-
ing density to a 24 well tissue culture plate and expand to 106 cells/
well. Do not fuse them all – keep some as an insurance against failure
of the backfusion.

(iii) Prepare mouse spleen feeder cell plates (Protocol 5.5).

(iv) Fuse the transformed cells with the mouse myeloma cells at a ratio
of 1/1 as in Protocol 6.2. The controls are particularly important in
more complex fusions and must be included.

(v) Assay as soon as clones appear.

(vi) Most of the resultant cells will be unstable so clone positive secretors quickly and keep recloning until every well with growth is also
positive.

7.5.3. Transformation followed by cloning of the antibody coding genes

This strategy is covered in Chapter 9, the essential technical problem
being to get a clone large enough to be amenable to genomic or cDNA
amplification by PCR. EBV transformation tends to favour the IgG1
(or IgA1 in the case of an IgA) subclass (Miyawaki et al., 1988) and
suitable homopolymer tailing or inverse PCR strategies using the
known constant region sequences could therefore be considered.

7.6. Transformation with oncogenes

This is still a comparatively young area. There is no doubt that certain
oncogenes, and notably the *myc* oncogene incorporated into random
sites in the genomes of transgenic mice can lead to in vivo occurrence
of B cell lymphomas (Nussenzweig et al., 1988) but the resultant lymphomas do not produce useful antibody. It has proved technically
more difficult to use oncogenes to transform B cells in vitro. The range
of oncogenes used is quite small and centred on *myc* and *ras* with the
occasional addition of *raf* and *abl* presumably on the principle that
the more oncogenes transfected, the greater the possibility of producing a stable transformed line (Kurie et al., 1990; Overell et al., 1989).

It is clear that both in vivo and in vitro there is a tendency for only pre-B cells to be immortalised and since these are at the stage where they make only heavy chain or small amounts of surface IgM, they are not suitable for antibody production.

There has also been some effort to immortalise T cells (Cattermole et al., 1989). Unlike T cells requiring IL-2 for growth, which is the current method of immortalising them, genuinely 'genetically' immortalised T helper cells might well secrete large amounts of known interleukins and also new interleukins. At the moment, the areas of research devoted to immortalising single B cells are largely dependent on lymphokines secreted by the mouse EL4 line with human help (see below).

7.7. Short term cloning of B cells in lymphokine enriched medium

It is not yet possible to expand single B cells into an immortal clonal population by application of defined purified lymphokines. However, the laboratory of Zubler (Zubler et al., 1987; Wen et al., 1987) has developed a less well defined system which can expand 90% of FACS sorted single primary B (CD19 + or CD20 +) cells into clones of up to 400 cells in size. The cells secrete IgG, IgM and IgA and sometimes combinations of these are found in the supernatant of a single clone indicating isotype switch. The tissue culture system uses a mutant of the well established mouse thymoma line EL4 (Hilfiker et al., 1981) called EL4 B5. This is irradiated and used as feeder layer together with conditioned medium from human T cells and macrophages and a small amount (typically 3 ng/ml) of phorbol myristyl acetate (PMA). The process is interesting not only as a method which works well in its own right but as an indication that it should soon be possible to grow human B cell clones in more defined medium without fusion in the same way as T cell clones can now be propagated in IL-2 without fusion.

CHAPTER 8

Selection and cloning

8.1. Early feeding and assay of fusions

Laboratory protocols vary widely in their recommendations about feeding. The following principles should be noted:

(i) Aminopterin inhibits many normal cell functions and should be removed from the feeding medium as soon as possible. The time to do this can best be judged by monitoring the dead myeloma control wells. In the rodent system, these are frequently dead within 7–10 days and it may never be necessary to feed a fusion with medium containing aminopterin at all. In addition, feeding at early stages is better performed (to avoid disturbance of emerging clones) if fresh medium is added without total removal of old medium and in consequence residual aminopterin will probably remain despite its instability. If the control cells are dead, it is recommended that the feeding medium should not include aminopterin. Conversely, aminopterin is one of the least stable components of the feeding medium and sometimes it is clear from the inspection of the myeloma cells at 4 days after fusion that it has not been effective. Medium with fresh aminopterin may be added at this stage. It is important to monitor the control wells at all times.

(ii) One single surviving myeloma cell in any culture is likely to outgrow the hybridomas. With less stable systems such as human fusions, this can be an important factor and human hybridomas are usually maintained in aminopterin or azaserine containing medium for some weeks after fusion.

(iii) After the aminopterin is removed, hypoxanthine and thymidine should still be supplied for at least a week. Not only may residual aminopterin remain in the medium, but the emerging cells may need time to adapt the pathways of purine and pyrimidine biosynthesis.

(iv) Fast growing clones are indicated by the change in pH (i.e., yellow medium). These should be fed.

(v) Every tissue culture operation increases the risk of contamination and may disturb the growing clones. Thus feeding should be as infrequent as possible.

(vi) All clones should be assayed and subcloned as early as possible.

(vii) Change of medium designed to feed the cells also removes the antibody they produce. This is important as the spleen cells die quite slowly and tend to make substantial amounts of antibody so that the small additional amount of positive antibody production from a growing clone is difficult to separate from background antibody production from the spleen cells.

It is quite obvious that most of these criteria cannot be satisfied by any feeding schedule as they are frequently in conflict. Published protocols vary widely in their advice on the care of clones at this stage as different weight is put on the main considerations described above. Most groups feed between 5 and 7 days with fresh medium. Some remove old medium to do this and others plate out the original fusion in smaller amounts so that there is room in the fusion wells for feeding without disturbing the cells. To a large extent the decision depends on the confidence of the operator. A beginner is probably better with minimal manipulations while an experienced operator can remove and add medium without disturbing the cells or increasing the risk of contamination. There are also different considerations for human fusions which tend to grow slightly more slowly than mouse ones. In consequence, the schedule given in Protocol 8.1 below should not be rigidly adhered to but rather should be adapted according to the rate of growth of the clones and considerations (i) to (v).

PROTOCOL 8.1: POST FUSION CARE OF HYBRIDOMAS

(i) Inspect the cells after 4–5 days. There should be extensive cell death and the tissue culture plate should be a scene of devastation. However, it should be possible to begin to see the development of small clear clones of developing cells in the test wells (Fig. 6.1). The control myeloma cells should be dead but the control spleen cells may still be viable. If the myeloma cells are not dead, it is possible to feed with fresh aminopterin but the fusion is unlikely to yield as many clones.

(ii) Between 4–5 days feed the fusion. The beginner's fusion in 24 well tissue culture plates can simply be given an extra 1 ml of fresh medium containing HAT. The standard fusion in 96 well plates should have 0.1 ml of old medium gently removed and replaced with fresh medium containing HAT. HAT is probably not necessary for mouse fusions at this stage (although it is for human ones) and one can obtain excellent clones by simply feeding with medium.

(iii) Between 7 and 10 days clones should be clearly visible. In a mouse fusion they are readily identified. In a rat fusion they are harder to detect as they tend to be more sprawling growth. However, since rat fusions are generally quite stable, there is less pressure to assay and clone early. Human clones are usually also quite clear but EBV transformants can be free floating in clumps which are not, in fact clones but rather aggregates of transformed cells. When clones are 100–200 cells (about 1 mm across) they should be screened. If one holds the plate up to the light, it should be just possible to see the off-white button of a clone. If this is visible, then screening should be immediate (same day).

0.1 ml of supernatant should be removed for assay and replaced with fresh medium (no HAT). It is important to assay the spleen cell control wells at this stage as they will give an indication of background antibody secretion from unfused spleen cells.

If a fusion shows no obvious growth after 14 days it can be fed again with complete medium (no HAT) but if it shows no growth after 21 days it is probably not worth keeping. While it has been known for groups to isolate clones as long as 6 weeks after fusion, it is far better to give up and do another one.

8.2. Failure of fusions

Fusions may fail for obvious reasons such as contamination or equipment failure. Poor aminopterin will lead to failure but this is readily detected by growth in the myeloma control wells. In some cases, however, protocols are faithfully adhered to, the control cells die, and no positive clones are obtained. Such failures divide naturally into two groups.

8.2.1. Failure where clonal growth is good

If a fusion showed good growth but gave no positive wells then both the immunising antigen and the assay used for antibody detection should be examined closely. It may be that both worked well to yield and detect antibody in polyclonal sera but not monoclonal antibodies. The differences in assay likely to be encountered are discussed in Chapter 2 but the most likely problems are:
(i) The antigen required is a very minor component of the main immunogen and the fusion has been dominated by stronger antigens. This means that the antigen must be further purified from the original immunogen for the next attempt or that some new selection procedure must be adopted. If the titre of the original animal was high, this is unlikely. If it was below 1 in 1000 this is a possible source of difficulty.
(ii) The assay (Chapter 2) may have been unsuitable for monoclonal antibodies. If the polyclonal serum gave a high titre then the assay system should be dissected in detail. If it is, for example, dependent on a high epitope density then it may not be suitable for Mab production. The second antibody may also be over-specific. Throughout this book, the use of γ-chain specific second antibody is advised so that only IgG antibodies are detected. Provided that the polyclonal serum was also assayed with this antibody, it should cause no problems. However, if the polyclonal serum was assayed with an antibody simply to IgG, then most of the serum titre may reflect binding to the constant regions of the light chains on IgM molecules (Table 2.2).

8.2.2. Failure with no clonal growth

Only rarely is this due to direct operator error and such a possibility can readily be checked out by reference to others in the lab also doing fusions.

Failure is also unlikely to be due to the reagents such as HAT or PEG unless an error has been made in calculating the amounts weighed and dissolved, for example, an error of one order of magnitude in thymidine concentration in either direction will almost certainly result in a failed fusion. In general, however, fusions are tolerant of small errors in technique or reagents from different suppliers and while these may affect the number of clones, they have to be drastically wrong to give no clones at all.

In the vast majority of cases where there is no clonal growth, the fault lies with the myeloma cell line. The major problem for every hybridoma technologist is mycoplasma (see Section 5.4 for full details). Myeloma cells can continue to grow apparently normally while harbouring mycoplasma and mycoplasma can come into a laboratory at any time through tissue, personnel or imported cell lines. If it is mycoplasma then it must be removed immediately from all the equipment and cell lines as instructed in Section 5.4.3. Even established hybridomas are at risk if you have mycoplasma as they gradually cease to secrete. Thus, until decontamination of all material is complete, no established hybridoma or older myeloma stocks should be brought up from liquid nitrogen. If it is possible that any of the stock in liquid nitrogen is also contaminated, then these should be brought up in 'quarantine' if at all. If there is back-up stock, then it is best to throw dubious stock out and clear the nitrogen vats.

It is, however, possible that the myeloma cell line is not mycoplasma contaminated but was not in sufficiently active growth for fusion to occur. This is not so much a question of cell doubling time for the myeloma line but rather a requirement that the maximum number of the cells be in active S phase at the time of fusion. The myeloma cells should have been subcultured 12–24 hours before the fusion into fresh medium rich in FCS for this to occur. They should also have been harvested from this medium just before fusion and not 2–3 hours before as cells removed from FCS into RPMI very quickly cease cycling.

8.2.3. How to cope with a fusion which is too successful

This is a common occurrence and relates to the fusion being above expectations on the original plating schedule. Protocol 6.2 is for 8×96 well plates which means an expectation of 700–800 clones. A good fusion against a strong soluble antigen can often give over 2000 clones so that in the 8 plates there may be $3+$ clones/well. At this stage, in a fusion, all that is possible is to assay the fusion immediately for positively secreting clones. If there are a small number of positives, clone immediately going below the usual figure of 0.3 cells/well (Section 8.3). If there are a large number of positives, then redo the assay with less antigen in the detecting system (always using a γ-chain specific probe) so that only the high affinity clones register as positive. An alternative is to measure immunoglobulin secretion to give a better estimate of affinity (Section 11.6).

It is necessary to be realistic over a too successful fusion. The notion that you have an army of antibodies to different epitopes is an old fashioned one not in agreement with current immunological thinking. The expense of cloning 2000 emerging wells is ridiculous and there is no known antigen for which 2000 hybridomas are required. If one has done one good fusion one can do another and it is best to start by selecting up to 20 of the high-affinity secreting wells, clone and stabilise these, and leave further investigation to another fusion if the selected 20 are not suitable for the final use.

The rat system rarely yields such inconveniently successful fusions and this makes it rather attractive. Rat hybridomas being largely stable, one can assay and expand at leisure and decide which are the most suitable clones to expand at a much later stage.

8.3. Cloning of hybridomas

Cloning in the mouse fusion system or human EBV transformation system must be as soon as possible after the detection of positives, preferably as soon as possible after assay data is obtained. The reasons are that:

(i) In the mouse system, fused cells which carry an initial double load of chromosomes tend to take longer to replicate. These cells lose chromosomes very fast and if these chromosomes include either mouse chromosome 12, which codes for the immunoglobulin heavy chain locus, or mouse chromosome 6 which codes for the κ light chain locus, the ability to secrete the appropriate antibody will be lost. Cells which have lost chromosomes tend to outgrow their neighbours. This is probably true for cells in emerging mouse clones as mouse hybridomas tend to have a very similar DNA content to the parent myeloma line. Nonetheless, some mouse parent lines such as SP2/0 (Section 3.4) carry an almost tetraploid DNA load in a quite stable manner and rat hybridomas, unlike mouse ones, carry an almost tetraploid DNA content years after being established. There are also cases of many human cell lines which grow well in culture despite an excessive chromosome load. In consequence, the above explanation would appear to apply mouse fusions but not as a general principle of tissue culture.

(ii) In a fully developed plasmacyte (mature B lymphocyte secreting antibody) as much as half of the protein synthesising apparatus may be occupied with the synthesis of antibody. Thus fused cells making detectable amounts of antibody divert so much energy into this process that they are presumed inevitably to have less energy left for multiplication and secretion. Consequently, the cells secreting antibody are at a disadvantage compared to those not secreting antibody. Again, this may be true in the mouse system.

Neither explanation is satisfactory and the process of immortalisation with or without chromosome loss probably lies in oncogene activities still be to discovered. There is no doubt, however, about the fact that mouse fusions and EBV transformants must be cloned as early as possible. Fortunately, this chromosome loss is restricted to the period after fusion and mouse hybridomas are as stable as rat ones in the long-term.

8.3.1. Cloning by limiting dilution

In the early days of hybridoma technology, it was thought important to prove that a Mab really was monoclonal by cloning to mathematically acceptable limits. The theoretical approach to cloning by limiting dilution is based on the Poisson distribution

$$a = e^{-b}$$

Where a is the fraction of wells with no growth, b is the number of clones/well and e has the customary mathematical notation.

Thus, as described by Goding (1980) if $b = 1$ then $a = 0.37$, i.e., if 37% of the wells show no growth then the probability is that those which show growth have true monoclonal hybridomas in them. Cloning efficiency, correctly interpreted, is the ratio of theoretical potential cell growth to that experienced practically, expressed as a percentage.

The practical approach has always been more pragmatic and these equations are probably irrelevant to the process. The potential hybridoma must be immortalised in a short period of time. Most mouse and human hybridomas are mutually adherent and tend to clone in aggregates whether distributed at an official level of 1 cell/well by a laboratory technician with a hand held pipette or a fluorescence activated cell sorter. Finally, if the clone is assayed early enough, then it will have a very small number of cells and one is wasting these in counting them. If a positively secreting clone survives the first cloning with continued secretion, it will probably be stabilised and can be subjected to more rigorous cloning at a later stage.

Once the decision to clone a clump of cells which appears to secrete an antibody of interest has been taken, the priority is to find the lowest dilution of cells which still gives a positive result.

It is perhaps worth noting that some of the early work on human

Mabs around 1982 did not use cloning at all – possibly one of the many reasons why it was unsuccessful.

PROTOCOL 8.2: CLONING BY LIMITING DILUTION

(i) Select positive wells by assay.

(ii) Lay down 96 well mouse spleen feeder plates (Protocol 5.5). Many people do this during incubation periods in the assay on the assumption that they will then want to clone immediately.

(iii) Aspirate the relevant clone from the fusion plate by holding the pipette tip vertically over it. If there are two clones in the same well, aspirate them independently.

(iv) Pipette the aspirate into 5 ml complete medium (20% FCS). This will be 20–200 cells/ml depending on the size of the clone.

(v) On a single feeder plate, plate out 100 μl of this into rows A and B. This will be 2–20 cells/well depending on the size of the original clone.

(vi) You should have a remaining volume of around 2.5 ml. Dilute this with 7.5 ml complete medium and plate out on rows C and D. This will be 0.5 to 5 cells/well depending on the size of the original clone.

(vii) Discard half the remainder to leave you with approximately 2.5 ml. Add 7.5 ml complete medium and plate out over rows E and F. This will be 0.125 to 1.25 cells/well.

(viii) Discard half the remainder to leave you with approximately 2.5 ml. Add 7.5 ml complete medium and plate out over rows G and H. This will be 0.03 to 0.3 cells/well.

(ix) The clones will give visible growth after 1–3 weeks. Assay them all and chose those which secrete the desired antibody at the highest level of cloning dilution (i.e., wells G and H will be better than wells A and B).

(x) Reclone using the same strategy. This is generally only a precaution. The clone should be stable after 3 weeks.

8.3.2. Cloning in soft agar

Soft agar cloning is very rarely used and has largely historical interest because the original fusions of Kohler and Milstein (1975) used this method. It works best if the desired antigen is naturally present on the surface of sheep red blood cells (SRBCs) so that they can immediately be used as an indicator reagent to detect positively secreting clones. It is difficult to place it as a technique with a major role in modern hybridoma technology. It presents technical difficulties in that it is necessary to have molten agar for suspension of the cells and the cells are obviously vulnerable to heat shock above 37°C. In addition, batches of agar are highly variable and some may be toxic. Civin and Banquerigo (1983) have described cloning in tubes of low temperature gelation agar which circumvents both of these problems and may prove more suitable than the conventional agar cloning described.

In soft agar cloning the cells are grown in an upper layer of 0.25–0.3% agar over a lower layer of 0.5% agar. Either layer can contain feeder cells and although this is not strictly necessary, it is recommended in Protocol 8.3.

PROTOCOL 8.3: CLONING IN SOFT AGAR

(i) Prepare a 1% solution of Bacto agar in distilled water. Autoclave, cool to 50°C and mix with an equal volume of 2 × RPMI. This preparation can be stored in 100 ml aliquots and FCS (10%) and P/S added shortly before use.
(ii) Prepare mouse spleen feeder cells at 10^8 cells/ml.
(iii) Melt 100 ml of stock agar from step (i), add FCS to 20% and cool. To 50 ml of this, once the temperature has fallen below 40°C, add the feeder cells. Plate immediately in 5 ml aliquots into several 6 cm diameter petri dishes. Allow to set.
(iv) Aspirate the positive clone into 5 ml complete medium as in Protocol 8.2. In a 24 well tissue culture plate, dilute serially one in four, i.e., 0.15 ml of aspirate plus 0.45 ml complete medium, 0.15 ml of re-

sultant suspension into 0.45 ml complete medium etc. across ten wells of the plate.

(v) Melt 3 ml stock agar sample (i) and when it is below 400 add to 0.5 ml of cells at each dilution and pour each dilution over a separate petri dish as prepared in (iii).

(vi) After 7–10 days select growing clones from the plate at the lowest dilution to show growth, transfer to tissue culture dish, grow for 3–4 days and assay.

8.3.3. Cloning by the fluorescence activated cell sorter (FACS)

Most cell sorters have an adaption which makes it possible to clone cells at 1/well. In the cases where this is done, it is usual to stain the cells with a B cell marker or antigen and perform positive selection. It is, however, taking a sledge hammer to a fly when limiting dilution cloning can be performed at much lesser expense. FACS cloning should be kept for specialised uses such as that in Section 7.7.

8.3.4 Cloning of human cells

This is covered extensively for transformants and their backfusions in Section 7.4. Protocols such as 8.2 may be used but human cells seldom clone readily and it is realistic to have wells at 10 cells/well in addition to lower dilutions. While complex feeder systems have been suggested, our laboratory has found mouse spleen as good as any of these.

8.4. Failure of cloning

8.4.1. Introduction

It is at the cloning stages that initial positive wells tend to be lost in mouse fusions. Sometimes this is unavoidable as the clone loses the relevant chromosomes at an early stage of growth but in general it is avoidable if the relevant primary well is identified and cloned early enough. In cross species fusions, chromosome loss is clearly a complex and selective process with different human chromosomes being retained in different cell types so that mouse fibroblasts differentially retain one set of human chromosomes while mouse myeloma cells differentially retain a different set (Croce et al., 1980). It is only rarely that a human mouse fusion gives stable antibody secretion although it definitely can happen.

8.4.2. Failure with no or little growth

This probably means that the starting material had very few cells. It could also mean that mycoplasma contamination crept in at the cloning stage. Slow growth of clones on the other hand may well relate to the positive secretors which tend to grow more slowly and a cloning plate should be kept and reassayed for at least three weeks.

8.4.3. Failure with growth

This could also be mycoplasma as mycoplasma infected hybridomas tend to lose secretion (Section 5.4.3). In general, however, it tends to indicate that cloning was undertaken too late and that the primary well was already overgrown with non-secretors which are assumed to grow faster. Any positive wells should be expanded and subcloned again. If the same phenomenon occurs, i.e., clones but little antibody secretion, then the hybridoma is unstable and the operator will have to make the decision as to whether the specificity is of sufficient value to keep continually recloning the few positives in the fairly slender hope of finally obtaining stable progeny.

8.5. Continuation of cloning

Most protocols suggest that two limiting dilution subclonings are adequate to produce a fully monoclonal antibody producing hybridoma. It is, however, advisable to reclone hybridomas every six months as a matter of good routine laboratory practice. In such cloning, every well with growth should be positive and a single negative is indicative of potential instability. In particular, lines should be checked to make sure that every cell makes antibody before they are put into expensive bulk production systems.

CHAPTER 9

The use of recombinant DNA methods

9.1. Background

There are several ways in which recombinant DNA methods have been developed to improve monoclonal antibody technology. Unlike the basic fusion technique, these ways and their possible applications are all patented (Section 1.17) as they involve new methods designed to overcome problems which are sometimes only perceived but sometimes genuinely experienced in various aspects of conventional mouse Mab generation and application.

Current recombinant techniques are based on two main concepts. The first is that conventionally generated Mabs may be improved by the application of DNA technology to alter the quantity or quality of Mabs which have been initially produced by the basic rodent fusion system. The second, is that the constraints on the classical fusion system may be circumvented by bypassing the fusion process entirely and generating random genetic libraries of heavy and light chains from which a wider range of Mabs may be produced. The main applications are outlined in Table 9.1 and analysed below.

The aims of the strategies in Table 9.1 are not always readily achieved. Aim (i) is useful but not necessary for a well organised laboratory which has good practice and a wide range of storage systems (Section 5.3.3). Aim (ii) ranges from desirable to obligate in the case of chronically unstable human hybridomas and is further expanded below. Aims (iii)–(v) have been achieved and shown to be technically successful in vitro, while extrapolation to in vivo systems has had limited clinical success. The research contribution of site directed mu-

TABLE 9.1
Applications of recombinant DNA technology to Mabs*

For established hybridomas secreting valuable Mabs

(i) To have a safe store of the relevant antibody coding genes of rodent hybridomas as a contingency against liquid nitrogen failure, rampant mycoplasma infection or other unforeseen disasters.

(ii) To give more stable expression/have a safe store of the relevant antibody coding genes for human hybridomas which are frequently unstable.

(iii) To alter the constant regions of the Mab so that it can be used in another species (e.g., man) with minimal rejection.

(iv) To alter the effector functions (constant regions) of the Mab in order to map them on the antibody molecule and/or to substitute a suitable subclass for effector function.

(v) To alter the framework sites within the variable regions of a Mab, usually in conjunction with (iii) above, so that it can be used in another species with even more minimal rejection.

(vi) To alter the Complementarity Determining Regions (CDRs – the genes encoding amino acids critical in antibody binding) in the variable region of a Mab in order to improve affinity or specificity.

(vii) To produce larger amounts of Mab in novel expression systems.

To establish immortalised antibody production by new methods

(viii) Amplification of the antibody coding genes from libraries of V_H and V_L genes of spleen, blood or lymph node cells, where each contributory cell may express different variable genes each coding for a different antibody binding capacity.

* See text for further analysis.

tagenesis is considerable in aim (iv) where, for example, the precise attachment sites of Fc receptors and the C1q component of complement can be mapped (Duncan et al., 1988; Duncan and Winter, 1988).

Aim (vi) was, until recently, only represented by the serendipitous success of Roberts et al. (1987), who predicted that binding of a Mab to lysosyme would be reduced or abolished by removal of two amino acid sequences considered critical. In the event, the removal of the two critical sequences unexpectedly increased binding 8 fold. A surprising number of embryonic protein engineers quote this contrary example to promote grant applications in the area of antibody engineering. However, more recently, in the specific case of catalytic Mabs, site directed mutagenesis techniques have been successful in increasing catalytic rate (Baldwin and Schultz, 1989; Iversen et al., 1990).

Aim (vii) depends on the Mab in question being required in larger amounts at lower costs than can be generated by the many bulk tissue culture systems available (Chapter 10). The systems described to date give apparently large yields but have not been fully tested in quality control procedures.

Aim (viii), essentially a 'shotgun' approach is by far the most radical departure from classical techniques and results directly from the application of polymerase chain reaction (PCR) technology. Aims (i) to (vii) covered alterations which could improve or stabilise established Mabs. Aim (viii) seeks to establish a new method of making Mabs by immortalising the variable regions from a high proportion of the B cells in the relevant tissue from the appropriately immunised individual. It is discussed further in Section 9.6.4.3.

Extensive technical protocols on recombinant DNA technology are now available and among these, the three volume compendium of Sambrook et al. (1989) which is the the 2nd Edition of the classic Maniatis laboratory manual, is currently the accepted text. Ironically, this invaluable book carries a brief single-page protocol on lymphocyte fusion together with most of the relevant experimental protocols for the application of recombinant DNA technology, but no guide to the specific applications directed to the unique nature of antibody genes. Bothwell et al. (1990) have also published a smaller but valuable technical manual, the relevance being that these authors have been heavily involved in work with antibody genes.

9.2. Antibody genes

9.2.1. Antibody genes are different from most other genes in that they undergo a series of well regulated rearrangements to create functional genes as the B lymphocyte differentiates

The DNA in most cell types in an individual is identical and most mammalian genes in man or mouse are flanked by the same sequences in any cell in the body. The genes of the immune system are different in that they undergo comparatively local but relevant rearrangements as the cells develop from stem cells to become mature lymphocytes. The precise specificity of any monoclonal antibody is a result of a long complex in vivo selection process, well described in general (Roitt, Brostoff and Male, 1989) and specialised (Hames and Glover, 1988) immunological texts. The salient facts are expressed in Fig. 9.1. In essence, the immune system rearranges to combine three different types of segment of DNA in the case of the heavy chain, and two in the case of the light chain to give a wide variety of possible combinations of variable genes. This development is precisely regulated and firstly any one of the 12 D_H segments is recombined with any one of the four J_H segments. As a second event, this fused DJ sequence is combined with any of the 200+ V genes. In the case of the heavy chain, further diversity is provided by the addition of 'N regions' which are added in an apparently random manner on either side of the D_H sequences

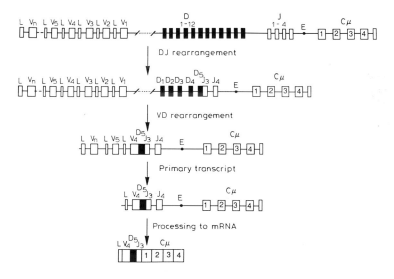

Fig. 9.1. The genetic basis of antibody heavy chain diversity in the mouse heavy chain. Note that further diversity is added during isotype switch (Figs. 4.1 and 4.2). E is the immunoglobulin heavy chain enhancer sequence.

during the the recombination process by the enzyme terminal transferase, the complementary sequence being added by the repair component of the DNA polymerase system (lacking in SCID mice – see Sections 3.6 and 4.19). The combined VDJ sequence is then transcribed into high molecular weight RNA and this is processed with any additional J sequences lying 3' to the J sequence involved in the recombination being removed along with the intron between VDJ and the constant region. As there are over 200 V_H sequences, 12 D_H sequences, 4 J_H sequences, and any number of N sequences, the potential number of heavy chain sequences is in the region of $200 \times 12 \times 4 \times$ an additional considerable unknown factor for N sequences. The potential diversity of the light chain is smaller, but still considerable. There are thought to be over 300 Vκ genes and 4 functional Jκ genes giving 1200 possible Vk genes. If any light chain can combine with any heavy chain, the combinatorial diversity of the two chains means that over 10^7 antibodies can, in principle be generated from gene rearrangement alone. Cells which have undergone successful rearrangement make IgM antibodies which are polyspecific and of low affinity but high avidity. These act as the first line of defence. If the intrusion persists through chronic or acute infection, or repeated immunisation, then they mature into IgG, IgA or (rarely) IgE secreting cells by isotype switch (Fig. 4.2).

There is a substantial 6 kb or greater intron which separates the rearranged VDJ gene from the constant gene in all antibody isotypes. Thus any strategy for cloning immunoglobulin genomic DNA must have the capacity to handle comparatively large pieces of DNA.

9.2.2. Additional variability is added during isotype switch

There is considerable, antigen driven, additional variability added as the antibody secreting cell matures, particularly as it undergoes isotype switching. This is somatic mutation in which bases in the complementarity determining regions but also in the framework regions of genomic DNA undergo point mutations which increase affinity for antigen. The mechanisms of isotype switching are covered in greater detail in Chapter 4. The somatic mutation process is random throughout the variable region and makes a nonsense of any attempt to assess the upper limit of antibody diversity. During this switch, candidate cells expressing IgM are thought either to undergo mutations which improve their affinity for antigen, in which case they are selected, or to experience mutations which fail to improve it in which case, they are not selected (Fig. 4.1). In addition, cells which bind to 'self' antigen are generally deleted.

It is worth noting that, as a result of somatic mutation, the design of suitable PCR primers (Section 9.6) for antibody gene amplification is very difficult. If they are biased towards unmutated genomic V gene sequences, they may only represent the early, low affinity, library.

9.2.3. Transcription

Transcription of the immunoglobulin heavy chain gene can occur without, but is greatly increased by, an enhancer sequence on the DNA which is situated in the intron between the J and C regions (reviewed by Atchison, 1988). This enhancer sequence is tissue specific, i.e., not activated in cell types other than B cells. There are two heavy chain enhancers, two κ light chain enhancers. The situation with the λ light chain is less clear as it is a minor locus in the mouse and a poorly characterised locus in man.

9.2.4. Translation and assembly

In the normal B lymphocyte, or myeloma cell line, several additional steps are required for antibody expression. Antibody heavy and light chains are assembled and glycosylated in a complex process specific to B cells. Correct assembly is necessary for recognition and glycosylation is necessary for various aspects of antibody function such as binding to Fc receptors.

9.3. Whether to make whole antibody, or its subfragments

Monoclonal antibody technologists work with whole antibodies. Recombinant DNA technology is better suited to fragments. As ever, the methods employed for this have to relate to the final intended use of the antibody or its fragment (Fig. 9.2; Table 9.2). The arguments for the various fragments or whole antibody are often highly conflicting and are summarised below.

(i) Whole antibody This is required for any mechanism which invokes accessory cells of the immune system in ADCC (antibody dependent

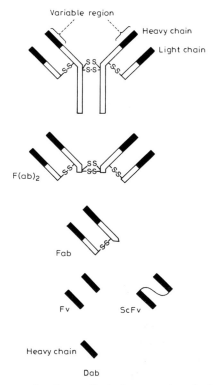

Fig. 9.2. The structure of various antibody fragments (see also Table 2.1).

TABLE 9.2
Applications of the various antibody fragments

	Whole Ab	(Fab)$_2$	Fab	Fv	dAb
Ab dependent cytotoxicity	Yes	No	No	No	No
Complement fixation	Yes	No	No	No	No
Affinity relative to whole Ab	100%	100%	1–10%	1–10%	10%*
In vivo half life** (mouse in human)	100%	10–50%	>10%	Unknown	Unknown
Best expansion vectors for genes	Bacterial	Bacterial	Bacterial	Bacterial	Bacterial
Possible expression vectors for genes	Eukaryote only	Eukaryote only	Eukaryote + bacterial	Eukaryote + bacterial	Eukaryote + bacterial

* One report only.
** For mouse Mabs in humans – there is a wide variation in biological half life for any Mab and this is only a compendium of analyses which compared fragments from the same antibody.

cell mediated cytotoxicity) which is generally considered to operate through Fc receptors, requiring no mediating molecules, or through complement mediated cytotoxicity which invokes the massive might of the cascade complement pathway. For some of these functions, it is preferable that the antibody be glycosylated normally. Both of these, and particularly the complement system can mean that the binding of a handful of antibody molecules to a much larger bacterium or eukaryotic cell, a situation analogous to the binding of barnacles to a submarine or battleship respectively, can lead to destruction of the target. In consequence, for an antibody to utilise the full destructive power of the normal biological systems which it has used throughout evolution, it should have a full constant chain region, preferably correctly glycosylated. This means that generally for in vivo use, whole antibody is preferable.

However, the very comprehensive function of whole antibody can also mean that unwanted and sometimes unexpected side effects can be encountered. There are several infectious diseases where a high serum antibody titre is known to exacerbate the condition, the most notable until recently being dengue and yellow fever viruses. It is now thought that this may also occur with HIV in certain situations (Section 1.12). Poor in vivo localisation of whole antibodies is often suggested to result from spurious binding to Fc receptors, even without such demonstrable pathogenic consequences, but this has seldom been proved and it is more likely that the antibody had a poor specificity profile to start with.

Unless one has a clear reason for using one of the antibody fragments (see below) or evidence that the enhancing effects described above are likely because of the nature of the virus and host cell, whole antibody is to be recommended. The considerable increase in avidity conferred by antibody bivalence is also a desirable feature.

(ii) F(ab)$_2$ fragments. These are not usually generated by recombinant DNA techniques. If a F(ab)$_2$ is required, it may be generated by treating the whole antibody with pepsin. This fragment will retain the advantage of the bivalence enhanced avidity and will not interact via Fc receptors. The amplification of the complement system will, however, be lost and consequently it is likely that much more F(ab)$_2$ than whole antibody will be required, mole for mole, to neutralise a virus, bacterium or affected cell. For in vivo use, it also has a shorter half life than whole antibody. It may, however, be effective to some degree with a toxin or radioisotope attached.

(iii) Fab. This fragment lacks the ability of whole antibody to kill cells by ADCC or complement, lacks the increased avidity conferred by bivalence, and has a very short half life in vivo. Positive reasons for using it which have been suggested include the fact that it may pass more readily into extravascular spaces, that it may be able to reach small holes or 'canyon sites' on viruses (although it can perform very little function when it arrives there) and that it can be generated more readily than whole antibody or other fragments in bacteria. The therapeutic use of a Fab is therefore very limited and by the barnacle on submarine analogy above, it would have to be present at high enough concentration to affect the progress or function of the submarine. On no in vivo application has a Fab been shown to outperform its parent Mab.

However, the fact that Fab can be generated by bacterial recombinant systems means that it is possible, at least in theory, to make a wide range. If the antigen is a simple one and the function of the required Mab is simple (e.g., catalysis, high-affinity binding only for biosensor construction) such that this wide range can be screened by simple methods designed for the task, Fab fragments will allow a much more comprehensive screening system to be employed. It would be quite possible to make such fragments into full antibodies using further recombinant methods should this be required later.

(iv) Fv. There is comparatively little data on Fv fragments, presumably because they cannot be assayed by the common methods, most of which involve a second antibody directed to the constant regions of the first. It is a very useful fragment for physicochemical studies such as NMR or X-ray crystallography which are suited to smaller proteins. Where these are produced in bacterial expression systems, they can be co-expressed linked by a flexible polyamino acid chain to give single-chain Fv (scFv) (Huston et al., 1988; McCafferty et al., 1990).

(v) dAb. This term (short for domain antibody) is used to describe binding molecules constructed with only the heavy chain variable domain (Ward et al., 1989). These fragments are reported to be able to bind to soluble protein antigens with moderate affinity but to tend to cross-react more readily than whole antibody (Section 9.6).

(vi) CDRs. CDR regions are the complementarity determining regions in the sequence of variable amino acids. Certain sequences in the variable region are basic to the framework of the antibody structure and vary little among antibodies directed to different antigens. The CDRs are clustered outside these essential framework regions and occur in three approximate groups on the primary sequence. Each heavy and light chain has three CDR regions and generally all six combine to form the antigen binding site. While it may therefore seem unlikely that any individual CDR could form a high-affinity interaction with antigen, they are considered to have potential in the field of rational drug design strategy and individual CDRs have been reported to show similar binding characteristics to the whole antibody from which they have been derived (Williams et al., 1989; Traub et al., 1989). In view of the fact that high-affinity binding requires most of the 6 CDR regions on a Mab (3 from each chain), it is likely that these will be required in concert.

9.4. The steps involved in cloning of antibody genes

These are shown diagrammatically in Fig. 9.3. The technical points involved in each step are discussed below.

9.4.1. The source of the cDNA or genomic DNA coding for H and L chains

The source of the cDNA is generally a hybridoma which is thought to be of value but which is unstable either in tissue culture growth or in antibody production. The functionally rearranged and somatically mu-

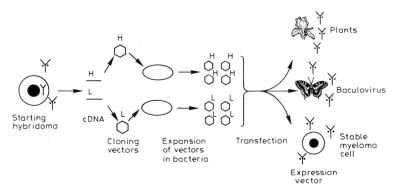

Fig. 9.3. Overall strategies for cloning and expression of antibody genes. The dot on the edge of the Mab implies glycosylation but not necessarily correct glycosylation.

tated variable genes from all hybridomas secreting any antibody of value should be stored as recombinant DNA since this removes the concerns and costs occasioned by cell storage in vulnerable liquid nitrogen.

9.4.2. Whether to clone genomic DNA or cDNA

This choice depends on two main factors:
(i) Whether PCR is to be used. Polymerase chain reaction (PCR – Section 9.6) can amplify a cDNA clone coding for an entire heavy or light chain including the constant regions. The cDNA for the heavy chain encodes around 2–3 kilobase pairs (kb), depending on antibody isotype, while the genomic DNA can encode up to 12 kb depending on the class of antibody and size of the intron between VDJ and the relevant constant reqion. In consequence, until recently, it was only possible to amplify genomic V regions, since the size of the intron between VDJ and C is such that it generally makes whole gene amplification beyond the range of current PCR technology. cDNA is a straightforward antibody coding sequence with no requirement for post transcriptional processing. It is comparatively easy to isolate.
(ii) The expression vector (Section 9.4.7). If it is to be a myeloma cell then the gene will perform best with the maximal accessory functional sequences. The use of genomic DNA means that the upstream eukaryote promoter sequence and also the enhancer sequence (Section 9.2.3) located in the intron downstream of the VDJ region are incorporated into the cloned sequence. In consequence, for myeloma cell expression systems, genomic DNA has advantages. However, the relevant enhancer and promoter sequences can be provided by the cloning vector or incorporated into the cloned gene. If the expression system is not a myeloma cell the enhancer, which is highly tissue specific, becomes irrelevant.

9.4.3. Methods of detecting antibody coding cDNA or genomic DNA

Antibody coding cDNA molecules are made from the poly(A)$^+$ cytoplasmic mRNA population utilising oligo(dT) cellulose or beads and reverse transcriptase (Sambrook et al., 1988; Bothwell et al., 1990). Full sized cDNA molecules have a predicted size range and libraries from the heavy and light chain, respectively, can be constructed and further identified with J or C region gene probes. If the class of antibody is known then it is generally the latter. It should be noted that although functionally rearranged immunoglobulin genes are encoded by only one sister chromatid, the locus on the other chromosome may also be rearranged and transcribed. Hence the presence of non-functionally rearranged sequences may complicate the detection. These will, however, usually be smaller since they generally lack the V region.

There are many published methods for making genomic DNA and several manufacturers market kits which are claimed to give high yield of good quality DNA. At the moment, these kits are quite expensive. Most established methods involve SDS and proteinase K to inactivate nucleases followed by extraction with phenol and precipitation in ethanol or isopropanol. The two main requirements are a high molecular weight product (which means that procedures should not incorporate shearing or freezing of the DNA) and a high yield. In the case of antibody genes, particularly where an unstable human hybridoma is involved, the latter is particularly important. The high salt extraction method of Miller et al. (1988) gives a good yield of high molecular weight material from a small number of lymphocytes. Genomic DNA cloning uses the fact that antibody genes rearrange so that it is possible to distinguish the functionally rearranged V gene from the other members of its family by its proximity to rearranged D or J genes. The relevant sequences of restriction nuclease digested genomic DNA can generally be identified by Southern blotting for the appropriate size differences using J region probes which will be unaltered in other cell types (e.g., liver) from the same strain of animal, but altered by the rearrangement in the hybridoma line (Fig. 9.4).

9.4.4. Manipulation of the antibody genes

The most common manipulation procedure used for antibody genes is the replacement of the rodent constant region with the human one,

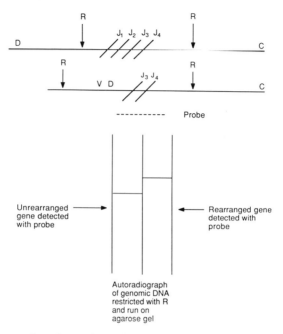

Fig. 9.4. The use of J region probes to detect rearranged genomic DNA. The restriction fragment in the rearranged gene is a different size (in this case larger) from the restriction fragment in the unrearranged gene.

or a series of human ones of different isotype (Fig. 1.7).The theoretical basis behind this concept relates to the difficulty of giving repeated doses of a mouse or rat Mab for in vivo use in any non rodent species including man. Such antibodies are frequently rejected by the human-anti mouse IgG response and their full therapeutic efficacy has therefore been impossible to evaluate (Section 1.12). The solution has been to tailor a classically generated mouse Mab so as to make it more suitable for therapy (see Morrison et al., 1988 and Shin and Morrison, 1989, for a technical description). The basic technique involves the replacement of the constant regions of the heavy and light chains of a mouse IgG Mab with the constant regions of a human myeloma protein Mab of chosen class and subclass. A variant on this involves additional replacement of the 'framework', largely invariant portions of the variable regions so that, apart from those amino acids which are intimately involved in the reaction with the antigen, the antibody is entirely human (Jones et al., 1986; Reichman et al., 1988; Junghans et al., 1990) and it is significant that the Reichman et al. (1988) found that some sequences within the 'framework' regions were also essential to establish full affinity. Since preliminary clinical studies with the more simple adaptation of using the entire mouse variable region have indicated very little rejection (Lo Buglio et al., 1989), this further sophistication may not be considered necessary. To a large extent, rejection will be dependent on whether the foreign variable sequences contain peptides which can be 'presented' to helper T cells (Chapter 4).

To date, only a handful of antibodies have been 'humanised' in this way and their long-term clinical value (Neuberger et al., 1985; Hale et al., 1988; LoBuglio et al., 1989; Hardman et al., 1989; Queen et al., 1990) remains to be evaluated. Surprisingly, some of these studies have proceeded to therapeutic trials involving large amounts of antibody with only limited characterisation of the antigen.

The large intron between the rearranged VDJ and the expressed constant region which offers a wide range of restriction sites, and each immunoglobulin constant chain is preceded by a conveniently large switch site containing many sequences suitable for restriction endonuclease digestion so that isolation of the VDJ encoding sequence becomes a comparatively simple operation.

New restriction sites, and where required, sequence alterations, can also be produced by site directed mutagenesis of the DNA. Kits for this are marketed by a wide range of firms and the technique is developing rapidly. The classical method of site directed mutagenesis requires (i) the cloning of the gene into the double-stranded form of a single-stranded bacteriophage (e.g., M13); (ii) the subsequent annealing of the single strand with a 17–20 base oligonucleotide containing the required mutation in the middle (Fig. 9.5); (iii) the subsequent extension of the mutagenic oligonucleotide by DNA polymerase to give a double-strand heteroduplex; (iv) the transfection of this heteroduplex into the appropriate E. coli host; (v) screening of the resultant

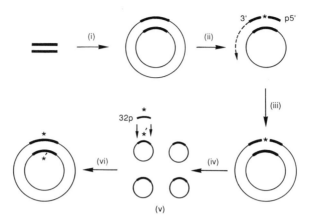

Fig. 9.5. Site directed mutagenesis. * indicates the altered sequence and *′ its complementary sequence.

bacteriophage plaques with radiolabelled probe to select the appropriate mutants; and (vi) recovery of the mutant sequences as double-stranded DNA from the intracellular replicative form of the bacteriophage.

Kunkel et al. (1987) have described a variation on this technique which greatly simplifies step (v) above. The M13 template to be used is first grown in a strain of bacteria which incorporate dUTP rather than dTTP into the single-stranded DNA, and after mutagenesis, the heteroduplex is transfected in a wild-type strain in which the uracil containing template replicates poorly. In consequence, the mutant strand, containing thymidine, is strongly selected and the majority of the plaques are positive. A more recent alternative strategy is to use smaller phagemids containing the origin of replication of the filamentous phage f1 (Stratagene). These, together with a helper phage, M13 K07, can yield single-stranded DNA from either strand for site directed mutagenesis and allow the avoidance of steps (i) and (vi) above. Finally, site directed mutagenesis can also be performed by manipulation of the PCR primers to carry the required mutation.

9.4.5. Vectors and systems for expansion of the antibody coding genes (shuttle vectors)

9.4.5.1. Choice of vector type

The vector can be either plasmid or viral. There are a wide range of commercially available plasmid vectors with the appropriate functions. Their transformation efficiency of *E. coli* is comparatively low (around 10^7 colonies/μg DNA) but if only the genes for a single antibody molecule (as opposed to a library) are being cloned, this is unimportant. Bacteriophage lambda (Section 9.6.4.3.) is used to create diverse libraries because of its high transformation efficiency (10^9 colonies/μg DNA) but requires 45–50 kb for efficient packaging. While it can be used for initial amplification of sequences in *E. coli*, it is only used for expression of antibody fragments in bacteria since the packaging requirements mean that it is not possible to achieve efficient transfection of the small percentage of antibody coding gene sequences within its genome in mammalian cells.

9.4.5.2. Necessary functions encoded by the shuttle vector

In order that an inserted antibody gene be expressed in mammalian cells, a vector requires a promoter sequence, an enhancer sequence, and a sequence to indicate poly(A) addition at the end of the transcript. In addition, as the DNA has to be propagated in a prokaryotic system in order to obtain large amounts for, say, transfection, then the relevant prokaryote sequences which facilitate such a procedure have to be incorporated in the vector. In further addition, marker genes which give selective growth advantage to only those cells which have taken up the relevant DNA are also required and these have to be put under the control of a suitable eukaryote promoter.

Figure 9.6 shows the simplest possible plasmid cloning vector for genomic DNA. It has to contain;

(a)   a bacterial origin of replication to allow the plasmid to replicate in *E. coli*.

(b)   a bacterial selection system to give selective growth advantage to the small number of bacterial host cells which have taken up the

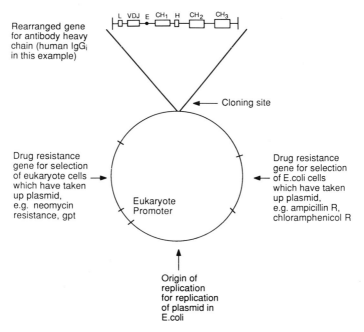

Fig. 9.6. The basic features of an antibody cloning vector for amplification in *E. coli* followed by expression in myeloma cells. In this case, the genomic DNA of the heavy chain is indicated in the cloning site.

plasmid – typically ampicillin resistance, tetracycline resistance or chloramphenicol resistance.

(c) a (usually) dominant eukaryote gene selectable marker for a gene which is transferred into the eukaryote cell along with the gene coding for antibody. This is essential as very few cells will take up the DNA and these must be identified. This is most commonly the neo R gene which can inactivate the aminoglycoside antibiotic G418, preventing it from binding to eukaryote 80S ribosomes (aminoglycoside 3′phosphotransferase, known as APH). Another well used system is the gpt gene which codes for guanine phosphoribosyl transferase. This is a bacterial enzyme similar to the eukaryote h(g)prt enzyme (Section 3.3), but with the additional ability to convert xanthine into GMP. The gene can function in eukaryote cells under the transcriptional control of an SV40 promoter. If all other routes to GMP synthesis are blocked by mycophenolic acid (MPA), then if aminopterin and adenine and xanthine are supplied, only cells which have taken up, and can express this gene will grow.

(d) a cloning site – many vectors have a wide variety of restriction nuclease sites clustered in a short region for ease of cloning of genes. This site is known as the polycloning or polylinker site.

If both expression of antibody heavy and light chains in the same cell is required (and this is usually the case), then the genes encoding light and heavy chains are generally transfected on separate vectors. While this is not essential for the bacterial propagation stage, it is easier for selection of eukaryote cells which express both chains (and both selectable markers, e.g., neo R and gpt as described above). In the baculovirus system (see below) both chains have to be in opposite orientations on the same vector.

9.4.6. Transfection procedures

While there are many reported methods for transfection such as calcium phosphate precipitation and protoplast fusion, undoubtedly the most efficient method is by electroporation. A brief electric pulse is used to make the recipient cells temporarily permeable to the DNA. The precise conditions for electroporation of myeloma cells can vary considerably from those more generally described for attached cells. Electroporation is interestingly like fusion in that one of the most important factors is to have the recipient myeloma cells in logarithmic growth.

The protocol given below should be varied where indicated in order to suit the cells used.

PROTOCOL 9.1: TRANSFECTION INTO MYELOMA CELLS

(i) Linear DNA integrates more efficiently than supercoiled DNA so it is necessary to treat the plasmid with a restriction enzyme that will cut once, but not in the immunoglobulin coding insert. About 10 μg linearised plasmid is required per electroporation. Linearise the plasmid, phenol extract, and wash in ethanol using conventional techniques. Resuspend in 1/10 TE (1 mM Tris-HCl, pH 8, 0.1 mM EDTA) at 1 mg/ml.

(ii) Grow non-secreting myeloma cells to logarithmic phase ($< 6 \times 10^5$ cells/ml) in a small plastic flask holding 7 ml of culture fluid. Harvest and wash twice with RPMI immediately before electroporation. Resuspend in RPMI at 10^6 cells/0.8 ml.

(iii) Add 5–10 μl linearised DNA to the 0.8 ml of cells, mix, transfer to a cuvette with an inter-electrode distance of 0.4 cm.

(iv) Apply electric field at 960 μF. A voltage of at least 200 V/0.4 cm will be required. This is, however, variable with cell line and may need to be optimised with several samples.

(v) Electroporation is at room temperature, there is no need for all DNA and cells to incubate before or after the pulse. Immediately after electroporation, return cells to complete medium (10% FCS) at 10^5 cells/ml and plate 100 μl into 96 well culture plates at 10^4 cells/well. Add 100 μl of selective medium after 48 h. 3–4 days later, gently remove 100 μl and feed with a further 100 μl of selective medium.

(vi) Inspect for clones after 7–14 days.

9.4.7. Expression vectors

9.4.7.1. Normal antibody gene expression

Antibody molecules undergo a complex series of steps in their final assembly within the normal B cell or myeloma cell lines. The leader sequences on the two chains are bound to a signal recognition protein which delivers them to a docking protein on the endoplasmic reticulum. Within the endoplasmic reticulum, the leader sequence is split off and the heavy and light chains are assembled together with the aid of the heavy chain binding protein, BiP, which binds to heavy chain in an ATP reversible manner, limiting its self aggregation until it can be correctly assembled to the light chain (Munro and Pelham, 1986; reviewed by Pelham, 1989). Assembly may also involve protein disulphide isomerase (Roth and Pierce, 1987). Heavy chains alone are neither expressed at the cell surface nor secreted and must acquire a light chain before they can proceed. Light chains, on the other hand, can sometimes be secreted alone.

The antibody is glycosylated within the endoplasmic reticulum to give a 'high mannose' structure which is then altered and trimmed in the Golgi apparatus (reviewed by Farquhar, 1985). Glycosylation is essential for the binding of antibody to C1q, the first component of the complement effector cascade and, while it is not clear precisely what sequence of sugars is necessary, many non-myeloma expression systems do not provide the correct sequence.

In consequence, the requirements for an expression system making whole antibody are that it assemble the heterodimer correctly, remove the leader sequences if they are present on the original construct, supply glycosylated sequences compatible with antibody function, and preferably, secrete the protein in substantial amounts. To date, few expression systems capable of all these functions have been described.

9.4.7.2. Expression in E. coli and yeast

E. coli is not a suitable host system for expression of whole antibody for reasons outlined in Section 9.5 below. It has, however, been extensively used for the expression of Fab or Fv fragments. Yeast cells have been reported to secrete whole glycosylated antibody molecules at very low levels (ng/ml) but these antibody molecules do not bind to C1q, presumably because the glycosylation pattern is inappropriate (Horwitz et al., 1988). Fab fragments can also be assembled in yeast, again at rather low yield and it is likely that the yeast modification and transport systems are different from those in a myeloma or primary B cell (Schekman, 1985).

9.4.7.3. Expression in myeloma cell lines

Successful expression to date has largely been in myeloma cell lines which are themselves non-secretors but which possess the apparatus to secrete. Early experiments involving only the heavy chain used the J558L myeloma line (Oi et al., 1983) since this is a myeloma producing light chains capable of allowing the transfected heavy chain to be transported to the cell surface. Standard fusion partners such as SP2/0 or 653 (Section 3.4) are now usually employed since it is customary to transfect both chains. Most cell lines which fuse well also transfect well and no special cell line is necessary. Recombinant antibodies or 'transfectomas' can be grown in mouse ascites without rejection. The yield in tissue culture is usually lower than the yield from a mouse hybridoma but can be up to 20 μg/ml (Shin and Morrison, 1989).

9.4.7.4. Expression in the baculovirus system

The baculovirus system is an insect system based usually on the infection of *Spodoptera frugiperda* (fall armyworm) cells with the multiple nucleocapsid polyhedrosis virus (MNPV) originally isolated from the nocturnal moth *Autographa californica*, which has the common name alfalfa looper. Other systems such as the nucleocapsid polyhedrosis virus of the silkworm *Bombyx mori* may also be used (reviewed by Miller, 1988). The basis of the system is that the polyhedrin gene, which is non-essential for the infection of cells in culture, is driven by a very strong late promoter and can be replaced by the genes encoding a foreign protein under the control of this promoter. Thus, late in infection 50–70% of the protein in the infected cell can be the foreign material. The system has the further potential for introduction into a variety of in vivo systems, most usually the larvae of the cabbage looper moth *Trichoplusia ni* to yield substantial amounts of low cost recombinant protein (Price et al., 1989) and has shown excellent results for a variety of monomeric recombinant proteins from the insect haemolymph.

Various groups have used this system to produce whole antibodies (zuPutlitz et al., 1990; Haseman and Capra, 1990). cDNA is always used as there is some doubt as to whether the insect cells can splice mammalian transcripts directly. Technically, the heavy and light chains are most readily transfected on the same vector. However, eukaryote systems do not handle dicistronic messages well and where two genes in the same orientation are introduced with two identical promoters, one or other is frequently lost due to homologous recombination. In consequence, heavy and light chains are introduced, each under the control of a separate polyhedrin promoter, but in opposite orientations. The system makes functional antibody which is glycosylated, although not trimmed by the equivalent of the processes taking place in the Golgi of normal B cells or myeloma cells (Section 9.4.6). The infected insect cells make substantial amounts of heavy and light chains and at least some of these are correctly assembled in that a positive ELISA assay with antigen is obtained. Haseman and Capra (1990) report recovery of 5 μg/ml from the insect cell culture supernatant. This is not a high yield in comparison to myeloma cells but substantially above yeast and *E. coli*. In addition, zuPulitz et al. (1990) report binding to C1q which would appear to indicate functional, albeit deviant, glycosylation.

9.4.7.5. Expression in plants

Plant cells are generally transformed by the bacterial vector *Agrobacterium tumefaciens* containing the sequences coding for the foreign protein. Hiatt et al. (1989) generated separate heavy and light chain transformant tobacco plants and then sexually crossed the two types of plant to obtain progeny which expressed both chains as 1.3% of the total leaf protein. Although the antibody was not secreted, the leader sequences were required for expression of chains either alone or together, presumably because these delivered the chains into the correct cellular compartment. The glycosylation status of such plant derived Mabs is not yet clarified.

9.5. Expression in E. coli

9.5.1. Introduction

E. coli has not been a suitable system for producing whole antibody to date. It can, however, be used to produce Fab or Fv fragments. These have severe limitations in many Mab applications (Section 9.3). The technical systems involved are reviewed by Plukthun and Skerra

(1989) and Better and Horwitz (1989). The complex system of anti-body assembly cannot be reproduced in the reducing environment of the bacterial cytoplasm and bacterial systems do not glycosylate. However, the antibody chains can be placed within a dicistronic mRNA, separated by a translational Stop sequence and then directed through the periplasmic space to secretion by the use of bacterial leader sequences such as that preceding the secreted enzyme pectate lyase (from *Erwinia cartovora*). In this process the light chain and the heavy chain fragments comprising the V_H and V_L are claimed to be able to reassemble to form an Fv while $V_H + C_H1$ and $V_L + C_L1$ regions are claimed to be able to assemble together correctly into a functional disulphide linked Fab. The yield is not high and the quoted levels of around 2 mg/l compare unfavourably with a myeloma expression system, especially in ascites, but the cost is quite low. Single chain Fv (scFv) fragments can also be produced by linking the V_H and V_L sequences with a flexible linker of 15 amino acids and an anti-digoxin Mab has been expressed in *E. coli* (Huston et al., 1988) while the scFv of an anti-lysozyme Mab has been expressed in the filamentous phage fd (McCafferty et al., 1990). There is little that the *E. coli* system can offer for bulk production of an individual Mab but it has advantages where fragments are required. Its main value may be the provision of PCR generated gene libraries (Section 9.6.4), especially if these prove to be adaptable to bacteriophage systems.

9.5.2. Sequences to be cloned

Since *E. coli* lacks the ability to assemble complex molecules such as whole antibody or $F(ab)_2$, it is essential to omit or mutate sequences which encode the disulphide bonds which cross-link the heavy chains, i.e., to cleave the sequence coding for the disulphide bonds before cysteine residues found at the hinge region around position 225 in the heavy chain. This used to be achieved by site directed mutagenesis (Section 9.4.4). The resultant amplification of the hybridised sequence gave both altered and mutant forms which had to be distinguished by hybridisation with the relevant oligonucleotide. In current times the process would be simplified by the manipulation of the PCR primers (see below).

The cloned sequences must also have a leader element which allows them to be secreted into the periplasmic space and/or the bacterial culture medium and so the leader sequence for pectate lyase (see above) is attached to both. To try and overcome the problem of differential production of heavy and light chains, heavy and light chains are frequently introduced on the same vector in the same transcriptional and translational orientation, but the two must be separated by a translational stop signal. An additional refinement is to introduce a peptide 'tag' coding sequence, usually at the end of the heavy chain which helps assay identification (Section 2.11).

9.5.3. Vectors for expression in E. coli

Essentially all that is required to amplify genes is the usual selection systems e.g. ampicillin resistance, chloramphenicol resistance, a suitable origin of replication, e.g., from pBR 322. Only if the gene is to be expressed in *E. coli*, rather than removed and put into a eukaryote system, is it necessary to have a strong promoter giving good expression. However, the final use of the Fab fragment should also be considered. Some vectors such as bacteriophage lambda will give higher transformation frequency in *E. coli* than others. Some, such as M13 or phagemids, are more suitable for sequencing (Section 9.4.5.1).

9.6. Recombinant techniques involving the use of PCR

9.6.1. Introduction to PCR

Polymerase chain reaction (PCR) has revolutionised recombinant DNA technology since its first reported use in 1985 (Saiki et al., 1985). PCR was a technique which was always conceptually possible but technically cumbersome and expensive until the discovery of the heat stable Taq (*Thermus aquaticus*) DNA polymerase, since fresh DNA polymerase had previously to be added after each heating and cooling cycle. The patent for the technique, although not all the applications of it, was originally held by the Cetus Corporation and is now held by Hoffman la Roche. A number of other (more) heat resistant DNA polymerases have come on the market since the original patent filing but it is the instrumentation that has been the focus of the Cetus patent application. The basic technique is shown in Fig. 9.7. A useful volume of practical PCR protocols has been published (Innis et al., 1990) and will doubtless be the forerunner of many others.

The essential power of the PCR technique is that it is possible to amplify any small segment of DNA (e.g., < 5 kb) if the 18–28 bp sequences at either end of the DNA sequence to be amplified are

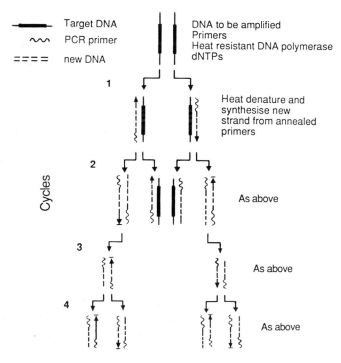

Fig. 9.7. Polymerase chain reaction. The basic concept.

known. In addition, ready changes can be made in the flanking ends of the amplified genes to introduce suitable restriction endonuclease sites without the need for the extra steps involved in site directed mutagenesis techniques.

9.6.2. General limitations of PCR

These are

(a) The size of fragment which may be expanded efficiently and accurately is currently small (>6 kb in most laboratories but increasing rapidly in size as the technology improves). This means that, for antibody genes, the technique has until recently been restricted to cDNA amplification for expressed genes or to variable region amplification in rearranged genomes. The size of the intron between VDJ and C in most hybridoma heavy chains (6–8 kb) makes amplification of large genomic DNA clones beyond this point technically more difficult.

(b) The fact that the Taq DNA polymerase has an intrinsic high error frequency means that only 30 replication cycles are currently possible before unacceptable random mutations occur and are amplified. Thus while amplification of the DNA from a single cell remains technically possible, it is a more complex process than is apparent from a single diagram. A series of 20 amplification cycles has to be followed by removal of the material for sequencing followed by further selection of unmutated sequences with a subsequent further series of 20 amplification cycles and so on. In this context, antibody genes are particularly difficult to assess, since they will be expected to contain point somatic mutations from the germline in any case and the mutations generated artificially by the PCR reaction will have to be distinguished.

(c) The purity of the reagents is important. Early PCR experiments were complicated by 'carryover' of primers from one experiment to another leading to amplification of unwanted sequences. The reagent vessels are now generally sterilised with UV light to inactivate any unwanted DNA. However, the reagents themselves, both DNA to be amplified and primers, must still be pure.

These technical difficulties are likely to be overcome as the technology develops. In particular, new thermostable DNA polymerases which are less error prone are being rapidly developed.

9.6.3. Additional problems experienced with the use of PCR and antibody genes

These all reflect the requirement for two specific 20-mer oligonucleotide primers able to anneal effectively to either end of the gene to be amplified. In the basic technique, these two sequences must be known before PCR is applied. Current methods of sequencing can be adapted to this but the requirement for a sufficient amount of cells to yield sufficient DNA to be sequenced so that the appropriate primers may be constructed remains and at least the 5' of these is likely to be specific to an individual hybridoma. This is particularly important for Mab production since somatic mutation during isotype switch (Chapter 4) can substantially alter key sequences involved in antigen binding throughout the VDJ region.

A persistent problem in PCR of antibody genes is the fact that aberrant rearrangements of the gene can occur and are often expressed as DJC segments lacking a V segment at the 5' end. This means that oligonucleotide primers directed to this area can amplify such sterile transcripts. These should be identified by their smaller size and avoided.

9.6.4. New possibilities for recombinant antibody production as a result of PCR

9.6.4.1. Cloning the cDNA or genomic DNA of an established hybridoma

For an established hybridoma which grows well enough to generate sufficient material for either cDNA cloning and sequencing, or protein sequencing, it is possible to determine the appropriate flanking sequences which can be used for the PCR induced expansion of the cDNA coding for both light and heavy chains without the need to

construct a cDNA library. Implicit in this approach is the requirement for some sort of sequence data so that although it can be demonstrated as experimentally feasible with a small number of cells, these
are generally cells from a well established and fully characterised hybridoma (Chiang et al., 1989).

A further method which has been used to amplify the receptor
genes of T cells, but not yet B cells, is 'anchored' PCR which utilises
the enzyme terminal transferase to attach a homopolymeric sequence
of G residues to the 5′ end, effectively in front of the original V region
(Fig. 9.8). The amplification primers are then a sequence of C residues
together with the specific primer in the J region of the molecule. While
this has been shown to work for T cells (Loh et al., 1989), it may be
important to remember that T cells do not undergo somatic mutation
in their J regions while B cells do.

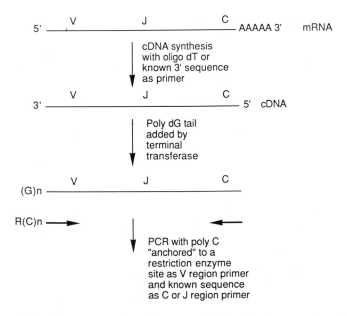

Fig. 9.8. Tailing of a sequence using polymerase chain reaction in a case where the sequence in the V region is unknown.

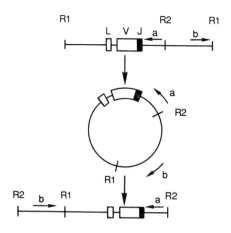

Fig. 9.9. Inverse PCR for an unknown V sequence.

In laboratories which have been able to extend the size of the amplified fragment to 5–6 kb, it is possible to use genomic DNA to amplify the variable region of an established hybridoma by the use of Inverse PCR (Fig. 9.9). This technique has considerable potential as the known constant region sequences are the only ones required for amplification (Zwickl et al., 1990).

9.6.4.2. Cloning the genes of an unstable hybridoma

A longstanding technical problem in human Mab technology which PCR can theoretically overcome is that encountered in all genuine 'human' hybridomas. PCR remains theoretically capable of amplifying the cDNA from a single cell and is practically capable of doing so within a small clone. Consequently, it has immense potential for the stabilisation of human hybridoma production which has been a major technical problem in hybridoma technology (Sections 1.9 and 3.6) for many years. Nonetheless, the relevant variable region flanking sequences must be known so that the appropriate flanking primers may be constructed and the 5' primer presents a particular problem.

While at first glance the relatively conserved leader sequence may seem to be appropriate for the 5' end primer sequence and indeed this has been used (by some groups), it is common to many other secreted proteins and not widely suitable. One possibility may be to use Kabat and Wu consensus variable region sequences (see below) for the 5′ end probes and constant region sequences for the 3′ probe only. The relevant variable region can be amplified by recombinant DNA methodology and expressed in other, more stable systems. Another is to use anchored PCR (Fig. 9.8). A third is to use inverse PCR (Fig. 9.9) on cDNA utilising a restriction site in the leader sequence together with one in the constant region. The antibody isotype carrying the appropriate constant region sequence can be determined on a single hybridoma cell by staining with isotype specific monoclonal antibodies.

9.6.4.3. PCR variable gene libraries

The construction of these involves amplification of the relevant genes from a major section of the repertoire of antibody producing cells of a (usually) immunised rodent or human by PCR and expression of the variable regions only, or variable and first constant region, in a bacterial vector system which is readily and economically screened on filters or ELISA. This type of technique dispenses with fusion procedures entirely (Fig. 9.10). The potential repertoire is considerable. A mouse spleen has 10^8 cells of which one third are B cells. Hence, if all these B cells offer a different specificity, this approach could offer an immense range. In contrast, a conventional mouse fusion will yield only 10^3 clones. Among the suggested advantages of the technique are the fact that genes which are not normally expressed because of binding to forbidden antigens such as 'self' may be immortalised (although these will only be low-affinity IgM variable regions).

Two main groups have constructed and patented such libraries. The Cambridge group (Ward et al., 1989) made M13 libraries from only the heavy chain variable sequences of genomic DNA from the spleens of immunised mice (dAbs – see Fig. 9.2). The Stratacyte group (Huse et al., 1989) used independently generated heavy and light chain variable gene libraries, also from the spleens of immunised mice to form bacteriophage lambda Fab libraries which contain the disulphide bond between heavy and light chains but stop short of the disul-

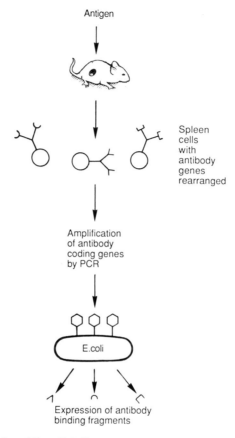

Antigen

Spleen
cells
with
antibody
genes
rearranged

Amplification
of antibody
coding genes
by PCR

E.coli

Expression of antibody
binding fragments

Fig. 9.10. Construction of Fv or Fab libraries in bacteriophage and expression in *E. coli.*

phide bond linking the heavy chains to each other. This second group have also created libraries from the peripheral blood B cells of human donors immunised with tetanus toxin (Mullinax et al., 1990). Subsequently, the Cambridge group produced scFv libraries using phage fd (Clackson et al., 1991).

While it may be immediately perceived that a library expressing both antibody chains is substantially superior to one only expressing the heavy chain, the two chain strategy has a technical complication.

Since the heavy and light chain libraries are amplified independently before recombination into Fab libraries, this means that the potential library created by the random combination is in the region of 10^{12}.

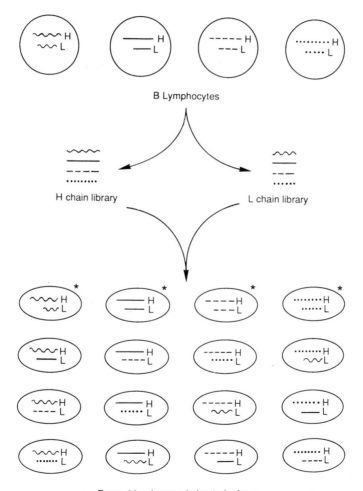

Fig. 9.11. The libraries constructed in Fig. 9.10 lead to 'scrambling' of the original Mab chains, increasing the screening load. * indicates original specificity.

However, the original heavy and light chain pairing precisely selected by antigen for each individual B cell is lost and 10^{12} clones must be screened to regain it (Fig. 9.11).

In the case of scFv dAbs, there is no constant region 'handle' for second antibody detection systems. However, for simple proteins or catalytic antibodies, these systems are probably adequate.

The amplification probes used have been the consensus sequences flanking the variable regions. These can be obtained from the extensive sequence information available in the Kabat and Wu databases. Huse et al. (1989), in generating Fab libraries, used a hinge region sequence to define the 3' end of the amplified product while Ward et al. (1989) used consensus J region sequences. In both cases, analysis of the resultant library with probes which detect variable gene 'families' suggests that the libraries cover all the main known families and therefore have the capacity to represent a considerable proportion of the repertoire, although it is difficult to estimate the extent to which the library may lack the highest affinity antibodies which have extensive somatic mutation in the variable genes.

9.6.4.4. Comparison of variable gene libraries with the conventional technique

At the moment, such techniques have several technical barriers to overcome before they replace the basic (unpatented – Section 1.17) fusion technique.

(a) The requirement for immunisation   By far the most formidable barrier is the nature of the immune system and its response to antigen. This requires an input from helper T cells in localised areas of immune tissue (Section 4.1) to achieve a high-affinity immune response. A low-affinity response, may be of limited value in a polyclonal antiserum (Section 1.5) but is of no value in a Mab which will inevitably cross-react. In consequence, such techniques can only be applied to hyper-immunised individuals, mouse or man. Unfortunately, these are the very situations in which classical techniques, even in man, can already provide high-affinity Mabs (Section 4.19). What would be of much

greater value, is a technique which could generate good Mabs without the requirement for immunisation. The SCID mouse may in due course provide such a system for both this novel approach and conventional Mab production procedures (Sections 3.6 and 4.19).

(b) Quality of library   It should be emphasised that these libraries are capable of detection of most of the known heavy chain gene 'families'. However, in essence, the PCR primers, selected as they are for consensus binding are likely to select against the highest affinity clones. It is likely that the polyspecific germ line IgM repertoire, rather than the randomly hypermutated IgG repertoire, will be selectively amplified. Even after hyperimmunisation, a large number of IgM Mabs will be produced by newly emerging lymphocytes which have encountered antigen for the first time at the final boost. In a conventional fusion, by selecting for IgG Mabs via constant region probes employed at an early stage (Chapter 2), these can be avoided.

(c) Affinity   The quality of the library also affects the affinity of the Mabs generated. The competitive filter binding methods originally used by some recombinant groups to determine 'apparent' affinity are of very limited validity in physicochemical terms (Section 11.6.2) as the molar concentration of binding fragment is unknown. It is technically quite simple to determine true affinity for the soluble protein antigens used in these PCR techniques (Section 11.6.3), and it is likely that this situation will soon be further clarified. At the moment, the preliminary data of Ward et al. (1989) and Clackson et al. (1991) using true affinity methods for a limited number of dAbs suggest medium range affinity values are adequate for physicochemical studies with pure antigen but capable of cross-reaction with contaminants when the antigen is a small component of the mixture.

(d) Screening methodology   Insofar as the screening systems rely on blotting or ELISA (Chapter 2) the technique cannot readily be adapted to generate antibodies to complex native antigens such as cell membrane proteins and so would appear to have limited potential for

the production of therapeutic Mabs or diagnostic Mabs to cell surface antigens which are generally selected by FACS or similar methods. Most of these, at the screening stage, involve a second antibody which cannot detect Dabs or Fvs since they have no constant region (Fig. 9.2). This problem could probably be overcome by new technology. At the moment, it is difficult to screen a conventional fusion with up to 10^3 clones by such a system. The barrier of expense in personnel hours and reagents for screening 10^8 to 10^{12} is formidable. The screening systems involved present a daunting challenge for scientists working with any but the most simple antigens. Comparatively few new commercially relevant antibodies can be detected on nitrocellulose filter blotting assays. Pooling screening strategies and/or more sophisticated assay systems would need to be developed.

(e) Fragment of antibody produced It is necessary in such a technique to express the antibody genes in *E. coli* and consequently whole antibody molecules cannot be generated (Section 9.5). This problem could be overcome by splicing on the appropriate constant regions at a later stage.

The main advantage of variable PCR libraries over conventional assays would appear to lie in areas such as catalytic Mabs where the main technical problem is that while many Mabs bind 'transition state intermediate' (Section 1.14), few of these catalyse the required reaction and screening by binding yields only a small proportion of catalytic Mabs. Logically, if only one Mab out of 50 which bind the intermediate is capable of catalysis, 100 out of 5000 will be able to do so and exponents of this technique emphasise extrapolations of this type. Most other applications of Mabs require high-affinity binding. In the unique case of catalytic Mabs, ability to catalyse a reaction may be more important than affinity (Benkovic et al., 1990).

9.7. Where recombinant DNA technology will be of value

In such a fast moving field it is difficult to predict future trends. The greatest potential of recombinant DNA technology seems in early 1991, to be in the production of 'genuine' human hybridomas from individuals who have a proven clinical response as a result of exposure to an antigen to which normal individuals cannot legally, ethically, or above all technically be exposed, e.g. mature IgG responses in tumour draining lymph nodes or mature IgG rheumatoid factors in joints. This is because these are areas refractive to the established non-patented technology. Many other uses seem to appear to be a technique looking for an application rather than a biological problem looking for a solution. However, the same could also have been said of conventional hybridoma technology in the mid-1970s.

CHAPTER 10

Antibody production and purification

10.1. Maintenance of cell stocks

At least 10 vials of healthy, mycoplasma free hybridoma should be laid down in liquid nitrogen as soon as it is established by a minimum of two clonings. Cells should be frozen from logarithmic culture, as with cells for fusion. Only a small percentage of cells recover from liquid nitrogen freezing and these are believed to be the cells which have been in the early stages of division. A culture destined for freezing should be subcloned 24 hours before (Chapter 5). Every 6 months, a vial of cells should be recovered and checked for viability. The quality of liquid nitrogen storage is surprisingly variable (Chapter 5).

A valuable hybridoma should be stored in at least two and preferably three different locations in case the primary source fails. The cells in these 'backup' locations should be checked every 6 months in the same manner as the cells in the primary source.

If the stocks in liquid nitrogen are running low, then one vial should be brought up into tissue culture in rich medium, propagated under conditions of exponential growth, and returned as several vials to liquid nitrogen.

If the hybridoma is of definite value, the genes should be cloned and stored as DNA, dry and less vulnerable to any tissue culture or nitrogen failure.

10.2. Expansion of hybridomas on a laboratory scale (1–20 mg Ab)

10.2.1. Introduction

Expansion is a different procedure from regular culture of hybridomas and no account should a cell population being expanded be regarded as the main stock for future work as this latter should be in liquid nitrogen. If the correct assay methods have been used, then all hybridomas produced may have potential use. However, a large number of clones from a single fusion may generate antibody directed to the same epitope and it is likely that only one or two clones secreting antibody of highest affinity and directed to the correct epitope will be required. In consequence, it is necessary to grow up enough of each stock of hybridoma to be able to characterise it further. For this task only 1–2 mg are required.

10.2.2. Expansion in vitro for preliminary characterisation (1–2 mg)

Expansion in vitro is a generally better system than the in vivo system described in Section 10.4, as it provides a more pure preparation of antibody. The only IgG contaminants are from the FCS which should not, in theory contain any antibody (but poor preparations can contain up to 1.3 mg/ml of bovine immunoglobulin (Underwood et al., 1983 – see Section 5.2.2) with no contaminating rat or mouse immunoglobulin which can make complicate purification from ascites fluid. Contamination may be further reduced by the use of the large range of serum free media available on the market which also contain protein but defined amounts of defined proteins which can be readily removed (Section 5.2.4).

In vitro, there are two strategies. Both assume that the cells destined for bulk production should be regarded as terminal and that the relevant clones are in the liquid nitrogen bank. Both also are based on the fact that cells in logarithmic growth do not make a lot of antibody while cells which have completed growth and are essentially terminal make and secrete 2–10 fold more antibody.

(i) A most effective approach for maximising antibody yield from a small flask is therefore to grow cells in 20% FCS in a small flask maintaining them at 10^5/ml or lower and then transfer them into medium alone, serum free medium or medium with < 1% FCS. The cells change from growth and division to antibody secretion and the yield of antibody can be up to 2 mg – more than enough for preliminary characterisation.

(ii) The alternative approach is based on the notion that cells must be 'adapted' to lower levels of FCS. They are given gradual expansion from 96 well cloning plates to 24 well tissue culture plates, to 25 cm^2 small culture flasks, 80 cm^2 medium culture flasks and 175 cm^2 large culture flasks with the cell density growing through the range of 10^5 to 10^6/ml at each stage. During this process, the FCS concentration is reduced to < 5% or the cells are introduced to serum free medium. Only after such expansion is the culture grown to exhaustion. The final yield is comparable to the first method (1–2 mg) but at much greater cost and effort, especially if several hybridomas at once are to be cloned.

Human hybridomas, as usual, are more difficult and require more precise schedules. For example strategy (i) will work well for a human mouse hybridoma but not a human EBV transformant. Serum free medium is particularly desirable for human Mabs destined for potential therapeutic use.

10.3. Expansion in vitro for more extensive characterisation

A wide variety of devices and systems are now available to increase antibody production to larger quantities. These can include a wide size range of 'spinner' flasks which have a central stirring arm and permit addition of medium or removal of cells by the side arm, and gassed roller bottles which are an inexpensive system for laboratories equipped with 37°C rooms. It is also possible simply to grow cells to exhaustion in large plastic culture flasks as described in Section 10.2.1.

Industrial scale culture may be required for antibodies which have wide diagnostic or therapeutic use and here the considerations are largely economic to balance yield against quality and cost. It is necessary to ask not only how much antibody the system can generate at a specific cost, but also what subsequent costs will be incurred by purification from other components of the generating system, whether the antibody will be correctly processed for function (for example, if it is glycosylated by the expansion system, is it correctly glycosylated?), and whether steps will be necessary to remove or inactivate transforming viral genomes which may contaminate the material. Among the large scale culture systems used have been hollow fibre reactors (Altschuler et al., 1986), large fermentors (Birch et al., 1985), and microencapsulation (Duff et al., 1985).

Genetic methods in prokaryotes or yeast have to date been largely unsuccessful in producing substantial quantities of correctly assembled Mabs and new recombinant DNA systems involving insects (Zu Pulitz et al., 1990, Haseman and Capra, 1990) or plants (Hiatt et al., 1989), are not yet fully evaluated (Sections 9.7.4 and 9.7.5).

10.4. Expansion of hybridomas in vivo

Expansion of a tumour cell line such as a myeloma in any animal is becoming increasingly less acceptable to governments under pressure from environmentalists and animal rights campaigners. In many countries licences are only issued for this work to experienced operators and under rigorous conditions. All animals used for ascites should be sacrificed before they are distressed. The environmental move away from ascites fluid is assisted by the fact that it yields commercially unsuitable antibody (see below).

10.4.1. Expansion in mice

Mice primed intraperitoneally with mineral oils tend to become susceptible to the development of Mineral Oil induced PlasmaCytomas

(MOPCs). The Balb/c line is particularly susceptible and it is by this method that the original P3K line (Section 3.4) was produced. The main active ingredient in such mineral oils is pristane (2,6,10,14 tetramethyl pentadecane) which has been shown to operate by depressing the normal immune function of the mouse so that internally produced or injected myeloma cells are able to grow without rejection (Freund and Blair, 1982).

Ascites fluid obtained from the peritoneal cavity of tumour cell injected mice or rats, is generally very like serum. It has irrelevant immunoglobulins, complement components, albumin and all the enzymes of the blood clotting cascade so that, if the cells are required, it must be collected, like blood, in anticoagulants. In consequence, ascites products should not to be regarded as a bag of pure antibody. While the fluid can contain very large amounts of specific antibody (10–20 mg/ml) at little effort and cost in comparison to tissue culture systems, this antibody is contaminated with irrelevant mouse IgG which is difficult to remove without antigen based affinity purification – a procedure suitable for simple protein antigens or haptens but unsuitable for more complex antigens. The distinction is important as, whereas in the in vitro system it is sufficent to demonstrate an SDS PAGE gel of pure IgG H and L chains in comparison to culture medium, in the ascites system, it is necessary to prove that these H and L chains are directed to antigen since normal mouse peritoneal fluid also has IgG.

Ascites fluid also has an important function in clearing infections from hybridomas (Section 5.4).

It is obviously necessary to use mice which are histocompatible to the hybridoma. In the normal event, these will be Balb/c. If a different strain of mouse has been used to elicit a better antibody response for the initial fusion, then an f 1 hybrid of Balb/c and the mouse used (Chapter 4). A pure Balb/c hybridoma, on the other hand, can be propagated in hybrid mice of any f 1 strain of which one parent is Balb/c and it has been suggested that better yields are obtained from certain of such hybrid strains than from the parent Balb/c (Stewart et al., 1989).

As in all expansion systems, success depends on the injected cells being in logarithmic growth.

PROTOCOL 10.1: PRODUCTION OF MABS IN MOUSE ASCITES

(i) Using a 21G needle, inject 0.5 ml pristane into the peritoneal cavity of 4 or more Balb/c mice, 1–4 months old, either sex. You will inject these with the hybridoma 10–20 days later. Do not keep mice beyond 30 days as they will be vulnerable to spontaneous (irrelevant) myeloma generation.

Most laboratories keep a continuous small supply of pristane primed mice ready and inject a few each week so inject a second set of 4 for potential further passaging after 7 days, 14 days etc. In effect, set aside an hour at a definite time each week for ascites work.

(ii) Grow the hybridoma in culture in 10–20% FCS to the point where you have $1-5 \times 10^6$ cells in logarithmic growth. (Proportionally more for more than 4 mice.)

(iii) When they are growing well, and within the 10–20 day time period for a group of available mice, harvest the cells and wash them thoroughly but speedily in RPMI at least 5 times. They will be heavily coated with BSA from the FCS and you will elicit a polyclonal response to BSA if you fail to remove this. Resuspend in 2 ml PBS (or RPMI) (more for more than 4 mice).

(iv) Using a 21G needle, inject each mouse intraperitoneally with 0.5 ml ($0.25-1.25 \times 10^6$ hybridoma cells). Obtain or prepare sterile capped 5–10 ml tubes coated with or containing anticoagulants such as heparin or EDTA. These are routine in hospital laboratories.

(v) Monitor the mice closely from 7–14 days post injection. Ascites tumours grow fast and the mice should be inspected every day. There are 3 possible outcomes – no growth, solid tumour growth, or free growing ascites. A solid tumour is visible as a localised bulge and a free growing tumour visualised by gross and mobile distension of the peritoneal cavity.

(vi) A solid tumour can only be obtained by killing the mouse. Many hybridomas form solid tumours at first passage but grow freely at second passage. The solid tumour is almost invariably associated with the mesenteric lymph nodes in the gut (Appendix 1) and can be removed and 'spilled' with a scalpel blade (do not puncture the gut) for immediate re-injection into a further group of pristane primed mice. The second time, it generally grows freely.

Free growing tumours can be obtained either by killing the mouse and extracting the hybridoma + antibody containing fluid into a heparinised tube or by 'tapping' the mouse, i.e., inserting a 21 or 18 G needle, draining the fluid into a heparinised tube leaving the mouse alive for more fluid to build up for subsequent 'tapping'. Most scientists prefer not to do this and, in the U.K., few have government licences to cover such a procedure.

(vii) Centrifuge the ascites fluid, store the supernatant in aliquots, assaying a portion and process the cells as in (viii).

(viii) Tumours from ascites bearing mice whether solid or free growing can be propagated again in culture but usually re-adapt slowly. Either type of tumour yields large numbers of cells and these should be (a) reinjected into a second set of mice, (b) frozen, and (c) regrown in culture.

10.4.2. Failure of in vivo expansion in mice

There are seldom any problems for an experienced laboratory to expand its own hybridomas in ascites. Most problems relate to hybridomas obtained from other laboratories.

10.4.2.1. Failure to grow
This is due to:

(i) The hybridoma being of incompatible origin, i.e., rat or non-Balb/c and this information not being correctly transmitted with the cell line.

(ii) Insufficient hybridoma cells of good health and in logarithmic expansion being injected.

However, if a persistent failure of a hybridoma to grow in ascites is experienced and the cell line is definitely from original Balb/c mice, it is possible to use f1 hybrids of Balb/c with another strain.

10.4.2.2. Growth but failure to secrete required antibody

This is due to:

(i) The hybridoma having been obtained from elsewhere and being used on a new assay system outwith its original selection system (Chapter 2)

(ii) The hybridoma being unstable at the start.

(iii) The hybridoma having been heavily infected with mycoplasma so that it has ceased to secrete (Section 5.4).

10.4.3. In vivo expansion in the rat

Rat hybridomas yield > 50 ml ascites fluid at 10–20 mg/ml and can therefore provide an impressive amount of antibody. As with the mouse, this is inevitably contaminated with irrelevant rat IgG. Unlike the MOPC induced mouse plasmacytomas, the original Lou/C rat hybridoma occurred spontaneously and one can readily produce rat hybridomas without any form of pre-priming of the animals. Also unlike the mouse, every rat injected with the hybridoma generates ascites growth both in solid and free floating form. The tumours tend to invade the liver and the rats are clearly distressed long before they are distended.

Bazin's group have suggested that production can be further enhanced by the use of pristane or complete Freunds adjuvant (Kints et al., 1989). Given that the unprimed animal responds well and that the procedure is already traumatic to the animals, this additional treatment would appear to be superfluous.

10.4.4. Expansion of human hybridomas in animals

'Transfectomas' producing 'humanised' recombinant chimaeric Mabs (Sections 1.9 and 9.4) can be produced in ascites fluid normally provided that the strain of mouse is compatible with the cell line used for expression. The fact that the antibody itself is foreign to the mouse is overcome by the rate of growth of the cells. In addition, the occasional stable heterohybridoma (from human cells fused with mouse human hybrids) has been reported to be capable of growth in the parent mouse strain, although there are few recent confirmations of early reports.

'Genuine' human hybridomas can be occasionally grown in selected strains of mice which are naturally immunodeficient or in more widely used strains of mice which can be made immunodeficient by radiation (400 rad). The nude mouse has little hair, but its relevance to immunology is that it also has no thymus. It therefore lacks the ability to educate both cytotoxic and helper T cells to recognise 'self' antigens as opposed to foreign antigens and abrogates the ability of the latter group to give lymphokines as 'help' to emerging B cells. These mice are reported to have a normal B cell response but this is almost certainly low grade IgM. The reported Natural Killer (NK) cell response is also probably polyspecific.

The SCID mouse lacks ability to repair DNA (Fulop and Phillips, 1990) and in consequence cannot supply the repair systems necessary for the production of N regions in immunoglobulin heavy chains (Section 9.2). Since these systems are also required for diversity generation in T cell receptors, the technical result is an immunodeficient mouse.

Colonies of either mouse are obviously very difficult and costly to maintain since they are highly vulnerable to environmental pathogens. Neither have yet produced useful amounts of a relevant human Mab and they compare poorly with in vitro bulk culture systems.

10.5. Storage of Mabs

10.5.1. Stability checks

All clone supernatants should be tested at an early stage by taking three aliquots, heating one to 50°C for 3 minutes, freezing and thawing another and keeping the third as control. The three aliquots are then assayed together to check that the antibody has a suitable stability for handling. Most antibodies are extensively disulphide bonded and survive in the mammalian body at 37°C for periods of days or weeks. They are also usually resistant to heating at much higher temperatures for short periods of time and ascitic fluid or serum is often heated to 57°C for 3–5 min to destroy proteolytic enzyme activity with very little effect on antibody titre. As with all other applications of Mabs, the occasional one may be unstable and prove either heat sensitive or sensitive to freezing and thawing. In either case it is unlikely to be a useful antibody and, unless it appears to have a singularly unique specificity, it is better to leave it and concentrate on other clones.

10.5.2. Storage and transport of Mabs

10.5.2.1. General storage

The method of storage depends on how and when the stored material is going to be used. If the antibody has been obtained as a sterile sample from tissue culture or from ascites fluid, there is obviously little chance of bacterial contamination and for short periods of time the culture supernatant can simply be stored at 4°C. If it is being stored for longer periods of time, it is usually frozen at −20°C, in suitably sized aliquots for use on thawing. Despite the fact that most Mabs are stable, it is better not to freeze and thaw them too often.

Some protocols recommend the use of low levels of sodium azide (0.01%) to stop bacterial growth and many commercial solutions of antibody will contain azide. If the sampling has been sterile, azide should not be necessary. It is also a serious problem if the Mabs are to be used in any assay involving enzymes such as horseradish peroxidase or for 'panning' of live cells. The last traces of azide are very difficult to remove.

Antibodies can be lyophilised but this leads to a strong tendency to aggregate, particularly in the case of IgG Mabs and should be avoided where possible.

IgM Mabs, with their more complex structure, usually store less well than IgG Mabs and are less stable to heat or freezing and thawing. However, as has been emphasised throughout this book, this class of Mab is best avoided.

10.5.2.2. Specific storage problems with ascites fluid

Ascites fluid can be contaminated with proteases and nucleases (the latter being less important). Most proteolytic activity can be removed by heating at 60°C for 3 minutes without damaging the antibody and this is in any case a good test for an antibody to be used in extreme field conditions. A small pilot heating experiment should be undertaken. If the antibody is heat sensitive but still valuable, protease inhibitors may be added. However, protease inhibitors do not cover the full range of serum protease activity and many such as PMSF are highly toxic so that a better strategy is to purify immediately or freeze and purify immediately after thawing.

10.5.3. Transport of Mabs and hybridomas

Mabs can be sent as sterile tissue culture supernatant in a small flask or universal container, wrapped in bubble plastic in a padded Jiffy bag to minimise the chance of breakage in the mail. This is also the most convenient method for international transfer. The customs laws in the U.S.A. are very strict with respect to the import of any antibody or cell which has been grown in FCS because of foot and mouth disease regulations and it is usually necessary to obtain an import certificate certifying the health of the FCS.

Mabs can also be sent frozen packed in dry ice but this makes for a much bulkier parcel, difficult to transport by air.

Hybridomas can be transported by taking a culture in logarithmic growth in a small plastic flask and filling this flask to the top with complete medium to minimise gas exchange. They can then be sent in padded containers by first class mail or special mail services, or carried in the pocket on an aircraft and will usually grow again after 3–4 days in the mail. While most airlines X-ray hand baggage, the dose is not sufficient to damage the cells.

One of the most convenient methods of transferring hybridomas between labs in the one country is to transport them in newly inoculated ascites mice. Animal import restrictions make this a less convenient method for moving between many countries.

10.6. Purification of Mabs

10.6.1. Introduction

Most main methods for Mab purification have been developed by commercial firms to encompass purification of large amounts of Mabs with a single method. At production level, a single step process is perceived to be more economical than a process requiring two or more steps. The approaches for pilot and large scale production are different (for example ammonium sulphate precipitation on a bulk culture would incur unacceptable expense).

For routine laboratory use there is no need to purify a Mab and each batch can be titred and used directly. However, most sophisticated uses of Mabs require that they be purified. Obviously extensive purification is required for all therapeutic uses but in addition, a pure Mab is a standard reagent whereas a tissue culture supernatant is not. Many of the more complex immunosensor systems (Chapter 12) require that the Mab be linked directly to a detecting agent such as an enzyme or fluorescent label and obviously this requires pure Mab to start with.

Commercial literature frequently suggests that Mabs can readily be classified for purification and that, for example, one single method will suit all mouse IgG1 Mabs. Unfortunately this is frequently not the case and our own laboratory has found it necessary sometimes to use completely different techniques to purify two different Mabs of the same class directed against the same antigen. The variable region has a substantial contribution to the overall charge of the protein and can therefore influence strategy. Nonetheless, it can be useful to have a knowledge of class and subclass (Chapter 11) before commencing purification.

10.6.2. Main likely contaminants

The main contaminants of any Mab grown in culture are likely to be from the FCS and will be largely bovine serum proteins, the most dominant being bovine albumin. If the culture was grown in 10% FCS, there may be up to 4 mg/ml albumin and only 100 μg/ml of the required Mab (less if it is a human hybridoma). FCS can also contain some bovine IgG which is more difficult to purify from the antibody. If the Mab has been grown in serum free medium (Chapter 5), then it is more readily purified.

The main contaminants in ascites fluid are mouse serum proteins including substantial amounts of mouse albumin. The most difficult contaminant to remove is irrelevant mouse IgG.

Immunoglobulin purification is extensively covered in many standard texts (Weir et al., 1986; Johnstone and Thorpe, 1987; Harlow and Lane, 1988). For any single Mab, a series of pilot systems should be run and the best of these can be combined in the final schedule. A general strategy which uses the simplest and most economical methods first is given in Table 10.1.

10.6.3. Concentration with ammonium sulphate or caprylic acid

Ammonium sulphate precipitation is a classic method for subfractionating serum proteins. While it may give slight purification, it is really mainly a method for concentrating antibody. It is convenient for reducing the Mab in a comparatively large volume of tissue culture supernatant to a much smaller volume which is more suitable for application to a column and removes some of the albumin. High-grade

TABLE 10.1
Strategy for purifying a Mab – in order of approach

First step: Concentrate with ammonium sulphate (optionally + caprylic acid) (Protocols 10.2 and 10.3). This will give concentrated and partially purified antibody.
Second step: Purify on DEAE, or Mono Q if you have FPLC (Protocol 10.4). This may give pure antibody.
Third step: Purify on protein A or protein G (Protocol 10.5). By this stage the antibody should be pure.
Fourth step: Purify by affinity chromatography (Protocol 10.6).

Note: 'Pure' implies a relative standard. If only antibody is visible on a silver stained polyacrylamide gel, then it is suitable for diagnostic use. For clinical use it must be shown to be free of pyogens and viruses and subjected to extensive testing.

AnalaR ammonium sulphate should be used as the lower grade material as it is frequently contaminated with heavy metal ions.

PROTOCOL 10.2: PRECIPITATION WITH AMMONIUM SULPHATE

(i) The simplest method is to prepare a 100% saturated (> 770 g/l) ammonium sulphate solution at pH 7. The solution will take some time to dissolve and should be stirred for several hours before use.

(ii) Do not use all the sample but keep a small amount aside for a comparative study. For a pilot study, 10 ml saturated ammonium sulphate are added to 10 ml tissue culture supernatant or ascites fluid very slowly with vigorous stirring. Stir for at least 2 hours at 4°C. A clear white precipitate should form.

(iii) Centrifuge at $3000 \times g$ for 30 min in toughened glass centrifuge tubes. Decant the supernatant into a flask and resuspend the pellet in one tenth of the original volume (1 ml). Dialyse this overnight in small bore dialysis tubing against three changes of PBS. The volume will increase dramatically and should be measured at the end of the dialysis. A sample of the supernatant should also be dialysed against the PBS in small bore dialysis tubing overnight.

(iv) The next day measure the increased volume of the two ammonium sulphate prepared samples and the absorbance at 280 nm (a 1 mg/ml solution of most IgG antibodies gives an absorbance of 1.35 at 280 nm against the appropriate reference solution). Perform an assay for antibody activity using these two samples and the original sample, taking account of the volume increase to find if the antibody has definitely been concentrated.

There are various possible outcomes:

(a) All the antibody binding activity will be in the pellet fraction and none in the supernatant in which case one can either proceed to scale up the purification or do a second pilot run to see whether all the antibody also precipitates at the lower level of 40% saturation, excluding more albumin.

(b) Substantial amounts of antibody remain in the supernatant in which case a second pilot run should be performed at 60% saturation. If most of the antibody activity remains in the pellet then only the protein which precipitates between 50 and 60% may be used.

(c) Both ammonium sulphate fractions show a lower titre in relation to the amount of antibody protein than the original. The usual reason for this is too short a dialysis time. However, if it persists with longer dialysis, ammonium sulphate fractionation is unsuitable for that Mab. Fortunately, this is rare.

Caprylic (octanoic) acid precipitates most other serum proteins at pH 4 but leaves most IgG antibodies in solution (Russ et al., 1983). It dilutes the Mab somewhat but it can then be concentrated by ammonium sulphate, free of most other serum proteins. The method works more frequently with ascites than with tissue culture supernatant (McKinney and Parkinson, 1987).

PROTOCOL 10.3: PRECIPITATION OF CONTAMINATING PROTEINS WITH CAPRYLIC ACID

(i) Obtain high-grade AnalaR caprylic acid.

(ii) As in protocol 10.2, keep a sample of Mab from the same batch for comparative assay. To 10 ml of ascites fluid or tissue culture supernatant add 30 ml 60 mM Na acetate, pH 4. The final pH should be 4.5.

(iii) Add 0.4 ml caprylic acid dropwise slowly with stirring and leave stirring for 1 hour. Centrifuge at $5000 \times g$ for 15 minutes.

(iv) Decant the supernatant and dialyse in small bore tubing overnight against PBS with three changes. Note the volume.

(v) Redissolve the pellet in 2 ml PBS and also dialyse overnight (this may not dissolve too readily).

(vi) The next day, measure the absorbance of all three samples at 280 nm (a 1 mg/ml solution of most IgG antibodies gives an absorbance of 1.35 at 280 nm against the appropriate reference solution) and assay both fractions alongside the original sample, taking into account the volume changes and assess the extent to which the antibody has remained in the supernatant.

(vii) Concentrate the antibody in the supernatant by ammonium sulphate precipitation (Protocol 10.2).

10.6.4. Mab chromatography

10.6.4.1. Mab purification kits

These are offered by all the main chromatography firms (Pharmacia, BioRad and others). In many cases they may work well although at some expense. However, they are based on the concept that the constant region alone dictates the relevant properties of an antibody for purification purposes and all too often they do not have the predicted results for a selected individual Mab. The variable region of an antibody contributes around one quarter of the protein and this can significantly affect the behaviour of any Mab on purification, and in consequence, such 'kits' only reflect the behaviour of a small number of antibodies of any species and class.

10.6.4.2. Chromatography matrices

Many ligands which preferentially bind antibody, or which preferentially bind major contaminants can be obtained attached to a variety of solid matrices including Sepharose, agarose, and acrylic beads. Cellulose is seldom now used as a matrix as it is susceptible to volume changes which alter column packing. Some of the matrices, notably agarose, Sepharose or the older Sephadex based matrices confer the original advantages of size differentiation for which they were developed. Acrylic based matrices are superior for their their physical stability and resistance to pressure on HPLC and FPLC. Large proteins are excluded from a beaded or cross-linked structure and eluted in advance of small proteins. This application is restricted to matrices with defined pore size. In the case of Mab production, the 150 kDa Mab will elute ahead of the major contaminant which is the 65 kDa BSA but only when the correct size defining matrix is used. Within the Pharmacia range, this is Sepharose CL-4B which separates molecules within the range of 30 kDa to 500 kDa or Sephacryl S-300 which separates molecules within the range 50 kDa to 1000 kDa. To a large extent attempts to separate by size alone are restricted to final purification. The method of choice should involve a fast flowing readily packed matrix containing the maximal number of antibody binding sites/ ml. It should also be economical to purchase and regenerate.

Superose 12 is a gel filtration medium designed for use with FPLC consisting of beaded cross-linked agarose prepacked in a reusable column. Obviously a laboratory with access to FPLC may prefer to use this as as several samples can be analysed at high resolution in a short period of time. The usefulness of FPLC is greatly enhanced by the availability of new FPLC columns with affinity matrices such as protein A – Sepharose 12.

10.6.4.3. *Fast protein liquid chromatography (FPLC)*

FPLC is the method of choice for antibody pilot purification. The prepacked columns are precisely defined for performance. Most FPLC instruments have a direct readout for absorbance at 280 nm and any individual Mab can be purified in 5–20 minutes on the correct matrix. It has limitations for large scale production. Simple pilot experiments can also lead to an indication as to how to best purify a Mab and give equally useful indications as to the method of large scale production.

10.6.5. *Purification with DEAE linked reagents*

DiEthylAminoEthyl cellulose has been used for many years in the purification of polyclonal IgG from serum. More recently it has been used attached to fast flow matrices such as Sephadex, Sepharose or acrylamide bead (see above). Additionally, QAE compounds with a higher density of positive groups have become available attached to similar matrices. In the case of laboratories with FPLC equipment, sealed columns containing similar matrices (Mono Q columns) are now frequently used.

The background to the basis for using positively charged matrices is that most IgG molecules have a comparatively low proportion of basic amino acids on the constant region. As a consequence, most IgG Mabs have poor binding to DEAE groups at low pH and ionic strength values whereas other serum proteins, and in particular albumin from most species, bind strongly. As bovine or rodent albumin is the main protein contaminant in most Mab preparations, this is a useful method. IgG Mabs either do not bind at all, or are recovered in the front fractions from a gentle gradient of increasing salt concentration.

While protein A has subclass specificity in its recognition, DEAE binding relates only to basic amino acid residues and there is less species and subclass variation. However, monoclonal antibodies can be very individual in their ability to bind DEAE and of any two from the same species and of the same class directed to similar antigens, one may elute rapidly from the column leaving all other material behind, and the other may elute slowly with increasing gradient and still have some contamination from other proteins.

The main advantages of DEAE over protein A is that extremes of pH are not necessary for purification as an ionic strength gradient rather than a pH gradient is used, that with all but the most maverick of Mabs, it removes the bulk of the albumin, and that it is a low cost procedure.

PROTOCOL 10.4: PILOT PURIFICATION ON MONO-Q OR DEAE

(A) FPLC on a Mono-Q Column
(i) Prepare 500 ml each of 0.1 M potassium phosphate buffer, pH 6.5 (A) and 0.4 M potassium phosphate buffer, pH 6.5 (B). Equilibrate column at the lower ionic strength.
(ii) Dilute ascites or culture fluid 1 in 10 with buffer A and filter sample through 0.45 μ filter. Alternatively, for low titre antibody, dialyse into buffer A. Filter through 0.45 μ filter.
(iii) Inject 100 μl of sample and elute at 2 ml/min with gradient of buffer A increasing to 100% buffer B. Collect 0.5 ml samples and measure ELISA activity of first peak and subsequent peaks.

(B) Simple laboratory DEAE-Sephacel purification of Mabs
(i) Pour an 8 ml column of DEAE-Sephacel (Pharmacia) into a small chromatography column (e.g., Pharmacia C10/10) or the barrel of an 8 ml pipette plugged with a glass wool filter and equilibrate with 50

mM phosphate buffer, pH 6.8. This will bind >1 g of albumin, the major contaminant of most Mab preparations.

(ii) The test sample used should have an assay titre of at least 1 in 100 and be dialysed into 50 mM sodium phosphate, pH 6.8. It should contain no more than 1 mg albumin (10% FCS has around 4 mg albumin/ml). The most usual application is to use dialysed ammonium sulphate concentrated material (Protocol 10.2).

(iii) Add 1 ml of sample to the column and allow it to flow in, washing with 50 mM Na phosphate buffer. Collect 0.5 ml fractions. Most IgG Mabs will not bind and be immediately recovered. Measure absorbance at 280 nm (a 1 mg/ml solution of most IgG antibodies gives an absorbance of 1.35 at 280 nm against the appropriate reference solution) and immunoassay by the usual method.

(iv) Gradually, using either stepwise or gradient elution according to convenience, elute the column with the same buffer at increasing ionic strength (50 mM Na phosphate, pH 8, with increasing amounts of NaCl up to 0.2 M). Most IgG elutes below 50 mM NaCl while albumin remains bound.

Collect 0.5 ml samples, measure absorbance at 280 nm and immunoassay all fractions.

(v) If the column is to be re-used, all the albumin must be removed, with 10 ml 2 M guanidinium chloride and the column regenerated with Buffer A.

10.6.6. Purification with protein A or protein G

Protein A is a 42 kDa protein found on the cell walls of *Staphylococcus aureus* which binds to the Fc region of a wide range of antibody subclasses from many species (Langone 1982a,b). It is available at low cost from many suppliers either alone or coupled to various matrices such as Sepharose (Pharmacia). The main advantage of protein A is that it is inexpensive and that it can be readily dissociated from antibodies in weak acid without denaturation of either antibody or protein A. Its main disadvantage to date is that it does not bind well to certain subclasses. In particular, it binds poorly to the mouse IgG1

TABLE 10.2

Binding of various IgG subclasses to protein A and protein G

	Protein A	Protein G
Mouse IgG1	Weak (1)	Strong (2,6)
Mouse IgG2a	Medium	Strong
Mouse IgG2b	Strong	Medium
Mouse IgG3	Weak	Medium
Rat IgG1	Weak (3,4,7)	Weak (2,6,7)
Rat IgG2a	Low	Strong
Rat IgG2b	Low	Weak
Rag IgG2c	Medium	Medium
Human IgG1	Strong (5)	Strong (2,6)
Human IgG2	Medium	Strong
Human IgG3	Weak	Strong
Human IgG4	Strong	Strong

References: (1) Ey et al., 1978; (2) Akerstrom and Bjorck, 1986; (3) Rousseaux et al., 1981; (4) Nilsson et al., 1982; (5) Duhamel et al., 1979; (6) Bjork and Kronvall, 1984; (7) Bazin, 1990.

subclass, the human IgG3 subclass and most rat Mabs (Table 10.2). For this reason, a second similar protein, protein G (molecular mass: 60 kDa) has been developed more recently to attempt to fill these gaps in the repertoire of protein A. It binds well to mouse IgG1 and human IgG3 but poorly to most rat isotypes. Thus, in general, the protein A/protein G method is unsuitable for rat hybridoma purification. There is still some dispute as to the extent of binding of different subclasses and this probably relates to the different experimental conditions of pH, ionic strength etc. at which the relative strengths of binding were evaluated. It is, however agreed that IgM and IgA antibodies seldom bind to protein A or protein G, the only exception being the human IgA2 subclass (Saltvedt and Harboe, 1976).

PROTOCOL 10.5: PILOT PURIFICATION WITH PROTEIN A (MOUSE OR HUMAN MABS ONLY)

Before attempting this it is best to determine antibody class and if it is, for example a mouse IgG1, replace protein A with protein G in the protocol.

(A) FPLC on a protein A-Superose column
(i) Prepare 500 ml each of 0.1 M citrate buffer adjusted to pH 7 (A) and pH 2.5.
   Mix 100 ml of 70% A with 100 ml 30% B (Buffer C) and equilibrate column. Dilute ascites or culture fluid 1 in 10 with Buffer C and filter sample through 0.45 μ filter. For low titre samples dialyse into buffer C.
(ii) Inject 100 μl of sample and elute at 2 ml/min with 40 ml gradient of starting buffer increasing to 100% buffer B. Collect 0.5 ml samples, examine elution profile at 280 nm, and measure ELISA activity of eluted and retained peaks.

(B) Simple laboratory protein A purification of Mabs
(i) Suspend 1 g of protein A-Sepharose Cl-4B (Pharmacia) in 200 ml PBS, pH 8, for at least 30 minutes. Use a small chromatography column (e.g., Pharmacia C10/10) or the barrel of a disposable 10 ml syringe plugged with a glass wool filter. Pour the gel gently trying to leave no discontinuities and a final flat surface. The column can be run at room temperature. If it is to be stored this should be at 4°C and this may alter its flow properties. For a small column this is unimportant. Larger columns intended for re-use should be poured and run at 4°C. Wash the column with at least 100 ml PBS followed by 0.1 M sodium citrate, pH 3, followed be re-equilibration with PBS, pH 8.
(ii) The test sample used should have an assay titre of at least 1 in 100 and be dialysed into PBS, pH 8. It should contain no more than 10 g of IgG from any source. The most usual application is to use ammonium sulphate concentrated material (Protocol 10.2).

(iii) Add 1 ml of sample to the column and allow it to flow in, washing with 5 ml PBS, pH 8, and collecting 0.5 ml fractions. These initial samples should be assessed for protein concentration by absorbance at 280 nm (a 1 mg/ml solution of most IgG antibodies gives an absorbance of 1.35 at 280 nm against the appropriate reference solution) and kept for immunoassay. If they are strongly positive then the antibody does not bind to protein A.

(iv) Elute the column with 5 ml 0.1 M sodium citrate buffer, pH 3.5, collecting 0.5 ml fractions as before directly into tubes containing 50 μl 1 M Tris-HCl, pH 8, to neutralise the solution. Measure absorbance at 280 nm and even if this is very low, keep for immunoassay.

(v) Assay all fractions. If the column is to be re-used, regenerate with 0.1 M Na citrate, pH 2.5.

10.6.7. Purification using affinity chromatography

Affinity chromatography is generally the last choice for a Mab which has a desired specificity but which is refractive to other approaches. The strength of affinity chromatography has always been for the selection of very minor antigens in a complex mixture and this is not the case with Mabs which form a significant although minor component of ascites and a larger component in most ammonium sulphate precipitates.

The reasons for affinity chromatography being a final resort include the extra manipulations and cost occasioned during the covalent attachment of the selecting protein to the matrix, the difficulty of attaching these selecting proteins to the matrix while maintaining their full binding affinity, and the leaching of these proteins from the matrix after initial attachment. All these factors make scaling up to bulk production with this method impractical.

The protocol given is for cyanogen bromide activated Sepharose but it should be noted that many other coupling methods are available and in particular, that the length of the 'arms' of the cross-linking molecules may alter the ability of the matrix to bind the selected protein. Cyanogen bromide reacts with amino groups and antibodies have a high proportion of these. The protocol given is for affinity selection of mouse IgG by a matrix bound polyclonal anti-mouse IgG antibody. However, if selection by antigen is required and this antigen has a small number of amino groups, then other types of activated Sepharose which will bind to acidic or cysteinyl(-SH) groups may be more effective.

To construct a matrix bound polyclonal antiserum for selecting a murine or human monoclonal antibody it is advisable to use an affinity selected polyclonal antiserum (Table 2.2) from rabbit, goat, sheep or other species. Alternatively, a high-affinity Mab directed to the appropriate mouse IgG class could in theory be used.

PROTOCOL 10.6: PILOT AFFINITY PURIFICATION OF MOUSE IgG

(i) Suspend 0.5 g CNBr activated Sepharose 4B and suspend in 10 ml 1 M HCl. Wash with 10×10 ml of 1 mM HCl on a sintered glass filter, porosity G3. Do not allow the gel to dry out.

(ii) Dissolve 5 mg affinity purified anti-mouse IgG (from sheep, goat, rabbit etc) in 1 ml 0.2 M $NaHCO_3$, 0.5 M NaCl buffer, pH 8.3 (Coupling buffer). Wash the gel with 2 ml coupling buffer and the immediately mix with protein solution either at room temperature for 2 hours or overnight at 4°C using gentle stirring or shaking but not magnetic stirring which may damage the beads.

(iii) Add 0.2 ml ethanolamine, pH 8 (blocking reagent) to neutralise reactive groups and mix gently for a further 60 min. Centrifuge at $500 \times g$ for 5 min and resuspend the gel in coupling buffer. Determine the amount of uncoupled antibody by measuring the absorbance at 280 nm (using coupling buffer as a reference). A 1 mg/ml solution of most IgG antibodies gives an absorbance of 1.35 at 280 nm against the appropriate reference solution. Less than 20% of the antibody should have bound. The remainder should be precipitated with ammonium sulphate and re-used.

(iv) Pour the gel into a small column (e.g., Pharmacia C10/10) or the barrel of a disposable 10 ml syringe plugged with a sintered glass filter. Wash with 50 ml of coupling buffer and a subsequent 50 ml of

0.1 M Na acetate, pH 4. At this stage, the column may be stored in 0.01% Na azide (but note that azide is highly toxic to cells and to many detection enzymes — Table 2.3). However, protein slowly leaches off most columns to which it is coupled and the column will have a limited lifetime whether in use or out of use unless stabilised by cross-linking (e.g., Protocol 12.5).

(v) Concentrate the Mab by ammonium sulphate (Protocol 10.2) and DEAE-Sephacel (Protocol 10.3). The elution conditions for a high-affinity Mab are quite extreme so perform a series of pilot experiments to test whether the Mab activity is reduced by 30 min incubation at room temperature in the common eluants:

(a)   3.5 M $MgCl_2$, 10 mM phosphate, pH 7.2,

(b)   distilled water,

(c)   100 mM triethlyamine, pH 11.5,

(d)   100 mM glycine, pH 2.5,

followed by immediate return to normal conditions of pH and ionic strength. Pick the one which gives the minimal reduction in activity to use in elution.

(vi) Pass the purified antibody into the column. Leave for 30 min. Then wash with PBS and retain the washings to assay and re-use by ammonium sulphate precipitation if it contains large amounts of specific Mab. Wash until the eluate is free of protein.

(vii) Elute with one or more of the eluants selected in (v) above. Measure protein concentration and Mab activity in all fractions.

10.7. Purification of IgM Mabs

It should be emphasised that IgM Mabs are poor, low-affinity, polyspecific reagents and the majority should have not been allowed to reach the stage of bulk culture and purification. If for some reason they are required for a specific application, then they are most conveniently purified by precipitation at low ionic strength. This is achieved by dialysis of the culture medium or ascites fluid containing the Mab into 2 mM sodium phosphate buffer, pH 6. The precipitate is then centrifuged at $5000 \times g$, washed with the same buffer and then resuspended in 10 mM Tris-HCl, 0.15 M NaCl, pH 7.2. Alternatively, the Mab may be purified on DEAE-Sephacel chromatography as described in Protocol 10.4, with each fraction being assayed for activity. Most IgM Mabs elute at higher ionic strength than IgG and are often contaminated with albumin. IgM Mabs should be further purified by gel filtration (e.g., Superose 12 on FPLC or Sepharose 6B equilibrated with 10 mM Tris-HCl, 0.15 M NaCl for simple laboratory use) since their molecular weight of 900,000 allows ready separation from IgG and albumin.

10.8. Purification of IgA Mabs

IgA Mabs are best purified on DEAE-Sephacel or agarose (Protocol 10.4) with assay for activity. Most elute at higher ionic strength than IgG (but lower than IgM) and have some albumin contamination. IgA molecules are larger than IgG (around 180,000) and can be purified from the main albumin contaminant by gel filtration (e.g., Superose 12 on FPLC or Sepharose 6B equilibrated with 10 mM Tris-HCl, 0.15 M NaCl for simple laboratory use).

CHAPTER 11

Characterisation of monoclonal antibodies

11.1. Introduction

The total characterisation of a monoclonal antibody is a long and complex procedure which varies widely with the intended use of the antibody. Characterisation goes hand in hand with the development of a Mab for its intended use and at any stage it may fail the increasingly stringent requirements placed on it. It should be emphasised that any single Mab is unlikely to proceed smoothly to the final use which is why there is a requirement for a panel of Mabs at early stages. Since it is expensive and tedious to continue to clone and expand large panels of Mabs, preliminary elimination procedures are required to reduce the size of the panel to a smaller group which can proceed to the next stage. The main preliminary questions are:

(i) What is the subclass of the Mab?

(ii) What is the affinity of the Mab?

(ii) Does the Mab react with different epitopes to other Mabs in the panel?

Subsidiary questions relate to final use:

(iv) Does the Mab react, at even very low affinity, with any major 'contaminant' in the final intended use? (Section 2.2.3(e)).

(v) Can the Mab be adapted/ bound/ crosslinked for final use without loss of antigen binding capacity?

The first three of these can be performed at an early stage with a small amount of Mab and the latter two only require slightly larger amounts.

An interesting difference between this edition and the 1984 edition is the requirement for proof of monoclonality. Cloning techniques are now so well established that this is seldom questioned.

11.2. Determination of antibody class

Apart from specific applications such as the ABO blood group antigens or precise requirements for IgA or IgE antibodies to study mucosal immunity or allergy, selection protocols for most uses should be for the IgG class only (Sections 1.3 and 2.2) and by the stage of determining class, the operator should have selected for IgG. Class specific anti-IgG antibodies are available for all species but they are often poor reagents for the minor subclasses, particularly rat IgG2c and human IgG4. Reagents for mouse and human subclass determination have improved considerably over the last 5 years but they do not represent a major sales outlet for any firm as a Mab is only class-typed once in a small experiment whereas large amounts of good antibody are required for screening and cloning.

It should be noted that class determination gives a much clearer result if tissue culture supernatant or its ammonium sulphate concentrate are used. Ascites fluid will have significant levels of irrelevant mouse or rat IgG, particularly IgG1 and this may lead to wrong identification.

11.2.1. Class determination by ELISA

Enzyme labelled IgG subclass specific second antibodies are available but at considerable expense so it is usual to use unlabelled ones as an additional layer on the ELISA sandwich. The ELISA system of subclassing involves plating, in sequence, antigen, the Mab supernatant, the polyclonal anti-subclass class antibody (usually rabbit), and polyclonal enzyme linked antibody directed against the immunoglobulin of the class specific antibody (i.e., goat anti-rabbit IgG) to give the final colour. Because subclass class specific antibodies tend to cross-react weakly with other classes it is usual to titre the Mab across the plate at several serial dilutions for each subclass specific antibody. Most firms sell kits which work in this manner.

Antibody characterisation of this type is a classic example of a situation in which a polyclonal anti-subclass specific second antibody, suitably absorbed, is actually preferable to a monoclonal one since it is desirable to have the antibody react with as many epitopes as possible.

11.2.2. Class determination by Ouchterlony immunoprecipitation

Class determination by Ouchterlony analysis is probably the simplest method to use to determine the subclass of an IgG Mab (Ouchterlony and Nilsson, 1986). It requires reasonable amounts of antibody to form a precipitate but takes little more than the ELISA with the extra 'sandwich'. It is undoubtedly less sensitive. Ouchterlony analysis is usually carried out on slides coated with 1% agar in which holes have been punched with a template to make a pattern of six outer wells in a circle with one central well in the middle of the circle. The agar is usually removed from the holes with a pasteur pipette by vacuum suction. The polyclonal subclass specific antibody and the Mab only form a precipitate under conditions in which neither is in excess. One slide is made for each of the four subclasses of IgG and two sets of template are punched on each slide. In one set 10 μl of the hybridoma supernatant (or preferably the ammonium sulphate concentrate) is placed in the middle with doubling dilutions of the subclass specific antibody around the outside and in the other the (undiluted) class specific antibody is placed in the centre with doubling dilutions of the hybridoma around the outside. The slides are incubated for 24 h at room temperature in a sealed plastic box on damp tissues to maintain a humidified atmosphere. The precipitate of Mab with subclass specific antibody is seen as a thin white line between the central and outer wells, best viewed in reflected light.

If no precipitate is seen after 48 h, the sensitivity of the reaction can be considerably increased by staining the slide with Coomassie blue (Section A.3.3). Failure to detect lines at this point indicates that either subclass specific antibody or hybridoma, usually the former, were in excess at all dilutions and a different range must be tried.

11.2.3. Class determination by agglutination of SRBCs

This method utilises subclass specific Mabs bound to the surface of sheep red blood cells. The Mab is mixed with each set of subclass specific SRBCs in a U bottomed mictrotitre plate. A negative reaction is shown by the SRBCs sinking to the bottom of the plate to form a button. In the positive reaction the Mabs cross-link the SRBCs to form a matrix which appears as a diffuse 'mat' across the microtitre well. Inexpensive kits containing all the appropriate reagents for this can be purchased from Serotec.

11.2.4. Class determination by electrophoresis of internally labelled antibody

Internally labelled antibodies subjected to electrophoresis on polyacrylamide gels containing sodium dodecyl sulphate (SDS-PAGE) give an indication of antibody class but do not permit subdivision of IgG antibodies into subclasses. It is particularly useful for the analysis of the relative rates of synthesis of various chains in complex fusions such as human fusions. An example is shown earlier in Fig. 3.6. The procedure involves the incorporation of radioactive amino acids into the monoclonal antibody by the growing hybridoma cells. It is usual to analyse both cytoplasmic and secreted antibody, since many myeloma and hybridoma lines differ considerably in their capacity to make and to secrete the antibody. The main difference among protocols relates to the choice of labelled amino acid for this purpose.

Almost any amino acid may be used but Galfre and Milstein (1981) report that lysine, arginine and phenylalanine are incorporated into the myeloma protein of the MOPC21 line at particularly high efficiency and this observation extrapolates to most IgG producing hybridomas. Leucine is also commonly used. However, the amino acid most frequently used for labelling is methionine. Amino acids can be obtained with ^{3}H, ^{14}C or (in the case of methionine), ^{35}S or ^{75}Se labels. The most economical is ^{3}H which suffers from the drawback of being a very weak beta emitter. ^{14}C amino acids are the most expensive. ^{75}Se-labelled methionine is reported to bind non-specifically to components of FCS (Gutmman et al., 1978) although it has the advantage of being a gamma emitter. The most common choice for labelling is [^{35}S]methionine which emits beta particles of approximately the same energy as ^{14}C and is less expensive and readily obtained at high specific activity. If the antibody is only to be labelled for class determination then ^{3}H-amino acids may readily be used. However, for further extended use in competition assays (Section 11.4.2) or in tissue localisation, it may be less suitable. One drawback of [^{35}S]methionine is the relatively short half life of ^{35}S (87 days) but this is quite long enough for most studies.

In order to label the protein it is necessary to have the cells growing in medium which has very little non-radioactive amino acid. Commercial supplies of medium without any particular amino acid are readily obtained. Some procedures advise the dialysis of the FCS into PBS as well but the amino acid concentration in FCS is usually small (in the order of 10 mg/l) and if FCS is used at low concentrations it will not dilute the medium significantly. Some protocols recommend labelling at high specific activity for short periods of time without any FCS present. If the specific activity of the amino acid is too low then very little will be incorporated into the monoclonal antibody. However, if the specific activity is so high as to make the amount of amino acid a rate limiting step in protein synthesis, then incorporation will also be poor and some protocols therefore recommend the addition of medium with 10% (around 3 mg/l) of the usual non-labelled amino acid concentration of the medium, particularly where the hybridomas are making large amounts of antibody. If the cells are growing well and making antibody, these are the only main factors which will affect incorporation.

PROTOCOL 11.1: INTERNAL LABELLING OF MABS WITH [^{35}S]METHIONINE

Note: Observe the usual precautions when working with radioactivity.
(i) Obtain sheep anti-rabbit IgG and rabbit anti-mouse IgG polyclonal antiserum and establish conditions where precipitation equivalence is optimal in a high detergent buffer (See (v)). Grow the hybridoma cells exponentially at a density of below 5×10^5 cells/ml. Before labelling, check that the viability is greater than 90%. At the same time, it is helpful, although not essential, to grow the parent myeloma line and any available marker cell lines known to secrete antibody under the same conditions and treat them in the same way as the hybridoma cells throughout the protocol.
(ii) Wash an aliquot of 5×10^5 cells in 5 ml RPMI minus methionine in a sterile conical universal container. Centrifuge at $400 \times g$ and decant the supernatant. Tap the pellet to loosen the cells and add 0.1 ml RPMI minus methionine containing medium containing 5% FCS and 100 μCi of [^{35}S]methionine at 37°C (800 Ci/mmol, Amersham)
(iii) Incubate at 37°C in a humidified CO_2 incubator shaking at 15-min intervals to resuspend the cells. After 90 min, remove 50 μl and transfer to 2 ml ice cold RPMI. Return the remainder of the culture to the incubator. Centrifuge the sampled material at $400 \times g$ for 5 min, discard the supernatant, and resuspend the pellet in 2 ml 0.1 M Tris-HCl, pH 8, 0.1 M KCl, 0.005 M $MgCl_2$ (TKM buffer). Wash twice with TKM buffer. When the cells are completely resuspended add 50 μl Triton X-100 in the same buffer and mix for 10 min. Centrifuge at $400 \times g$ for 10 min to pellet nuclei. Decant supernatant, discarding the pellet, and add 50 μl 10% sodium deoxycholate, 5% SDS in the same buffer. The radioactivity in this material represents the antibody being synthesised within the cell. Aliquot in 100 μl portions and store at 4°C until the material from step (iv) is ready for analysis.
(iv) 3–5 h after the start of the incubation add 350 μl unlabelled cold RPMI and centrifuge at $400 \times g$ for 5 min. Decant the supernatant into a polytube tube containing 10% Triton X-100, 10% sodium deoxycholate, and 5% SDS all dissolved in TKM buffer. Discard the pellet. The antibody in the supernatant fraction represents the secreted antibody.

(v) Precipitate both synthesised and secreted antibody with rabbit anti-mouse IgG followed by goat or sheep anti-rabbit IgG, already titred to give a precipitate (see (i)).

(vi) At this stage the samples may be frozen at $-70°C$ before analysis by SDS-PAGE and autoradiography or fluorography.

   Notes: (a) The two samples of cellular and secreted antibody may be subjected to SDS-PAGE and autoradiography or fluorography without further purification. On the stained gel, the background of other protein material will be low in the case of secreted antibody but contaminated with other proteins in the case of the cytoplasmic antibody. This should be minimised by the immune precipitation.

(b)   While in theory only a second antibody should be necessary for immune precipitation, the exact amount of antibody synthesised by the hybridoma under the incubation may be variable and it can be difficult to obtain correct conditions for 100% precipitation. The use of the third antibody ensures that all the labelled Mab is precipitated.

Failure to detect any radioactivity in the autoradiography may be due to

(1)   The methionine being of the wrong specific activity. This problem is discussed above and if controls of myelomas or hybridomas of known secretion capacity have been included at the same cell density as suggested in (i), these should also show no bands if the methionine is at fault. If the controls are positive then it is possible that the cells under test are not making or secreting antibody. This is a common occurrence in the human system.

(2)   The second or third antibodies may not precipitate the first antibody. If the second and third antibodies have been correctly pretitred to give a precipitate, this should not happen. It is best tested for by subjecting the cell culture supernatant to SDS-PAGE followed by autoradiography or fluorography and looking for bands in the appropriate molecular weight range, indicating that incorporation has occurred.

(3)   There are more bands than expected. Two light chain bands are generally observed in rat fusions which have used the rat Y3 line

since the endogenous kappa often shows slightly different mobility. In the case of the heavy chain, differential glycosylation of the antibody molecules can often show two chains close together. Human hybridomas fused with a secreting partner, show two chains because the cell makes two chains (Fig. 3.6). Human hybridomas also frequently have a completely different profile of synthesised and secreted antibody.

11.2.5. Light chain analysis

In the mouse and rat, most antibodies carry the kappa light chain and a lambda producing Mab is very rare. However, Bazin (1990) has noted that the rat kappa light chain has two allotypes (constant region sequences which differ between inbred species) and can supply antibodies which detect either of these. In the human system where 40% of the cells are lambda producers, the light chain is usually typed by either ELISA or Ouchterlony.

11.3. Proof that the antibody is monoclonal

This is now seldom required. If the hybridoma has been fully and correctly cloned it is probably unnecessary. If it is required then isoelectric focussing of internally labelled antibody is the only way. Isoelectric focussing can also give an indication of the heterogeneity of antibody production where human fusions between two cells which both secrete antibody has been employed (Fig. 3.6).

11.4. Epitope analysis

One of the earliest questions which is asked of a panel of hybridomas is the extent to which they are directed at the same or at different epitopes. This enables expansion of only those antibodies which bind to different determinants and can save much tissue culture time. Analysis of cross-reactivity between the antigen and other similar antigens is usually required early in the analytical process and Western blot (Section 11.4.5) will identify the antigenic protein in a complex mixture. However, where several Mabs clearly all bind to the one protein, they have to be characterised for comparative epitope specificity.

11.4.1. Strategies based on synthetic peptides

A strategy for epitope mapping of proteins, sometimes called mimitope mapping, has been extensively promoted by manufacturers of synthetic peptides but is of very limited value. The general idea is that a series of peptides can be constructed, each varying in one amino acid and that these will lead to elucidation of the epitope. However, crystallography has shown that most Mabs have natural conformational epitopes which involve amino acids distant from each other on the primary structure (See Section 2.2.1 or Laver et al. (1990) for a review). Synthetic peptides tend to be presented to the antibody at very high molar concentration and very low-affinity binding can occasionally be obtained with one among a group of related peptides presented to the Mab. These usually bear no relation to the epitope on which the Mab was originally selected and represent non-specific binding under excessively artificial laboratory conditions. This can be checked by exposure of the Mab to the peptide under conditions of lower local molarity. As with many approaches, this one is confused by the outdated view that a Mab has a single linear epitope, and forced up against it, will identify it. In reality (Sections 1.3, 11.6.2 and 2.2) a good Mab has a complex biologically relevant epitope and will only bind to small peptides under artificial conditions. A poor Mab will bind several antigens.

11.4.2. Determination of overlapping epitopes

Redundancy among a panel of Mabs to a simple protein is usually quite high. If a successful first fusion has led to the production of a Mab or Mab panel directed to one epitope or set of epitopes, then these can be purified and labelled directly with isotope or enzyme and

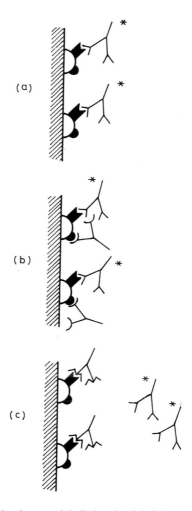

Fig. 11.1. Direct competition between labelled and unlabelled Mabs. (a) The labelled Mab is bound directly to the solid- phase antigen. (b) a second unlabelled Mab directed to a different epitope fails to compete and the bound signal remains unchanged. (c) A second unlabelled Mab directed to the same epitope displaces the first labelled Mab and the bound signal is reduced.

used in competition assays with the Mab supernatant being tested for its ability to compete out the labelled Mab (Fig. 11.1). The precise antigen concentration of the epitope (or the antigen on the surface of a cell) is obviously important and it is essential that this be fully saturated with the labelled Mab for the unlabelled to compete. A preliminary experiment to check full saturation of the labelled Mab is then employed. The supernatants from the emerging clones can then be added and tested for their ability to reduce the signal strength from the test system with purified Mab. This can be applied to the majority of assay systems. It also gives a quick affinity ranking if the Mabs are to the same epitope as the labelled Mab since they can be tested for their relative abilities to dislodge it.

Positive competition indicates that the two Mabs share the same epitope, that they bind to epitopes sufficiently close as to be mutually exclusive, or that the binding of one causes a change in antigen structure so that the second cannot bind. Lack of competition indicates either that the epitopes are distinct, or that the hybridoma supernatant contains too little antibody to give effective competition.

Direct competition studies between two unlabelled Mabs at an earlier stage of selection (Fig. 11.2) is also possible. It has been used in ELISA (Friguet et al., 1983). The basis of this assay is that the signal strength will increase with a combination of two Mabs to different epitopes but not with two to the same epitopes. As above, it is essential that each Mab alone is capable of fully saturating all the epitopes presented in the assay at the concentration used by checking that further addition of the individual Mab does not enhance signal strength whereas addition of the second Mab does. This method is less definitive and requires low antigen concentrations or substantial amounts of Mab in many cases. However, it can be used at first screening and before Mab purification.

11.4.3. Determination of antibody specificity among a group of antigens

The most obvious method of performing this particular task is to assay the antibody independently on each antigen and this is indeed

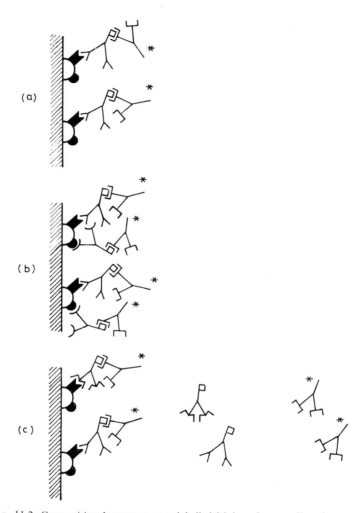

Fig. 11.2. Competition between two unlabelled Mabs using a radioactive or enzyme linked polyclonal detection system. (a) The reaction system with a single Mab. (b) Competition with a second Mab directed to a different epitope. The amount of detecting antibody bound is increased. (c) Competition with a second Mab directed to the same epitope. The amount of detecting antibody bound is not increased.

the usual method of screening where antigens on material such as tissue sections are involved. With soluble or suspension antigens, it is however possible to test a Mab which has been labelled with isotope or enzyme by reacting it optimally in the test system and then with competing antigen. The ELISA example is shown in Fig. 11.3 but the method can be adapted for dot-blot analysis and more complex assay systems such as FACS. The key positive control for this experiment is to compete with the known antigen at an amount which clearly alters the nature or strength of the signal in order to establish the correct assay system. Competition with other molecules or cells can then be tested in a series of separate experiments.

This method has a variety of uses. One of these is to test that free

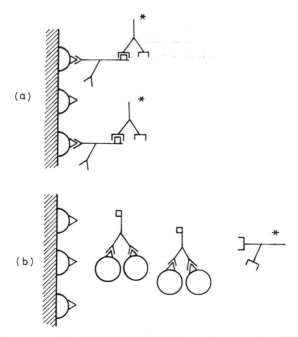

Fig. 11.3. Antigen competition ELISA. In (b) the free antigen competes with the plate bound antigen so that the signal is reduced. This is essentially a specialised example for Fig. 1.9.

antigen behaves in the same way as plate bound antigen in ELISA since plate binding can expose epitopes which are inaccessible in a native antigen in solution (Section 2.6.2). However, it should be noted that absence of competition does not necessarily indicate that the Mab does not bind at all to the competing antigen. There are several situations where it can be shown to bind competing antigen in a direct assay but not in a competition assay if the affinity for the competing antigen is lower.

11.4.4. Analysis of epitope specificity by antigen modification

In principle, antigenic specificity may be analysed by modification of any of the amino acid residues on the antigen in the same manner in which enzymes are inactivated with standard reagents to analyse their active sites. This can give information relating to the amino acids involved in the structure of the binding epitope. However, this is of comparatively small value in the analysis of cross-reactivity among antigens. The analysis of carbohydrate is, on the other hand, frequently relevant in hybridoma technology. This is because carbohydrate antigens frequently dominate a fusion with glycoprotein, glycolipid or bacterial antigens. While carbohydrate structures can have wide diversity and may be the most suitable for the final intended use of the Mab, on molecules such as glycoproteins or mucins, they show limited structural diversity and are likely to lead to cross-reactivity.

The first indication that the epitope may be carbohydrate is usually the antibody subclass. If it is IgG3 in the mouse or 2b in the rat, the epitope is very probably carbohydrate. A further approach is to compete with sugars at high concentrations (0.1–0.2 M) or with lectins of known carbohydrate binding specificty at lower concentrations. The two will often give different results since sugars frequently do not compete effectively while lectins in binding to carbohydrate epitopes, may also block protein epitopes.

It is also possible to use chemical or enzymic reagents which will alter the glycosidic residues. Periodate oxidation at low concentrations (10 mM) and neutral pH will oxidise sialic acid residues. At 50 mM concentrations and, pH 3, it will modify most other carbohydrate residues which have cis-hydroxyl groups. The altered antigen can then be used in a competition assay (Section 11.4.2) to determine whether it competes as effectively as the unmodified antigen. Enzymes used to remove carbohydrate include neuraminidase, galactose oxidase, and endoglycosidases of various types. Failure of these enzymes to remove antigenic activity does not indicate that the epitope is not, at least in part, carbohydrate but they are comparatively simple to perform and a positive result can give a quick indication of carbohydrate involvement.

If the antigen is a complex mixture of proteins then a competition assay among partially purified fractions of this mixture may quickly eliminate antigens of no interest and require only small amounts of the partially purified fraction. If it is a purified protein, then partial digestion with trypsin, chymotrypsin or cyanogen bromide followed by gel filtration chromatography can provide fragments for use in a competition assay or direct assay (Piershbacher et al., 1981). However, antigenic sites are frequently composed of conformational rather than linear epitopes and digestion of a protein may destroy these.

11.4.5. Analysis of epitope specificity by Western blot (Immunoblot)

A Western blot, in common usage, refers to the electrophoresis of the antigen on SDS-PAGE (Section A.3.3) followed by its subsequent transfer to nitrocellulose or other types of paper. The paper is then incubated with specific antibody followed by labelled polyclonal second antibody. The name originates from the use of Southern blots (Southern, 1965) for the analysis of DNA fragments from gels with labelled RNA (or cDNA) probes and the subsequent development of an inverse system for the analysis of RNA molecules from gels with DNA probes called 'Northern' blotting and has no political or climatic origins. Western blotting was originally developed by Towbin et al. (1979) with polyclonal antibodies and has proved an exceptionally valuable tool in hybridoma technology (reviewed by Stott, 1989). All the techniques have as their basis the transfer of electrophoretically separated material to (usually) nitrocellulose paper where the various bands can be assessed for binding to a probe which is labelled with enzyme, isotope or fluorophor. In the case of nucleic acids where the gel is usually a wide pore size agarose, difficult to manipulate, the transfer is usually by passive overlay and the probe is also nucleic acid. In the case of Western blotting, where comparatively small protein molecules are to be transferred from a narrow pore sized gel, the transfer is usually electrophoretic and the probe is an antibody.

Immunoblotting can, however, be technically more complex and less definitive than Northern or Southern blotting which involve nucleic acids, readily separated on the basis of their natural negative charge. The denaturants involved in SDS-PAGE may destroy the (mainly) conformational epitopes of most Mabs and they may renature poorly during the transfer to the paper. Thus while almost all polyclonal sera immunoblot well, Mabs frequently fail to immunoblot efficiently or bind non-specifically to major protein bands in the blot.

11.4.5.1. Is blotting an appropriate technique for Mabs?

The answer to this is often in the negative. Blotting is a low-resolution technique. Polyclonal antiserum, given very highly defined detection conditions, can detect an antigen which is a minor component of the electrophoretically separated mixture but the conditions for each antiserum have to be established and most sera, allowed to proceed beyond the optimal detection endpoint will identify a wide variety of antigens in the mixture. The same is true for many Mabs. It is not precise specificity which can be defined but rather selective affinity within a mixture of complex antigens.

However, at early stages, the operator is not certain of the affinity of the Mab and there is an obvious requirement to determine the molecular weight of the major antigen(s) detected. There is a limit to the amount of material which can be loaded onto SDS-PAGE to give clean bands. If the antigen is under 0.1% of the mixture (i.e., cell surface proteins in a whole cell lysate), and the Mab has been selected for binding to the cell surface, then it may not be able to detect the small amount of specific antigen on the electrophoresis track, which may in any case, not be in the native state. For Mabs, it is definitely preferable to probe as pure a preparation of antigen as possible at the start and then to expand the range of irrelevant antigens within which it is required to operate in stepwise fashion (e.g., membrane preps, then whole cells, then whole tissues). Many Mabs directed to cell surface proteins may also bind proteins within the cell, but this is irrelevant to their selected function. The problem only arises when an individual scientist, inexperienced in Mab technology tries to use a Mab outwith its selected context. To give a practical example, many useful anti CD Mabs (Table 1.3) are capable of detecting irrelevant intracellular proteins on complex immunoblots. Yet they are invaluable and specific detection reagents when faced with whole live impermeable cells.

11.4.5.2. Types of blotting equipment

The two basic types of blotting equipment are 'wet' and 'semi-dry'. Most manufacturers supply both. The 'wet' systems are vertical ones which generally use a platinum electrode and transfer antigen slowly with considerable heat generation. A cassette containing the gel and paper with supports of filter paper and plastic grids containing holes or slots to allow free access of buffer (Fig. 11.4), is immersed in a tank of buffer and the protein in the gel transfers to the paper placed on the anodic side. The main disadvantage of such systems is that they use a substantial amount of transfer buffer which has expensive ingredients.

The faster transfer 'semi-dry' systems, on the other hand, are horizontal, usually with graphite electrodes and the source of buffer is saturated pads of filter paper. It is possible to obtain transfer to paper from several gels stacked above each other in a single run, provided that each transfer system of gel and paper is separated from the neighbouring ones by dialysis membranes (Kyhse-Andersen, 1984). More important, the cost of buffer is reduced and most 'semi dry' blotting systems quickly recoup their capital costs by saving on glycine which is a major component of transfer buffer.

'Mini-gel' apparatus can be purchased for either system but has limited utility in cases where the antibody has to distinguish between closely spaced bands since transfer can broaden bands and any detection system involving photographic film further broadens bands.

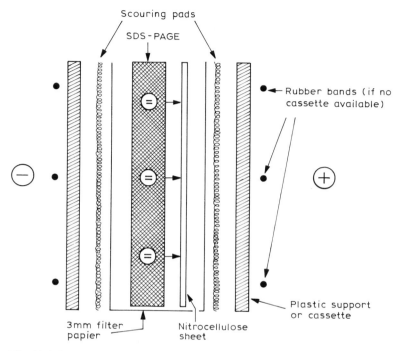

Fig. 11.4. Western blot apparatus for SDS-PAGE. Wet gels are usually blotted vertically and semi-dry gels horizontally.

11.4.5.3. Transfer of proteins from non-standard gels

Transfer can also be effected from isoelectric focussing gels which do
not use SDS, or indeed from PAGE with no SDS, but in this case,
it is necessary to pre-equilibrate the gel in 1% SDS/20% glycerol. If it
is definitely necessary to omit SDS, then transfer can still be effected
if the pH of the transfer buffer is raised to 8.8 (Stott and McLearie,
1986).

11.4.5.4. Membranes and transfer buffers

The membrane is usually nitrocellulose which has a high protein binding capacity. For rare proteins, it would obviously be convenient to
be able to reprobe a membrane from a single immunoblot several

times with different Mabs as is possible in the parallel nucleic acid systems. Unfortunately, such membranes as have been produced for this purpose to date, (Hy-Bond, Zeta-Probe) tend to bind protein nonspecifically and cannot be suitably saturated with blocking reagent. Nitrocellulose is inconveniently brittle and new types which incorporate nylon 'backing' to reduce this are also available.

The buffer used for transfer is generally the original buffer of Towbin et al. (1979) which is 25 mM Tris-HCl, 192 mM glycine, pH 8.3, containing 20% methanol. This last is essential to avoid expansion of the gel during electrophoretic transfer. The 'semi-dry' blotting system can be performed with less buffer and also with a lower molar concentration of glycine, its most expensive constituent.

11.4.5.5. Blocking and detection systems
After transfer, handling of the nitrocellulose bound antigen and detection systems are similar to a dot-blot (Protocols 2.3 and 2.4). There are, however, four major differences. The primary one is that in dot-blots the antigen concentration is chosen and known. In a complex mixture after electrophoresis, the antigen concentration may fall below the detection limits of the Mab. Only high-affinity Mabs can detect antigen if it is 0.1% of a complex mixture. The second, is that in dot-blots, the antigen structure has not been disrupted by SDS. Proteins may renature poorly in transfer, particularly if they are in small amounts. The third difference is that in dot-blot, the spacing between wells is chosen, whereas in electrophoretic separation it is possible to obtain two bands very close together and this can affect the choice of detection system. The choice of detection system, in turn, affects the choice of blocking system. The final difference is, that for Mab blots, it is essential to visualise the protein bands which have blotted. If a major protein band dominates both protein stain and blot, there is a suspicion that polyspecific binding of the Mab (or the polyclonal 2nd antibody) to common household cytoskeletal proteins has occurred. This requirement for a matching protein stain presents a problem for most protein blocking reagents as these saturate the filter paper and make it impossible to distinguish the original bands.

In consequence, the procedure of Batteiger et al. (1982) was developed. This procedure can only be used effectively if radiolabelled probes arc employed in tandem as it is highly inhibitory to most enzymes. It uses Tween 20 as blocking agent, and the original report used 0.5% which is fairly drastic. The highest affinity Mabs survive this but for a first attempt it is probably better to use a lower concentration. The other interesting development of the Tween system is the use of India ink (Glenney, 1986) which, in solutions containing Tween 20, binds to protein-bound nitrocellulose but not nitrocellulose itself. Blots can therefore technically be stained before blocking and subsequent detection with isotope (but not enzyme). Enzyme staining is sel-

TABLE 11.1

Detection and blocking systems to use for Mab blotting

Strategy	Result
(i) Duplicate the tracks in two halves of the gel. Stain one half for protein and the other for Mab binding using any method of blocking and staining.	Poor alignment of immunoblotted bands
(ii) Block with 0.1–0.5% Tween 20, then stain with Mab and isotope labelled polyclonal 2nd Ab or protein A. Autoradiograph. Finally stain with Amido black or India ink.	Tween is a rigorous test of a Mab. Start at 0.1% and work up. Final protein stain can be aligned with immunostain
(iii) Stain with India ink, block with either protein reagents or Tween 20. Detect with isotopes.	Good alignment. India ink is only specific in 0.2% Tween. Only difference from (ii) is that staining is at start.
(iv) Block with standard protein blocking reagents (BSA, blotto etc. – see Table 2.1). Detect with enzymes – coloured substrate	No alignment of immunostain with protein stain BUT resolution of closely spaced protein bands. Widely used for polyclonals. Seldom suitable for Mabs.
(v) Block with standard protein blocking reagents. Detect with enzymes (chemiluminescent substrate with enhancers (Table 2.3))	No alignment of immunostain. No resolution of closely spaced bands.

dom suitable for Mabs as its detection limits, even with chemiluminescent substrates, are much less sensitive than isotopic methods. On the
other hand, enzyme detection systems do give better resolution between closely spaced bands. There is no perfect system and Table 11.1
summarises some of the factors which affect these decisions.

PROTOCOL 11.2: WET IMMUNOBLOT OF SDS-PAGE

(i) If the antigen has been selected by any method other than dot-blot
(Protocol 2.4) then test its sensitivity to the Mab on dot-blot. A substantial number of antibody antigen systems do not transfer to dot-
blot, particularly those involving live cells (cell membrane protein) as
antigen. If they do transfer, they do so at low sensitivity.
(ii) Make up 1 litre transfer buffer (25 mM Tris-HCl; 192 mM glycine;
0.002% SDS, pH 8.3, plus 20% (v/v) methanol). Wearing gloves, cut
a piece of clean 0.45 u nitrocellulose paper and two Whatman 3 mm
pieces of filter paper equivalent to the size of the gel.
(iii) Perform the electrophoresis (Section A.3.3). Wearing gloves, wet
the sheets of nitrocellulose and filter paper thoroughly in transfer
buffer and lay first the support pad, then one sheet of Whatman 3 mm
paper, then the nitrocellulose sheet down in one half of the cassette
keeping wet at all stages. Remove the gel from the electrophoresis apparatus and place it on the sandwich keeping it wet at all stages. Still
wearing gloves, and washing the system with a jet of transfer buffer,
gently smooth out any air pockets so that the gel is directly aligned
with the paper. Cover the gel with the second sheet of Whatman 3
mm paper soaked in transfer buffer, the second support pad and the
second arm of the cassette.
(iv) Place in the transfer tank with the nitrocellulose membrane closest
to the positive (red) electrode. The recommended voltage gradient is
6 V/cm/h (Towbin 1979) but higher voltages may be used, preferably
with some form of cooling system. This is usually 400–500 mA current. The exact time for transfer depends on the percentage of the
polyacrylamide gels and the size of protein to be transferred. Proteins
above 100,000 in molecular weight are particularly difficult to blot un-

less they are in low percentage gels. A time of 2 h for a protein of 50,000 molecular weight is a reasonable guide.

(iv) Switch off the power and remove the nitrocellulose sheet. Mark the orientation with respect to the original gel by nicking a corner of the paper. Stain the gel with silver or Coomassie blue in order to determine the efficiency of transfer. At this point, the blot may be stored dried between two sheets of Whatman 3 mm filter paper for future blocking and staining.

PROTOCOL 11.3: SEMI-DRY IMMUNOBLOT OF SDS-PAGE

(i) If the antigen has been selected by any method other than dot-blot (Protocol 2.4) then test its sensitivity to the Mab on dot-blot. A substantial number of antibody antigen systems do not transfer to dot-blot, particularly those involving live cells (cell membrane protein) as antigen. If they do transfer, they do so at low sensitivity.

(ii) Make up 1 litre transfer buffer (25 mM Tris-HCl; 40 mM glycine; 0.04% SDS, pH 8.3, plus 20% (v/v) methanol). Wearing gloves, cut a piece of clean 0.45 μ nitrocellulose paper and six Whatman 3 mm pieces of filter paper equivalent to the size of the gel.

(iii) Perform the electrophoresis (Section A3.3). Wearing gloves, wet the sheets of nitrocellulose and filter paper thoroughly in transfer buffer and on top of the bottom electrode lay three layers of soaked Whatman 3 mm paper, then the nitrocellulose paper, then the gel. Still wearing gloves, and washing the system with a jet of transfer buffer, gently smooth out any air pockets so that the gel is directly aligned with the paper. Cover the gel with three layers of Whatman 3 mm paper soaked in transfer buffer, the second support pad and the second arm of the cassette. Then place the upper electrode on top.

(iv) Connect the electrodes, the anode (red) is usually at the bottom. Transfer for 1 hour at 400–500 mA current. The exact time for transfer depends on the percentage of the polyacrylamide gels and the size of protein to be transferred. Proteins above 100,000 in molecular weight are particularly difficult to blot unless they are in low percentage gels.

(v) Switch off the power and remove the nitrocellulose sheet. Mark the orientation with respect to the original gel by nicking a corner of the paper. Stain the gel with silver or Coomassie blue in order to determine the efficiency of transfer. At this point, the blot may be stored dried between two sheets of Whatman 3 mm for future blocking and staining.

NOTE The semi dry system can be used to transfer several gels at once in which case each 'set' of gel and nitrocellulose sandwiched between Whatman 3 mm filter paper should be separated by a sheet of dialysis membrane.

PROTOCOL 11.4: BLOCKING AND STAINING FOR ISOTOPE BASED DETECTION

(i) Wearing gloves, immerse the nitrocellulose paper in PBS containing 0.1% Tween 20. Incubate with rocking (not shaking – Tween is a detergent) for 1 hour. Wash for 3×30 min in PBS (1 ml /cm^2 of paper).

(ii) Incubate for 4+ hours or overnight with specific Mab at 10–50 times the concentration necessary to give a good positive on other assay systems (Immunoblotting is not a sensitive technique). Wash for 3×30 min in PBS (1 ml /cm^2 of paper).

(iii) Incubate with 10^8 cpm of either Protein A (Section 10.6.6) or affinity purified polyclonal second antibody (Table 2.2), labelled with ^{125}I by the method described in Protocol 12.1 for 2–4 h in minimal volume of PBS (ideally a sealed plastic bag).

(iv) Wash for 3×30 min in PBS (1 ml/cm^2 of paper).

(v) Cover the blot in Clingfilm and expose to X-ray film for 2–5 days. Develop the film. It is usual to obtain several exposures at different times in order to assess major and minor bands.

(vi) Stain the residual paper with either

(a) 0.1% Amido black, 45% methanol,10% acetic acid

(b) 1/1000 (v/v) genuine India ink / PBS containing 0.3% Tween 20

(vii) Align the stained immunoblot and exposed film. Scan both by reflectance densitometry if appropriate.

Note India ink with Tween 20 can also be used before step (ii) so that the protein bands may be visualised to see if they are worth staining with antibody and isotope.

PROTOCOL 11.5: BLOCKING AND STAINING FOR ENZYME BASED DETECTION

(i) Wearing gloves, immerse the paper in a protein blocking reagent such as Blotto, 5% serum or 10 mg/ml BSA (Table 2.1). This can contain 0.05% Tween 20 to stop non-specific interactions. Tween 20 sticks to the paper and more may inhibit the enzyme and/or precipitate the substrate solution. Wash for 3×30 min with shaking in PBS.

(ii) Incubate for $4+$ hours or overnight with specific Mab at 10–50 times the concentration necessary to give a good positive on other assay systems (immunoblotting is not a sensitive technique). Wash for 3×30 min in PBS (1 ml /cm^2 of paper).

(iii) Incubate for 1–4 h with horseradish peroxidase (HRP) labelled polyclonal second antibody (γ-chain specific) at $5 \times$ the concentration recommended for ELISA (blotting is less sensitive), diluted in 1% serum or BSA. Wash for 3×30 min with shaking in PBS.

(iv) Incubate with substrate – 3 mg/ml of 4-chloronaphthol in methanol, stored for up to one month in a dark bottle. Dilute with 5 volumes PBS and add H_2O_2 to 0.01%. It is important that the H_2O_2 be added immediately before use. Positive bands are dark blue /purple.

(v) Wash paper and store/photograph. Bands fade slightly but improve when wet. Scan by reflectance densitometry if appropriate.

Note: HRP has various chemiluminescent substrates which can be used, together with enhancers in conjunction with X-ray film to give an autoradiograph. Alkaline phosphatase also has such substrates (Table 2.3). These give higher detectability but lack the precise resolution of direct enzyme blots as two closely related bands, distinct on chemically stained blots, can be merged by the pathlength of light of X-rays on the film. While these higher detectability systems have high sensitivity, they also have high backgrounds.

11.4.6. Failure of blotting

While this can be due to technical failure, it is more often due to over-optimism on the part of the operator. An antigen which comprises a tiny percentage of total cellular protein is unlikely to be detected by this system without some sort of pre-purification. It will most certainly not have been originally selected by immunoblotting since no high quality Mab ever has been selected in this way. The main problem with this is experienced by labs who have obtained a Mab selected against a purified or 'restricted access' antigen (e.g., selected on whole live cells) and then try to use this Mab in whole cell or tissue extracts. As described in Sections 1.3 and 2.2, Mabs are never totally specific and when they are faced with an alternative dominant antigen at overwhelming concentrations, may well bind this at low affinity. The commonest situation in which this is encountered is where Mabs selected to cell surface markers or receptors are then tested against whole cell lysates. Cytoskeletal proteins such as the actins (MW 40–50K) form > 90% of the proteins in such a lysate and tend to dominate any whole cell blot. The true antigen, which may be a useful target, is only detected where it is at least a visible band on the matching protein blot.

11.4.6.1. Technical failures of blotting (rare)

(i) The antigen has not transferred.
This can be checked by staining the gel after transfer.
(ii) The detection system has not functioned/ or the antigen is not present in sufficient quantities to be detected.
This can be checked by dot-blot of antigen directly onto nitrocellulose paper without any electrophoretic step (Protocol 2.4).
(iii) The cell supernatant produces no Mab. This is typical if mycoplasma has entered the system and often true of cells imported from other labs. If it has happened, the hybridoma will grow well but cease to secrete, even in ascites. It is checked by using the original assay.
(iv) The Mab is of too low affinity and has been removed by the rigorous blocking and washing procedures. (IgMs often fail to blot for this reason.)

affinity in situations where the antigen is multivalent and the definition of multivalent includes cell surface antigens since these are immobilised in a largely two dimensional matrix. In addition, IgG bivalence
(there is no point in determining the affinity of an IgM) will raise the
affinity constant by up to two orders of magnitude as discussed in Section 2.2.3. However, the affinity constant should be measured where
possible if only to give a clear comparison with other reagents directed
to the same epitope. This affinity constant can be expressed in two
ways as discussed in Section 2.2.2. this depends on whether the lab
involved habitually does antibody or ligand binding studies.

$$K_{eq} = (Ab - Ag)/(Ab)(Ag) \text{ and is measured in l/mol or } M^{-1}$$

$$K_D = (Ab)(Ag)/(Ab - Ag) \text{ and is measured in mol/l or } M$$

It will be evident that one is the inverse of the other, and that a K_{eq}
of 10^{-9} M^{-1} is identical to a K_D of 10^9 M (or 1 nM). For the first,
the lower the value the better the antibody affinity and for the second,
the higher the value, the better the antibody affinity. Most Mab technologists only look at the power of ten involved and a few laboratories have dropped into the 'data massaging' habit of expressing affinity constants to look as good as possible. For example, while both
mean the same, an equilibrium association constant of 5×10^{-9} looks
better than an equilibrium dissociation constant of 2×10^8.

11.6.1. Quick affinity ranking of a panel

This can be achieved by using most assay methods and reducing the
amount of antigen available to a group of Mabs. For a good fusion,
early screening should not aim for quantity but rather quality. If high
affinity is the main target, then it is advisable to screen for clones
which detect the minimal amount of antigen at an early stage. Thus
if 100 positives are obtained coating an ELISA plate with 1 μg of antigen, a rescreening at 0.1 μg of antigen may only detect 20 positives
but they will be higher affinity.

As an additional refinement, if the supernatant is assayed for rodent IgG as well as antigen binding, then the two can be correlated. Only those cultures giving the strongest signal at the lowest IgG concentration should be expanded.

For washing assays such as ELISA, simply wash 2–3 more times. This is quite possible to do on ELISA plates which have already been developed once (Protocol 2.2)

11.6.2. Methods which do not measure affinity but may appear to do so

Good binding systems always emerge from the commercial mass of modern biotechnology and bad ones fail to do so. It is, nonetheless, useful to be able to anticipate this event and assess whether affinity constants suggested in the literature are valid. There is a disturbing new trend of data presentation which is suggested to indicate affinity but does not do so. The commonest is to use a quasi competition assay dislodging labelled bound antigen with unlabelled competing antigen. The implication is that the molar concentration which dislodges the labelled antigen represents the affinity constant. In an unconfined system where the antigen may be in vast excess (for example, washing a nitrocellulose filter in 10 ml buffer containing the appropriate antigen concentration), this does not indicate any parameter relevant to the affinity constant. The refinement of comparing the binding of a Mab of known affinity against the test Mab on the same filter, both being exposed to excess antigen, is only relevant where the comparative molar protein concentrations of both Mabs are precisely matched.

11.6.3. Affinity determination for Mabs directed against soluble antigens

11.6.3.1. By immunoprecipitation
This is best performed by classical methods involving either radiolabelled antibody or radiolabelled antigen. The most convenient isotope is ^{125}I, a gamma emitter with a medium range half life of 60 days. Io-

dine labels primarily tyrosine residues with the occasional histidine residue. It has the disadvantage that if the labelling is too extreme, tyrosine and/or histidine residues involved in interaction may be damaged. This is not usually a problem with whole antibody which has a large number of tyrosine residues (depending on antibody class) in the constant region. It should, however be noted as a potential problem in the labelling of Fab or Fv fragments (Section 9.3).

PROTOCOL 11.6: DETERMINATION OF THE AFFINITY CONSTANT FOR SOLUBLE ANTIGENS

(i) The endpoint for this protocol is the separation of Mab bound antigen from free antigen. This can be by 50% ammonium sulphate, 35% PEG, or 10% (v/v) Protein A beads. Select the system and check that the antigen alone is not precipitated/ does not bind to these. If Protein A beads are used, check that the antibody alone binds to them.

(ii) Radiolabel the antigen to 0.2–1 μCi/μg protein (and no higher) using the iodogen or iodobeads method (Protocol 12.1).

(iii) Use high titre antibody (preferably pure) from ascites or high producing bulk culture. It must be in excess to antigen.

(iv) In duplicate sets of 10 microtubes with lids, set up antigen dilutions over a range of 10–200 μg antigen in 100 μl of PBS. To each of one set of tubes add the Mab in 50 μl of PBS at a concentration of 200–300 μg/ml. To each of the other set add the relevant control (tissue culture supernatant, irrelevant ascites fluid, PBS if the Mab has been purified) as control.

(iv) To each tube add an equal volume of 100% ammonium sulphate, 70% PEG, or 20% (v/v) protein A beads, according to their suitability as determined in (i) above. Centrifuge at $600 \times g$ ($400 \times g$ for Protein A beads). Retain both supernatant and pellet, noting any relevant dilutions.

(v) For each antigen concentration, estimate the total molar concentration of antigen in both pellet and original supernatant before dilution. Subtract the radioactive counts from the precipitates in the control series of tubes from those in the test series and express this in terms of μg specific antigen bound in moles/l. The concentration of residual free antigen is then the difference between total antigen and bound antigen.

For example, if the original antigen was at a concentration of 10 μg/ml and had a molecular weight of 100,000, the total original concentration was 10^{-7} M. If the original aliquot of this gave 200,000 cpm and the bound antigen, after subtraction of the control value, gives 10,000 cpm then the concentration of bound antigen is 5×10^{-9} M and free antigen is 9.5×10^{-8}M. In this manner, obtain a series of results for bound (b) and free (c) antigen at all the concentrations employed.

(vi) The data may be plotted in two ways (Fig. 11.5). If the antibody concentration is not exactly known then according to the equation

$$1/b = 1/Kc(\text{Ab}_{\text{tot}}) + 1/\text{Ab}_{\text{tot}}$$

a plot of $1/b$ against $1/c$ gives a measure of Ab_{tot} which may be compared to the known concentration of Mab. The equilibrium affinity constant, K, is the value of $1/c$ when exactly half the total Mab is bound to antigen.

An alternative approach is to use the Sips plot (see Steward, 1986 for derivation)

$$\log b/(\text{Ab}_{\text{tot}} - b) = a \log K + a \log c$$

Thus if $\log (b/(\text{Ab}_{\text{tot}} - b))$ is plotted against $\log c$, $k = 1/c$ when the ordinate is zero. In this equation 'a' is the 'heterogeneity index' which should be low for a Mab.

11.6.3.2. Affinity determination by a quick ELISA method

The method developed by Friguet et al. (1985) has been widely used for affinity ranking of Mabs. It relies on the concept of plate bound antigen being identical to free antigen which is a wrong assumption in many cases. However, it is a very simple method for preliminary ranking of the affinity of a group of Mabs. It does not require pure

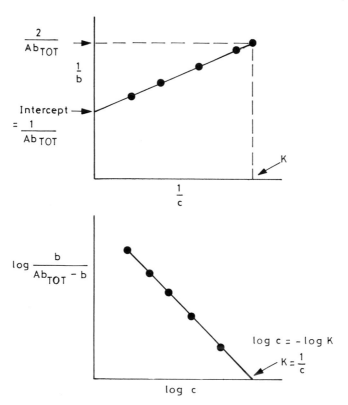

Fig. 11.5. Graphical plots for the determination of Mab affinity. Top, by the equation $1/b = 1/Kc(Ab_{tot}) + 1/Ab_{tot}$. Bottom, by the equation: $\log b/(Ab_{tot} - b) = a \log K + a \log c$. ($b$ = bound antigen in mol/l; c = free antigen in mol/l.).

Mab. It may be necessary to do the assay twice, firstly over a wide range of antigen concentrations and then homing in over the smaller concentration range which is relevant.

PROTOCOL 11.7: QUICK ELISA FOR AFFINITY DETERMINATION

(i) Set up the standard ELISA assay with the Mab using 1 μg pure antigen/well. Perform doubling dilutions of the Mab preparation to check that absorbance is linear with concentration through the operating range. Note the dilution of Mab which gives the absorbance at the top of the linear plot and use this for part (ii).

(ii) In a series of polytubes set up a range of antigen concentrations from 10^{-7} M to 10^{-10} M. Incubate overnight with the antibody concentration which gave top linear absorbance in (i).

(iii) In duplicate, pipette 100 μl from each polytube onto an ELISA plate coated with 1 μg/well of antigen. Include a sample of antibody alone at the same concentration. Incubate for 1 hour. Wash the plates as in a normal ELISA assay (Protocol 2.2), incubate with second antibody and develop colour by the usual system. Measure absorbance.

If the absorbance of the tube with antibody alone is A_0 (no competing antigen in the first incubation) and the absorbance at each concentration of competing antigen is A, then for each antigen concentration compute $A_0/(A_0 - A)$. Plot this on the ordinate against $1/(\text{substrate})$. This should give a linear plot, intercept should be 1, and the affinity constant will be given by the slope.

11.6.3.3. Affinity determination by fluorescence

Fluorescence methods depend either on the presence of endogenous tryptophan residues in antibody or antigen or on the use of a reporter molecule attached to the antigen. In both cases, it is necessary for the antibody antigen complex to have different fluorescence intensity from the additive fluorescence of antibody and antigen alone. Sometimes the fluorescence is quenched by the interaction and in other cases it is enhanced (reviewed by Parker, 1978). These methods are comparatively insensitive, as the difference in fluorescence is usually small and the method of measurement has a high statistical variation.

11.6.4. Affinity determination for Mabs directed to cellular antigens

There is an expanding requirement for methods which can measure this accurately as cell surface antigens become increasingly relevant targets in many labs. Cell surface affinity measurements still, however, fail to correlate with classical single molecule measurements and one major reason is the amplification (which may be important in vivo) of affinity by presentation on the surface of the cell of antigens in a comparatively local manner. This is therefore an 'avidity' rather than an affinity measurement (Section 2.2.2).

The 'cell' can also be a bacterium or virus and the former can be detected well on the FACS. However, most bacteria and viruses have too high an epitope density and limited cell surface antigen representation to give a valid result. They tend to indicate very high affinities where alternate assays indicate that this is not the case. The most reliable protocols are FACS protocols but it is also possible to determine cell bound affinity by quite simple methods.

11.6.4.1. Affinity determination using the FACS

There are several protocols for this and some are more rigorous than others (Sklar and Finney, 1982; Sklar et al., 1984; Chatelier et al., 1986; Griswold, 1987). Protocol 11.8 is adapted from Chatelier et al. (1986) and is designed to detect affinity values within the range of 10^{-9} M^{-1} (or 10^9 M) – see 11.6.1 above. It uses mg amounts of Mab and some hours of FACS time.

PROTOCOL 11.8: DETERMINING AFFINITY BY FACS

(i) Purify the Mab (Section 10.6) and label with fluorescein (Table 2.4). Store in the dark.

(ii) Prepare a series of six identical sets of four tubes (A1–4 to F1–4) each set (all As etc) containing 200 μl target cells at a range of $6 \times 10^5/$ml (all four A tubes), $2 \times 10^5/$ml (all four B tubes) up to to $3 \times 10^7/$ml (all four F tubes).

This can also be expressed as moles of cell per litre by dividing the number of cells per litre (6×10^8 to 3×10^{10} in the above case) by Avagadro's number (6×10^{23}), i.e., the final concentration being 1–50 fmol cell/l.

(iii) In the dark, or in covered containers, prepare 1 ml solutions each of fluoresceinated Mab in the range 1–50 μg/ml (e.g., 1, 5, 10, 20 and 50 μg/ml).

(iv) To tube A1 add 200 μl PBS and, using the usual 'red for dead' selection, measure the maximal fluorescence level set on the FACS with linear collection of FITC fluorescence. Do the same for tubes B1 to F1 to obtain the appropriate autofluorescence controls throughout the range of different cell densities.

(v) To tubes A2–F2 add 200 μl of the lowest concentration of Mab, incubate for 10–30 min, and repeat the exercise. There is no need to wash – Ag and Ab should be in contact at the correct concentration at as close a time to the measurement as possible. Measure the average fluorescence channel for the cells (F_t) and note the final Mab concentration Mab_{tot}.

(vi) To tubes A3–F3 add the second to lowest concentration of Mab, incubate for 10–30 min, and repeat the exercise. There is no need to wash.

(vii) Repeat this process for all other cell and Mab concentrations.

(viii) You should now have a range of F_t values for cells at the same dilution differentially illuminated within each range of antibody concentration.

Plot F_t (y-axis – ordinate) against Mab_{tot} (x-axis – abscissa) (plot 1).

This will give a series of curves each representing a single cell density, which flatten out at higher Mab concentrations.

(ix) Take a single F_t value and run a horizontal line across the above graph at the points where the curves are still linear. This will intersect with a series of data points representing different cell numbers (molarities). Note the values of Mab_{tot} required to obtain this at each cell concentration and do the same for several other F_t values in the linear range

(x) Replot the data to represent cell molarity (C) (see (i) above) on the abscissa (x-axis) against total Mab concentration (Mab_{tot}) on the ordinate (y-axis) (plot 2).

According to the equation

$$Mab_{tot} = Mab_{free} + Mab_{bound}$$

where $Mab_{bound} = $ moles Mab bound/cell $(r) \times$ molar concentration of cells (C)

$$Mab_{tot} = Mab_{free} + rC.$$

Thus the slope of each of these plots gives an r value for each different combination of antibody and antigen. The intercept gives free antibody.

(xi) The classical Scatchard plot of r/Mab_{free} against r can then be constructed (plot 3). The slope gives the affinity constant. Frequently the slope is bi (or multi) phasic.

Bator and Reading (1989) above have devised a simpler protocol for testing affinity on whole cells, similar to that used for pure antigens in Protocol 11.7 and, in contrast to Protocol 11.8, a FACS is not required. The difference is that cells are inadvisable as antigens in ELISA assays (Chapter 2) and in consequence, unbound antibody (rather than bound antibody) is assayed by a double polyclonal sandwich assay akin to Fig. 1.8 but with a polyclonal antibody on each side. This is not an ideal detection system and the antisera employed have to be carefully selected to give a reliable standard curve of Mab concentration. In addition, any dead cells in the system will bind the antibody non-specifically and have a strong effect on the results.

The cells are interacted with the Mab and then centrifuged to remove bound Mab. Unbound Mab is then assessed by its relative concentration in the ELISA supernatant. In principle, this method can be used by varying either cell or antibody concentration.

11.7. Karyotype analysis of hybridomas

Karyotyping is a skilled and complex technique and is probably best performed by medical genetics laboratories who undertake this task routinely. It should be performed on all cell lines from external sources, particularly human ones. Cultures are readily taken over by fast growing cell contaminants and there are many incidences of laboratories attempting to fuse and clone with cells which are not only of the wrong phenotype but also the wrong species. Karyotyping is also useful in the examination of the chromosome number of hybridomas and in the determination of which chromosomes are present in a cross species fusion. A very high-quality microscope is required.

The theoretical background to such techniques is based on the known effects of colchicine which inhibits microtubule polymerisation during mitosis. A consequence of this is that a high percentage of mitotic cells may be produced by treatment of the culture with colchicine. However, too much colchicine results in overcontracted chromosomes which are less readily identified and stained. There are a great variety of stains which may be used to identify human chromosomes in particular but the most generally employed one is Giemsa which gives very characteristic bands for each mammalian chromosome. The dye is not readily accessible to the chromosomes because of their protein coating which is more dense in the contracted state. Trypsin is therefore used to increase accessibility. However, too much trypsin releases the chromosomal DNA from its contracted condition and results in large diffusely stained chromosomes.

If only the number and general morphology of the chromosomes is required then the procedure given in Protocol 11.9 is comparatively simple. However, banding techniques are more complex. The Giemsa banding technique in Protocol 11.10 is dependent on the level of trypsinsation of the cells. Too much trypsin allows the chromosomes to expand so that their identification becomes difficult. Too little gives minimal access to the stain. Banding techniques also require expertise in identification. The protocols given below are for lymphoblastoid and suspension cultures and differ from protocols used for fibroblasts.

PROTOCOL 11.9: PREPARATION OF CHROMOSOME SPREADS

(i) Subculture 10 ml of cells at a density of 2–5×10^5/ml in 25-cm^2 flasks 24–48 h before karyotyping to make sure that they are in logarithmic growth. Prepare colchicine (Demecolcemid, Sigma) in 0.25 ml aliquots at 80 μg/ml in distilled water. This may be stored at $-20°$C.

(ii) Add 25 μl of the stock colchicine solution for each 10 ml of cells in culture. Incubate for 90 min (a shorter time will produce less contracted chromosomes) and centrifuge for 5 min at 400 × g in siliconised tubes. Pour off the supernatant and wash the cells in 0.14 M NaCl 5 mM KCl, 0.5 mM EDTA, 0.2% (w/v) phenol red, pH 7.4, recentrifuge and remove all but 2 ml of supernatant. Gently resuspend the cells in this by tapping the tube. Add 10 ml 0.075 M KCl at 37°C.

(iii) Incubate for 10 min at 37°C. Centrifuge for 5 min at 400 × g. Remove all but 0.2 ml of the supernatant and gently resuspend the cells by tapping the tube. Add 1 ml 3:1 methanol: acetic acid fixative (Freshly prepared and cooled to 4°C) slowly with shaking and then a further 9 ml. Seal the tube and place at 4°C for at least 30 min and several hours if this is suitable.

(v) Using a siliconised Pasteur pipette held close to the ear, drop the cell suspension onto a wet glass slide held at arms length. Dry the slide and examine at low magnification.

Note. If there are problems due to cell clumping then the 10 min incubation in 0.075 M KCl in step (ii) may be replaced by the addition of 6 drops of fixative followed by immediate centrifugation. This may reduce the quality of the spreads.

PROTOCOL 11.10: GIEMSA STAINING OF CHROMOSOME SPREADS

(i) Prepare a solution of trypsin (Difco-Bacto) in 10 ml normal (0.9%) saline. Aliquot in 0.5 ml portions and store at −20°C. Use aliquots as required and do not re-freeze. After thawing, dilute samples of 0.4 ml to 25 ml with normal saline.

(ii) Place the dried slide in a slide rack in a covered container with 2 × SSC (0.3 M NaCl,0.03 M Na citrate, pH 7). Incubate at 60 °C for 2 h. Remove the slide rack to containers with firstly 0.15 M NaCl and secondly distilled water to rinse.

$\rightarrow$

Fig. 11.6. G banded karyotype of normal human cells.

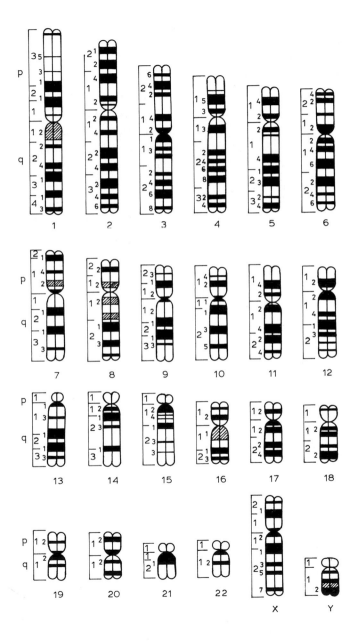

(iii) Dehydrate the slides by moving the slide rack sequentially for 2 min intervals to 50%, then 70%, 90%, 95% and 100% ethanol and air-dry.

(iv) Place a trial slide in the diluted trypsin solution for 70–80 s and rinse immediately in normal saline. Stain the slide in a fresh solution containing 4 parts BDH, pH 6.8, buffer (BDH Gurr code 33199) and one part Leishman's stain (0.15 g Leishman's powder in 100 ml methanol stirred cold for 2 h and filtered before use) for 3.5 min and rinse in pH 6.8 buffer immediately. Dry the slide on a hot or warm plate.

(v) Examine the slide under the microscope. If the chromosomes show little stain in the bands then increase the time in trypsin for a few seconds. If they appear bloated and diffuse then decrease it. If the banding is visible but of an unsuitable intensity and the chromosome morphology is normal, then alter the time in the stain accordingly. It is likely that the two variables (trypsin and stain time) may have to be altered several times to obtain an ideal identification.

(vi) Photograph the slide, cut out and pair the photographs of the individual chromosomes, and compare with the normal human karyotype (Fig. 11.6).

CHAPTER 12

Immunosensors

12.1. Biosensors

A biosensor is generally defined as a device which utilises a biological sensing element connected to a transducing system which leads to the output of an electronic signal, the strength of this signal usually being proportional to the concentration of a molecule or set of molecules detected by the biological sensing element. The general philosophy behind biosensor technology is that it should not require any human manipulation between probe and result.

The biological sensing element can be an enzyme, a biological receptor molecule, a whole organism such as an environmentally sensitive bacterium, all or part of a whole cell such as a squid axon and, in principle, even more complex biological systems such as whole tissues. It can also be an antibody and this chapter is directed solely to current applications and realistic projected applications in the immunosensor field. Methods in early stages which require complex equipment have not been considered suitable for coverage.

While immunosensor technology is an area of considerable interest to Mab technologists, it is also a difficult area to study in the literature because many of the potential applications are commercial and consequently the best methodology can remain unpublished until fully developed and marketed. Where it is published, complex optical and electronic systems are frequently involved and it is difficult for the Mab technologist to understand the precise nature of the signal transduction mechanism. Conversely, electrochemists or optics specialists generally test out a technique using polyclonal antibodies and haptens, assuming that all antibodies, including Mabs are precisely equally and exquisitely specific up to infinite detection limits whereas the immunologist knows their strengths and limitations. The task for the Mab technologist is to be able to produce a Mab (or panel of Mabs) compatible with the system to be used and able to give maximum detectability and sensitivity. Their task is often also to educate electrochemists or specialists in opto-electronics in the limitations as well as the potential of the immune system. This Chapter explains the basic concepts behind biosensor systems and describes how Mabs may best be generated to use them to their full potential.

12.2. Enzyme biosensors using enzymes as sensing elements

Direct enzyme biosensors convert a substrate into products which can make contact with the transduction system, either directly, or through a mediator such as ferrocene. The best characterised systems are in the oxidoreductase field where the product electrons can be passed directly to mediating molecules such as ferrocene (Fig. 12.1). Ferrocene and its derivatives are particularly well suited to this task as the aromatic rings can be coupled to a variety of derivatives which render it insoluble and capable of binding to graphite electrodes. It also has a low 'overpotential', i.e., it is readily regenerated at the electrode (Cardosi and Turner, 1987). Such 'mediator' molecules interface the bio-

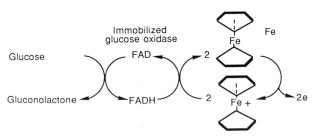

Fig. 12.1. The glucose oxidase enzyme based amperometric biosensor for detection of glucose.

logical and electronic components of the sensor leading to a direct current reading reflecting the glucose level in the test solution (Cass et al., 1984) and can be adapted to give implantable in vivo biosensors (Pickup, 1989). A commercial system based on this has been marketed and the success has led to speculative production of a variety of different immunosensors based on adaptions of the basic ideas behind the system.

12.3. The difference between enzyme based sensing elements and antibody based sensing elements

12.3.1. The specificity of the reaction

Enzymes have been designed throughout evolution to have specificity of binding which is reinforced by the proximity of one or more independent catalytic groups so that a reaction subsequent to binding can take place to yield product. Antibodies, on the other hand come from a necessarily brief period of local evolution within an individual animal and have less highly defined specificity since their normal role is to act in concert. In consequence, unless very carefully selected, any individual antibody is unlikely to have the same unique specificity for its antigen that an enzyme has for its substrate.

12.3.2. The kinetics of the reaction

Enzymes, in order to perform their natural function efficiently, have a rapid turnover of substrate so that a single enzyme molecule can convert up to 10^6 substrate molecules to product every second. Evolution has designed enzymes to release products readily in order to free the active site for a further substrate molecule. As a consequence most enzymes have a highly dynamic relationship with both substrate and product so that it is only on the occasional binding of substrate that the dynamic enzyme conformation is suitably placed to catalyse the reaction. The necessity for the binding to generate this optimal catalytic conformation adds to the precision specificity of enzymes. The ease with which it is possible to obtain pools of potentially catalytic Mabs which bind transition state intermediates (Section 1.14), in comparison to the difficulty of finding any one of these Mabs capable of catalysing the reaction, illustrates the case. Antibodies bind but the variable region has been selected for no other function. The kinetics are frequently different with a high-affinity Mab having a low K_{diss}. A single antibody molecule binds one or two molecules of antigen and thereafter tends to stay bound, generating no further signal.

In consequence, Mabs are unlikely to be able to compete with enzymes in situations in which a convenient and inexpensive enzyme assay system which can use the putative antigen as a specific substrate is available.

12.3.3. The use of an antibody sensing element with an enzyme as part of the transducing system

One of the commonest errors in biotechnology/immunoassay is to assume that if an enzyme gives a good lower limit of detectability in an assay, an antibody linked to that enzyme will do the same. At first consideration, attachment of an antibody to an enzyme should increase its sensitivity or lower the limit of detection (Chapter 2). In practice, this procedure abrogates the ability of the enzyme to detect substrate as a monitor of its concentration and the result only reflects the amount of antibody bound. Since many antibodies bind non-specifically, at low affinity, the result is that the attached enzymes can also amplify this signal in an indiscriminate manner (Fig. 12.2). The signal/noise ratio depends largely on the affinity of the antibody.

The ultimate detection limit of any immunosensor system is based on the overall intrinsic affinity of the Mab (or panel of Mabs) to the molecules under test.

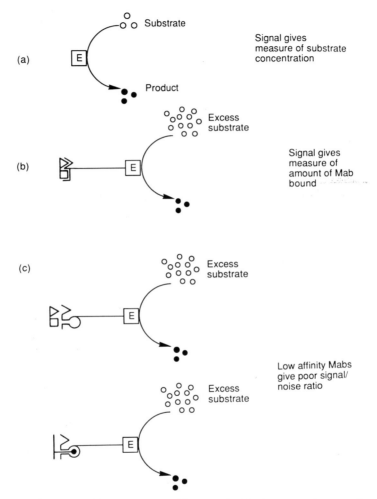

Fig. 12.2. Basing a Mab kit on an enzyme biosensor. In (a) the enzyme is measuring substrate concentration as in Fig. 12.1. In (b) a high-affinity Mab (see Fig. 1.3) is used and will measure antigen concentration within the capacity of its affinity for antigen. In (c) and (d) a low-affinity Mab is used and can measure true antigen to less acceptable detectability limits while also being able to bind to irrelevant material. The signal/noise ratio in (b), (c) and (d) depends on the Mab and not on the enzyme.

12.4. Requirement and potential application of antibody based immunosensors

12.4.1. Potential applications

The requirement for immunologically based biosensors is generally considered to be in the diagnostic field and particularly in the home diagnostic field (Section 1.11.6). Examples such as detection of contaminants in food or water are the most obvious application. One should, however, be aware at the start that this general approach has limitations. Home diagnostic kits for potentially epidemic infections frequently cannot legally be put on the open market. Thus kits detecting bacteria causing venereal disease cannot be sold in countries where this remains a 'notifiable' disease and home testing kits for the HIV virus are still banned in many countries. Projected applications in the clinical laboratory will have to prove superiority either in detection limits or in cost effectiveness to gain acceptance and the same is true for forensic or military use. With these caveats, it is possible to envisage a multitude of biological applications such as personal detection alarms for allergy sufferers, probes for detecting food additives or contaminants, and self monitoring systems for patients with chronic autoimmune conditions to allow them to administer drugs only when appropriate in the same manner as diabetic patients can monitor their current blood glucose level and take insulin only when appropriate. At the moment, this requirement being approached by the use of conventional diagnostic systems and the immunosensor adaption is largely in the area of electrochemical immunosensors.

Another requirement is for a different market which is perceived to be smaller but still significant. This is continuous monitoring without the need for any operator action or any need for regular input of enzyme substrates, fluorescent materials etc. This monitoring may be within the human body or in process control in industry or continuous environmental monitoring for water supplies or air conditioning plants. For these some of the optical systems (see below) may have greater potential.

12.4.2. Ideal immunosensor properties

The properties of the ideal immunosensor are listed in Table 12.1. Some requirements are expanded below with references to the many projected uses for which antibodies are well suited.

Stability

Antibodies are usually very stable molecules as a consequence of their disulphide bonded structure and, if kept in a protease free environment, can last for months (Section 10.5). They are designed to operate freely and are not altered in structure when separated from cell membranes as are many receptor molecules.

Economic

Mabs can be produced economically in large amounts (Section 10.2). These are substantially larger pure and functional yields than can be obtained for competitor molecules such as cell surface receptor molecules. In consequence Mabs may form part of a 'throwaway' detection system which can be regenerated or a renewable tip attached to the probe.

TABLE 12.1
Properties of the ideal immunosensor

(i) Sensitive
(ii) Specific
(iii) Small
(iv) Stable – i.e., long shelf life*
(v) Simple to use
(vi) Economical
(vii) Reusable or capable of continuous monitoring
(viii) Insensitive to minor environmental changes (Temp, pH etc)*
(viii) Able to sample a defined volume*
(ix) Homogeneous in use*

* See text for further detail.

Sensitivity to the environment

While antibody binding is sensitive to the environment, it is not as grossly sensitive as most enzymes, particularly with respect to temperature. A $10°$ change in temperature can affect an enzyme activity by several orders of magnitude but seldom affects antibody binding more than 5 fold. Obviously, any individual Mab should and can be selected during screening for a lack of excessive temperature dependence.

Homogeneous or heterogeneous immunosensors

A heterogeneous biosensor requires that either an operator or an instrument performs a function such as the washing away of unbound material or addition of sequential reagents. A homogeneous one gives a direct reading after binding without any further manipulations. Antibodies can be adapted to homogeneous assays but many which were selected on heterogeneous assays (washing, centrifugation of beads – e.g., ELISA – Section 2.6) will not operate efficiently in this context without selection for such use.

12.4.3. Possible defects in antibody based immunosensors

These lie with the quality of antibody employed. Antibodies are much more prone to non-specific binding than enzymes as discussed above. Since this binding is usually at comparatively low affinity, it can be removed by washing type assays and can be largely overcome if, ideally, sandwich (Fig. 1.8) assays using two Mabs to different epitopes on the antigen are employed since the chances of both Mabs binding non-specifically to the same antigen in the contaminant are greatly reduced. The less ideal but functional simple competition assays used for smaller antigens (Fig. 1.9) also incorporate washing or separation steps.

However, homogeneous assays such as those envisaged in many of the projected applications of optical immunosensors which employ a single Mab and incorporate no washing or separation step to remove low-affinity bound material will be vulnerable to nonspecific binding of irrelevant molecules in the sample, especially if these are present at high concentration. The use of panels of Mabs will overcome this to some extent.

12.5. Classification of immunosensor systems

Immunochemical systems have been classified largely according to their electronic transduction systems. Immunologically, almost all of them involve competition assays (Fig. 1.9) with labelled antigen being competed out by unlabelled antigen in the test sample. This is a less ideal system than the sandwich system as discussed in Section 1.11 and is likely to have limits on detection range further imposed by kinetic and mass transport constraints (Eddows, 1988).

12.5.1.1. Electrochemical

Such systems generally depend on the ability of enzyme linked to antibody to catalyse a reaction giving a product which can transfer a signal to the transducing agent. Electrochemical assays are further divided into potentiometric and amperometric ones. Potentiometric systems measure potential difference with respect to a reference electrode. The relationship between concentration and signal is logarithmic. In principle, if an antibody is absorbed onto the electrode and then interacted with an antigen, it will change in electrical charge and this can be measured with respect to the reference. In practice, such simple systems are prone to non-specific binding of antigen to the electrode. More recent potentiometric systems use antibodies or antigens linked to enzymes which produce ammonia (Gebauer and Rechnitz, 1982) or carbon dioxide (Fonong and Rechnitz, 1984; Keating and Rechnitz, 1985) for which standard electrode systems are developed, or ion selective electrodes (Keating and Rechnitz, 1984). This is an effective competition assay where the antigen from the sample dislodges the antibody from the antigen coupled enzyme so that the enzyme is free to function. An essential feature of most of these systems has been the immobilisation of the enzyme and/or antibody within the vicinity of the electrode. Methods for achieving this are reviewed by Barker (1987) and Tor et al. (1989).

Amperometric immunoassays are based on a change in current and frequently use oxidoreductase enzymes to yield electrons which can be directly transferred to the transducing agent. The relationship between concentration and current is linear. The enzyme based glucose detection system referred to above is amperometric. As in the case of potentiometric systems, competition assays are generally set up and in this case they can also involve attaching the antibody to transducer molecules such as ferrocene (Weber and Purdy, 1979) (Fig. 12.1) or labelling the antigen with metal ions (Wehmeyer et al., 1982; Doyle et al., 1982). The amperometric system is generally more readily miniaturised and easier to translate to use outside the laboratory environment. Both systems are reviewed by Green (1987a,b).

The success of the ferrocene based glucose enzyme based kit led to many attempts to adapt this to a 'competition' kit for low molecular weight antigens. It is possible to cross-link the enzyme itself (for example glucose oxidase – Fig. 12.1) to antigen so that it is inactive when specific antibody is bound to the attached antigen but active when the hapten is dislodged by free antigen from the sample under test. Similarly, a small antigenic hapten can be attached to the transducer molecule preventing it from functioning properly until the hapten bound antibody is dislodged by the free antigen from the sample under test. In this case, the enzyme is only acting as a reporter molecule under conditions of excess substrate and the resolution of the system is dependent on the affinity of the antibody as described above.

Electrochemical systems of this type also present difficulties for large antigens. The enzyme is generally confined to the region of the electrode by some sort of semi-permeable membrane through which small molecules can pass and further developments in membrane technology are required. Selective membranes which only allowed small proteins to pass such as those developed by Damon Biotech, would be particularly useful in the case of polypeptide antigens.

12.5.1.2. Piezoelectric

Piezoelectric systems depend on the vibration of a (usually) quartz crystal in response to a (usually) gold electrode. The vibrational frequency changes when the crystal is coated with protein and the magnitude of the change reflects the amount of protein adsorbed to the crystal (Karube and Gotoh, 1987; Guilbaut et al., 1988). Thus the vibrational frequency changes when antibody is adsorbed, and changes again when is adsorbed antibody binds antigen. Unlike most immunosensor systems, this one has been used to detect large bacterial or cellular antigens.

12.5.2. General optical systems

Optical systems have advantages over electrochemical systems in that they can operate at a distance from the reagent phase and do not require to be in direct physical contact with the biological receptor system. In principle, they have the additional advantage of being able to operate at several wavelengths at once and consequently being suitable for simultaneous assays of several antigens. They have the disadvantage of being difficult to miniaturise (Seitz, 1987). Most optical systems are based on optical fibres which have total internal reflection of the light entering the fibre so that the beam is guided along the length of the fibre. This is achieved by the cladding of the fibre core with material of lower refractive index than the material in which the beam is travelling (Fig. 12.3). The beam can be delivered into a membrane covered chamber at the end of the fibre where antibody is interacted with (for example) fluorescently labelled low molecular weight antigen haptenated to an inert protein in order to remain membrane impermeable. The fluorescence emission can be conveyed back up the fibre through optical filters to remove incident light. Test antigen can then diffuse in and replace this. Most of such systems are still in early stages of development but they do offer interesting possibilities for continuous monitoring at a distance (reviewed by Schultz, 1987a,b).

12.5.3. Internal Reflection Spectroscopy (IRS) optical systems

These systems are based on the ability of a reflected wave of light to differentiate between antigen molecules which are attached to a layer of antibody molecules bound to a reflecting surface and antigen molecules which are free in solution. The measurement can be either of the intensity of the reflected light or the angle of its detection. The IRS

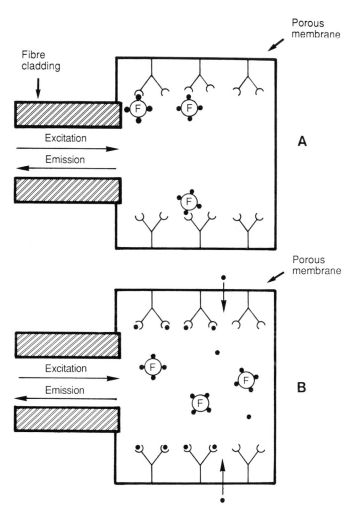

Fig. 12.3. The measurement of a small antigen at long range through the use of an optical fibre. This is a competition assay where the antigen can diffuse in and displace fluorescent labelled antigen haptenated onto a protein. The fluorescent label is then detected by the light beam.

systems include Attenuated Total Reflection (ATR), Total Internal Reflection Fluorescence (TIRF), Surface Plasmon Resonance (SPR) and the Fluorescence Capillary Fill Device (FCID). ATR,TIRF and SPR are reviewed by Sutherland and Dahne (1987) and FCFD by Badley et al. (1987).

ATR and TIRF both depend on the concept of evanescent light waves which penetrate only around 10–40 nm, depending on refractive index differences into the solution containing the antigen while the main beam is reflected back into the medium of higher refractive index. Thus, if the antibody (an IgG molecule is approximately 10 nm in length) is attached at the interface, the evanescent wave effectively only detects bound antigen molecules. ATR measures the loss in light energy due to absorption of the evanescent wave and TIRF, which is more suitable for Mab use, measures the fluorescence emitted by bound fluorescently labelled antigen molecules (Fig. 12.4). These systems can, at least in theory be coupled with fibre optic systems to produce homogeneous immunosensors which require no regeneration of reagent and can operate at a distance (Andrade et al., 1985). It is possibly worth noting that the evanescent wave range is very much smaller than the dimensions of large particles such as bacteria.

Surface plasmon resonance (also called surface plasmon oscillation)

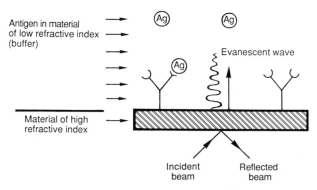

Fig. 12.4. Diagrammatic representation of the evanescent wave which can only see bound antigen on the edge of an optical interface.

also involves evanescent waves (see above) and is essentially an adaption of ATR. There is no requirement for a fluorescent label. However, it is not the light energy but rather change of the angle of the reflected light which is observed. The sample is adsorbed to a thin film of a conducting metal such as silver. At a precise angle of incidence, the evanescent wave is able to set off resonance oscillations in the electrons of the metal and the light energy is dissipated so that the intensity of the reflected beam drops dramatically. The process is sensitive to the refractive index of the material adjacent to the metal film. Consequently, if the metal has a protein adsorbed to its surface, the angle at which the resonance oscillation can occur is slightly altered. If this protein is further bound by another protein or bacterium, the angle is altered again (Fig. 12.5). SPR systems are also still in early stages of development but have been shown to be capable of resolution to nanomolar levels in immunoassay (Mayo and Hallock, 1989). At the moment, the equipment is complex and requires laser optics.

The Fluorescence capillary fill device (FCFD) is an optical system which also relies on detection of light at different angles but in this

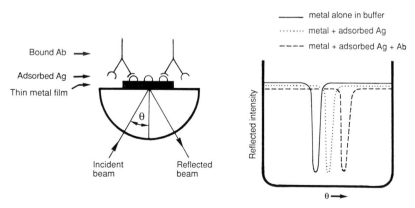

Fig. 12.5. Surface plasmon resonance. The angle at which the intensity of the reflected beam drops due to resonance with the electrons in the metal depends on the amount of protein attached to the metal. Note that the changes in angle are small and all within 1–2°C. The method may suit large antigens.

case it is fluorescence emission. The sample collection system (Fig. 12.6) consists of two glass slides held together to form a cell. The

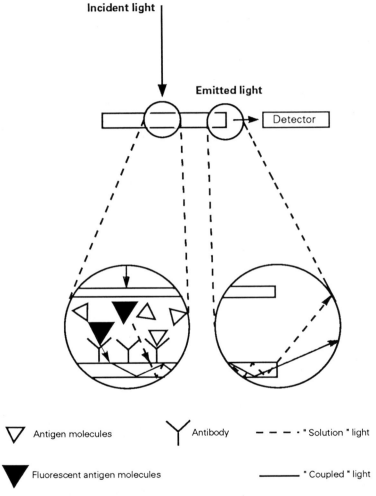

Fig. 12.6. The fluorescence capillary fill device. This is a competition assay. Unlabelled antigen molecules from the sample under test compete with fluorescent labelled antigen for binding to the Mab which is attached to the lower glass plate. The angle of the emitted fluorescence is different for free floating and bound antigen.

lower half of the top slide is coated with dried fluorescent antigen and the upper half of the bottom slide has antibody firmly attached. The sample can then be introduced by capillary action and dissolves the layer of fluorescent antigen. If there are no competing antigens in the sample, the fluorescent antigen will diffuse down and bind to the antibody on the bottom plate. Measurement is on the basis of the fact that the 'coupled' light emitted from bound fluorescent antigen is guided along the slide and emitted at a low angle while light from antigen in solution is reflected at much wider angles. The difference in angle is much greater than in SPR where it can be only a fraction of a degree. The advantages of the device are that it controls its own sample volume and is simple to operate. Since the slide systems can be made and distributed with minimal expense and then used with comparatively simple optical components, it may, should it show comparable detection limits to the more classical systems, find a place in the market more readily than the other optical systems.

Many optical systems require that the Mab be bound to glass/ quartz or other materials of precisely known refractive index in order to maintain the correct characteristics of the evanescent wave. In addition, 'capture' antibody systems must not extend too far so that the antigen is beyond the range of the evanescent wave. If the components of the system are to be reused, then good dissociation systems are also necessary. Suggested protocols are given in Section 12.7.

12.5.4. Chemiluminescent/bioluminescent systems

Chemiluminescent and bioluminescent systems sit uneasily in the biosensor field since they are currently laboratory based assays. They are, however, developing rapidly. They are more simple and economical to perform than many of the complex biosensor assays and could be developed fairly readily into automatic systems.

Most bioluminescent systems are currently too expensive to introduce as a component of any Mab based biosensor and although the bacterial luciferase gene has been cloned (Baldwin et al., 1984) the enzyme does not fulfil the requirements for enzyme immunoassay systems in terms of stability and lack of requirement of other co-factors. Its use in the biosensor and immunosensor field is reviewed by Daniliv and Ismailov (1989).

12.5.4.1. Homogeneous chemiluminescent systems

These have largely been developed for small antigens and have been used extensively for steroid assay (Messeri et al., 1989). The antigen is attached to a chemiluminescent probe which has enhanced light production when bound within the hydrophobic environment of an antibody (Fig. 12.7a). This is another competition assay for small antigens where free antigen can dislodge the bound labelled antigen. A competitive assay involving chemiluminescent antigen and fluorochrome labelled antibody has also been described (Campbell and Patel, 1983 – Fig. 12.7b). In this case the fluorochrome is excited by the wavelength of light emitted by the chemiluminescent molecule and emits at a different wavelength. These systems are intellectually attrac-

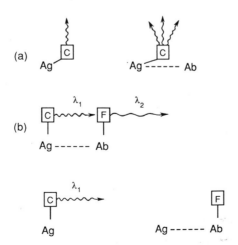

Fig. 12.7. Two homogeneous assays. In (a) the chemiluminescent signal is increased when antibody binds to antigen. In (b) the chemiluminescent molecule attached to the antigen emits light which excites the fluorophor attached to the Mab which then emits longer wavelength fluorescent light. If antigen from the sample displaces the chemiluminescent labelled antigen, the light energy transfer is lost.

tive but difficult to incorporate in full time monitoring or field use. One major disadvantage is that the light emission is transient and of comparatively low intensity.

12.5.4.2. Heterogeneous chemiluminescent systems

The heterogeneous assays are usually enzyme based assays where antibody in a sandwich assay (Fig. 1.9), or antigen in a competition assay (Fig. 1.8) are labelled with an enzyme with a chemiluminescent substrate. In consequence, these usually require a washing or separation step to remove unbound enzyme. Chemiluminescent substrates are available for many enzymes. Horseradish peroxidase, for example, has a variety of luminescent substrates of which the most commonly used is luminol with enhancers such as iodophenol to increase the strength and prolong the duration of the signal (Sections 2.6 and 2.7; Table 2.3). Alkaline phosphatase has the chemiluminescent substrate AMPPD as its only requirement, which may prove attractive for field kits because of the instability of the hydrogen peroxide in HRP substrate solutions. Thus any enzyme based system can be converted into one which yields light rather than colour and this light can be detected by a monitoring system and converted into a signal. The concept of a biosensor is to remove any need for operator and as such, most of these applications currently belong in immunoassay systems (Chapter 2). However, this is largely due to the fact that laboratory luminometers have only recently been developed and luminometers which can be employed in field use have yet to be designed. As photographic film can detect light emissions, the technology could also be developed by this route. If a passport photograph can be delivered in 3 minutes by a machine in a railway station, a chemiluminescent assay result should be capable of further refinement and automation by similar systems. A camera style luminometer has indeed already been designed (and patented) (Kricka and Thorpe, 1986).

12.6. General rules for adapting a Mab or panel of Mabs into a biosensor system

12.6.1. Affinity and epitope density

The Mab(s) must be of high affinity (Sections 1.3 and 2.2 for importance and screening, Section 11.6 for assessment) and to different epitopes if a pool is used. Almost all current biosensor pilot systems use polyclonal Mabs to haptens (i.e., several large molecules all able to bind to different parts of a single small one). With Mab technology, the starting point is a single molecule able to bind to a single antigenic epitope on, what is in many cases, a large molecule or particle.

12.6.2. The nature of the antigen

In particular, the size of the antigen is important. Most electrochemical systems have been developed for small and readily diffusable antigens and few optical systems have attempted to detect any large antigen. A large antigen would not diffuse through the membranes essential to electrochemical systems and the major part of a large antigen will not be detected by an evanescent wave on optical systems. Large antigens such as bacteria and viruses are refractive to many biosensor strategies although piezoelectric and SPR ones may have potential (Section 12.5).

12.6.3. The size of panel of Mabs to be used

While a single antibody may detect antigen, it may also detect irrelevant antigens at low affinity. This is unlikely but possible with a high-affinity antibody. If a second high-affinity antibody is involved in the detection the chances of it reacting with the same non specific epitopes are vanishingly small. Any assay system which involves two or more high-affinity antibodies is naturally superior, particularly if they are used in tandem (see for example the sandwich assay in Fig. 1.9).

12.6.4. Homogeneous or heterogeneous systems

Many Mabs which have been isolated by heterogeneous (i.e., washing) systems such as ELISA may not be suitable for homogeneous detection systems because of low-affinity binding to other materials in the sample which is removed by the washing. Conversely, Mabs selected by homogeneous systems such as agglutination may bind at too low an intrinsic affinity to maintain contact with antigen if a large number of washing steps are involved. It is undoubtedly better to make Mabs for the task. If other Mabs must be used, it is advisable to check their original screening and selection systems and either reject them, or be aware from the start that they may not perform as expected.

12.6.5. Alternative detection systems

Almost all current candidate immunological biosensor systems are tested on small haptens and these generally involve competition type assays. Large particles such as bacteria and viruses (100–1000 times the size of an antibody molecule) are refractive to many of the present candidate systems. They bear high-density cell surface markers and so generate low-affinity Mabs. They are invariably 'washed off' by hydrodynamic forces since only a small amount of the surface is antigen bound. In the barnacle and submarine analogy, however high the local affinity, adhesion will be limited with locally attached antibody as opposed to free floating antibody.

12.6.5.1. Polymerase chain reaction (PCR)
For any particle which contains any form of nucleic acid, PCR (Section 9.6) is potentially a much more sensitive alternative detection technique. At the moment, it is a laboratory based technique, but the technology is safe and simple, the procedures are simple and the main reagent (heat resistant DNA polymerase) can readily be produced in large amounts. In consequence, PCR is likely to move into wide diagnostic use potentially encompassing home and field use. While PCR cannot (at the time of writing) amplify the DNA from a single cell,

it can amplify the DNA from an ever decreasingly small number of cells. Analysis of bacteria and viruses within and without the clinical laboratory may well be replaced at lower cost by PCR. However, PCR cannot replace immunoassay for proteins, peptides, steroids, drugs etc. It is this latter market that may have the greatest potential for immunosensors.

12.6.5.2. Current simple diagnostic systems for proteins

Most of these are not technically immunosensor systems in that an electronic signal is not the final outcome although they could be adapted to give one. Yet, unlike many other immunosensor systems, they encompass most of the requirements in Table 12.1 and have proven success in the commercial market. These 'dipstick' kits involve a sandwich in which the matrix linked inner layer binds on one antigenic epitope and the enzyme linked outer antibody binds to another (Fig. 1.9). If the antigen is not present to link the two systems, a negative result is obtained. An ingenious variation of this is to have the first matrix as a coloured bead which can move up a porous stick in a version of thin layer chromatography carrying the relevant antigen (Fig. 12.8). A strip of absorbent material containing a second Mab directed to a different epitope on the antigen then retards the antigen bound beads and allows the remainder to continue and finally be trapped on a second strip containing anti-mouse immunoglobulin to serve as a positive control. If both first and second bands are visualised, the result is positive. If only the second band is visualised, the result is negative and the user has correctly followed the instructions. Inexpensive systems of this type are currently marketed by Unipath and are impressive in their ability to detect small levels of protein antigens such as human chorionic gonadotrophin (hCG) in urine of newly pregnant subjects down to picomolar concentrations.

In consequence, although the more sophisticated immunosensor technology systems can add to the possible range of applications of Mab technology, with their potential to encompass continuous use for in vivo or environmental monitoring or industrial process control, most complex systems are unrealistic with high equipment costs and

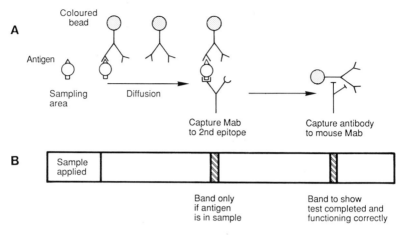

Fig. 12.8. The basis of one step sandwich type dipstick kits. A, what is happening. B, what the tester observes. The antigen attaches to the coloured bead and moves up the stick by thin layer chromatography. The coloured bead can only be attached to the second Mab if the antigen is there to cross-link it. Otherwise the bead continues until it is captured at the second point by a general anti-mouse IgG.

low detectability and sensitivity. Simpler systems are likely to prove better on both counts. Mab technologists should not assume that a complex detection system will improve this situation.

No immunosensor based project should be taken beyond the development stage unless the Mab (or panel of Mabs) involved have been shown to have detection limits comparable with other known immunoassay methods.

12.7. Labelling Mabs and their antigens

12.7.1. Labelling with ^{125}I

12.7.1.1. Labelling soluble proteins

Iodine has several isotopes and proteins are labelled with these according to the function required. ^{123}I is used for immunscintigraphy (Section 1.11.7), and ^{131}I, which emits powerful beta rays destructive within the millimetre range, is used in antibody targetted therapy. [125]I, which emits weak γ- and X-rays, is used in laboratory based diagnostics. It has a half life of 60 days. Most methods involve the oxidation of NaI to molecular iodine leading to tyrosine iodination with some iodination of histidine also occurring. If the Ab or Ag to be labelled lacks tyrosine, then various amino group labelling reagents can be purchased from suppliers such as Amersham International. The molecular iodine intermediate sublimes readily to contaminate the operator. The iodogen method described in Protocol 12.1 is strongly recommended, being is comparatively safe since the iodination which occurs on the bead surface is bound to the bead.

The level of iodination depends on the specific activity required and the extent to which the antibody or antigen can tolerate iodination without damage to the amino acids involved in binding. In this, as in many other labelling procedures, the Mab should be tested for biological activity before use.

PROTOCOL 12.1: MAB IODINATION (IODOBEADS METHOD)

This protocol can be used for other molecules over 10,000 in molecular weight.

Note: All work with isotopes must conform to local health and safety regulations.

(i) Purchase ready coated iodobeads (Pierce). (It is also quite simple to coat a glass bijoux bottle with iodogen (1,3,4,6-tetrachloro-3,6-diphenylglycoluril) by dissolving it at 1 μg/ml in chloroform, pipetting 100 μl into the bottle, and evaporating the chloroform. In this case, Step (iv) below would be omitted.

Either purchase ready poured PD-10 gel filtration columns (PD-25 will also be suitable for Mabs) or pour a gel filtration column of exclusion limit 20,000 to 50,000 in the barrel of a 5 ml syringe plugged with glass wool at the tip. Equilibrate the column with PBS.

(ii) Place 0.1–1 mg protein solution in a glass bijoux bottle in 0.5–1.0 ml of PBS, pH 7.2. Place in a lead pot.

(iii) Put on disposable gloves. In a well ventilated fume cupboard, and behind a perspex shield, add 500 μCi of carrier-free Na^{125}I, and allow to equilibrate for 15 minutes at room temperature.

(iv) Still in the fume cupboard and behind the shield, add 1 or 2 beads, and allow the reaction to proceed for 5–15 minutes in the hood depending on the extent of labelling required.

(v) Aspirate the solution and, still keeping it within the fume cupboard and behind the shield, apply to the gel filtration column pre-equilibrated with PBS. Elute with PBS.

(vi) Collect 1 ml fractions (approximately 10 fractions for proteins of molecular weight $> 10,000$), and count 5 μl aliquots. (^{125}I-protein is usually in fractions 2 to 4.)

(vii) Pool protein-containing fractions, determine specific activity and aliquot and store in lead sheets or pots.

12.7.1.2. Labelling cell membranes

If the antigen is a membrane protein then it is often convenient to label the proteins themselves and then precipitate them using second and third antibodies as described in Protocol 11.1. This is performed by gentle enzymatic oxidation using lactoperoxidase (Schlager, 1980).

12.7.2. Labelling with enzymes

The methods of labelling antibodies with enzymes are discussed at length in many other texts. With Mabs, as usual, the optimal method for one Mab may not be the optimal for another. Since enzymes also differ in their coupling methodology, there are a wide range of methods. The choice of enzymes and their substrates is discussed in Section 2.6.7 and tabulated in Table 2.4.

12.7.2.1. Labelling of horseradish peroxidase (HRP)

The method which is almost universally agreed to be the most successful for coupling HRP to enzymes is the periodate method of Wilson and Nakane (1978). The comparative efficiency of this method is probably one of the major reasons for the popularity of HRP as an enzyme label. The carbohydrate on the HRP is linked to the amino groups on the protein via Schiff base formation. It works well, because HRP has a high percentage of carbohydrate residues which are not too intimately linked to the active site. With the possible exception of glucose oxidase, the method is not generally suited to other enzyme labels. A more efficient protocol for large amounts of IgG can be found in Tijssen (1985) but this is less suited to laboratory quantities of Mab.

PROTOCOL 12.2: LABELLING OF MAB WITH HRP BY THE PERIODATE METHOD

(i) Dissolve 2 mg HRP in 0.5 ml distilled water. Add 0.1 ml freshly made up 10 mM $NaIO_4$ and shake gently for 20 min at room temperature.

(ii) Dialyse overnight at 4°C against 1 mM Na acetate buffer, pH 4.4.

(iii) Prepare 2 mg Mab solution in 0.25 ml 20 mM sodium carbonate, pH 9.5, and add to the dialysed HRP. Shake gently for 2 h at room temperature. Only unprotonated amino groups form the Schiff bases so a high pH is important.

(iv) Add 0.05 ml fresh sodium borohydride (4 mg/ml) to stabilise the conjugate. Stir for 2 h at room temperature. Shake gently at room temperature for 2 hours.

(v) Dialyse against PBS. Purify on FPLC with Superose 12 or gel filtration columns separating within the range 100,000 to 400,000. Assay both the protein and the antibody activity of each peak. HRP has a molecular weight of 44,000 and an IgG Mab of 150,000. Typical molar conjugation ratios are around 3:1 from this protocol. A molar concentration of 1:1 can be achieved by using less HRP but in that case less Mab will be conjugated.

Note Step (iii) can be improved in efficiency by increasing the local protein concentration. Pour the two protein solutions into a pasteur pipette with a heat sealed tip and add 15 mg dry Sephadex G-25. Elute at the end of the two hours with a few drops of 20 mM Na carbonate buffer, pH 9.5, and adjust the sodium borohydride addition to 1:20 of the eluted volume.

12.7.2.2. Cross-linking of Mabs to enzymes by bifunctional reagents
Glutaraldehyde is the main protein cross-linking reagent although
there are a wide range of other bifunctional reagents which attach to
amino, carboxyl or sulphydryl groups with a range of spacer arms.
If glutaraldehyde gives persistently poor results, these should be inves-
tigated on a pilot scale.

The glutaraldehyde method works poorly for HRP as a basic method although there are adaptations which improve efficiency. The commonest methods used for cross-linking of Mabs to alkaline phosphatase are adaptations of the protocol of Avreamas (1969). Generally
the calf intestine alkaline phosphatase (Section 2.6.7) rather than the
E. coli one is used. This has a molecular weight of around 85,000 and
to achieve 1:1 conjugates and avoid self polymerisation of the two reagents or the formation of large aggregates, the two should be combined at a weight ratio of 2:1 Mab/enzyme at concentrations no
higher than 10 mg/ml enzyme.

PROTOCOL 12.3: LABELLING OF MAB WITH ALKALINE PHOSPHATASE BY
THE GLUTARALDEHYDE METHOD

Note Glutaraldehyde should be handled in a fume cupboard.
(i) Mix 2.5 mg Mab with 5 mg alkaline phosphatase from calf intestine
in a total volume of 1 ml and dialyse extensively against 0.1 M sodium
phosphate buffer, pH 6.8. If either has been purified by ammonium
sulphate precipitation, it is essential to remove the ammonium ions.
(ii) Transfer to a small glass bijoux bottle with a magnetic stirrer and
slowly add 25 μl electron microscopy grade glutaraldehyde (i.e., in 5
μl aliquots). Leave for a further 2 h at room temperature without stirring and then, stirring again, add 50 μl of 1 M ethanolamine to block
reactive groups. Switch off and leave for a further 1 h at room temperature.
(iii) Dialyse extensively into 0.1 M NaCl 10 mM Tris-HCl, pH 8. Remember not to use PBS, as phosphate buffers inhibit alkaline phosphatase.
(iv) Remove any aggregates by centrifugation at 40,000 × g and purify

on FPLC with Superose 12 or gel filtration columns separating within the range 100,000 to 400,000. Free alkaline phosphatase should be at 80,000, free IgG Mab at 150,000, a 1:1 conjugate at 230,000 and higher levels of conjugation may also be seen. Assay for immunoreactivity as well as protein.

β-Galactosidase can also be conjugated to Mabs by the steps described above. It is a larger enzyme, of 460,000 in molecular weight with four subunits. Cross-linking on the basis of whole enzyme molecular weight means that it should be used at a weight ratio of 3:1 with respect to Mab. On the basis of the subunit molecular weight, this should be 0.8:1. The cross-linking reaction tends to yield aggregates very readily. In contrast to alkaline phosphatase, PBS buffer may be used in dialysis and purification.

Glucose oxidase has a molecular weight in the range 150,000 to 180,000 depending on source so that it should be used in equal milligram amounts to Mab for a 1:1 ratio. The commonest source is Aspergillus. This enzyme has 12% carbohydrate and can therefore be linked to Mabs by the periodate method (Protocol 12.2), although with lower efficiency than HRP. It can also be linked to Mabs by the glutaraldehyde method although with lower efficiency than alkaline phosphatase.

12.7.3. Biotinylation of Mabs

Biotinylated detection systems are discussed in Section 2.6.7. The advantage of biotinylation is that the same Mab preparation can then be used with a variety of different streptavidin labelled reagents – for example enzyme labelled histochemistry and FACS analysis. The disadvantage in comparison to directly labelled Mab is that an extra step is involved and the technique is not recommended for low-affinity Mabs. The commonest procedure is that of Bayer and Wilcheck which cross-links the N-hydroxysuccinimide ester of biotin to the free amino groups on the Mab. A variety of esters with different spacer arms may be obtained. However, it is possible to obtain biotin labelling reagents reactive with groups other than amino groups (Bayer and Wilcheck, 1980).

As with all cross-linking methods, over-biotinylation will reduce activity and the Mab should be checked in conventional assay at the end of the procedure.

PROTOCOL 12.4: BIOTINYLATION OF MABS

(i) Dialyse 1 mg Mab solution in 1 ml into 0.1 M Na borate, pH 8.8.
(ii) Dissolve 5 mg biotin in 1 ml dimethyl sulphoxide. Add 10 μl of this to the antibody solution. Mix well and incubate at room temperature for 4 h.
(iii) Stop the reaction by adding 20 μl 1 M ammonium chloride. Dialyse into PBS over 24 h at 4°C with several changes.

12.7.4. Labelling of Mabs with fluorochromes

The main methods for labelling Mabs with fluorochromes are listed in Table 2.4 and discussed in Sections 2.8 and 2.9. Fluorescein or rhodamine are readily attached to Mabs (Johnson and Holborow, 1986). Some of the large fluorochromes such as phycoerythrin are more difficult to attach and different labelling strategies are required. These usually involve the attachment of disulphide bonded cross-linking agents (Hardy, 1986) and it is possible to purchase sulphydryl group ready linked phycoerythrins for this purpose (Molecular Probes, Oregon).

12.7.5. Binding Mabs to solid surfaces for assay

12.7.5.1. Binding to beads
The binding of Mabs to polyvinyl chloride or polystyrene based ELISA plates and binding to nitrocellulose are discussed in Section 2.6.1, since these are the solid matrices in most regular screening use. Assay use can also involve these supports. However, many routine immunoassay methods require the binding of a Mab to specially activated beads. The beads together with bound antigen can therefore be removed in a centrifugation or chromatographic step (for example Fig. 12.8 above).

There are several strategies for this. Mabs can be directly bound to activated beads, linked to the beads by a sandwich layer of polyclonal anti-mouse IgG antibody, linked by protein A, or in the case of mouse Mabs which bind weakly to protein A, linked by a double sandwich of protein A–anti-mouse IgG. It is convenient to purchase the beads already optimally labelled and so protein A beads are very frequently used.

PROTOCOL 12.5: BINDING OF MABS TO PROTEIN A BEADS

(i) The Mab does not have to be completely pure but should obviously be a substantial proportion of the protein bound to the Protein A beads. Mix 1 ml of 1–2 mg/ml Mab with 2 ml wet beads and rock gently at room temperature for 1 h.

(ii) Add 20 ml sodium borate, pH 9 (high pH is necessary to remove the charge from the amino groups) and centrifuge at $2500 \times g$ for 5 min. Wash with a further 20 ml sodium borate and centrifuge again. The Mab should be bound to the protein A non-covalently at this stage.

(iii) Resuspend in 20 ml sodium borate, pH 9, and add dimethyl pimelimidate to give a final concentration of 20 mM. This will cross-link the bound Mab and protein A. Rock at room temperature for 30 min. Centrifuge at $2500 \times g$ and wash the beads in 0.2 M ethanolamine. Resuspend in PBS. Do not freeze but store at 4°C in the presence of 0.01% merthiolate.

Note 1. For Mabs which do not bind to protein A (Table 10.2), Protein G may be used. Alternatively, affinity purified (Table 2.2) anti-mouse IgG may be bound to the same volume of protein A beads with one washing step to remove unbound IgG, in a preliminary step before the start of the protocol to act as a capture antibody.

Note 2. The beads may also be used to purify antigen which can be eluted by the procedures described in Protocol 10.6, Step (v) onwards.

12.7.5.2. Binding to glass or quartz
Optical or piezoelectric immunosensor methods frequently require the binding of a Mab to glass or quartz. These are low-capacity surfaces in comparison to ELISA plates, nitrocellulose and activated beads.

Binding to glass is generally enhanced by the use of dichlorodimethyl silane to give a hydrophobic surface which will bind proteins (Elwing and Stenberg, 1981). In analogy to other binding systems, this can in many cases be amplified by the use of a capture polyclonal antibody as the first component bound to the glass while remaining within the range of the evanescent wave. Other systems include direct glutaraldehyde cross-linking to the solid surface (Shons, 1972) and polymer coupling with polyethyleneimine (D'Souza et al., 1986). Guilbault (1989) tried several methods for immobilisation of antibodies to *Salmonella* in a piezoelectric system and found polymer coupling to be the most reliable method. Where glutaraldehyde or other cross-linkers are used to bind the antibody to the solid surface, it is often possible to regenerate the antibody bound material while removing the bound antigen to allow for re-use (Blanchard et al., 1990).

PROTOCOL 12.6: BINDING OF MABS TO GLASS

(i) Wash standard soda glass slides thoroughly in 30% hydrogen peroxide in concentrated sulphuric acid for 10–15 min. Wash in distilled water, blow dry with compressed nitrogen gas, and dry over a 90°C hot plate for 10 min.
(ii) Immerse the slides in a 2% solution of dicholorodimethyl-silane in trichloroethylene and blow-dry with compressed nitrogen gas.
(iii) Coat the slide with the Mab solution at 0.1 mg/ml in PBS and leave overnight in a humidified box. Wash and rinse gently with PBS.

Appendix 1 – Animal handling techniques

A.1.1. Introduction

Detailed information on animal handling may be found in texts such as Williams and Chase (1967) and Herbert (1973). However, most of the procedures relevant to rodent hybridoma production are described below.

A.1.2. Requirement for animal handling licence

In many countries where appreciation of animal rights is increasing and groups active against research on animals are active, there are strict licensing requirements for laboratory workers using animals. In the U.K., under the Animals (Scientific Procedures) Act 1986. Each person who handles animals must have both a personal licence and a series of project licences covering the procedures to be undertaken. The animal, route of injection, method of killing etc. must be specified in detail. If methods of dubious value which cause trauma are to be used (for example intraperitoneal Freund's complete adjuvant), they will have to be justified. Most Home Office inspectors will advise on the detailed specifications necessary in an application for such a licence.

A.1.3. Handling

A.1.3.1. Identification

Individual animals in the same cage will often need to be identified for repeated immunisations or other procedures. The most satisfactory permanent methods for identifying mice and rats are by ear clips or by dyeing the fur. The system of ear clips illustrated in Fig. A.1.1. uses three positions on each ear.

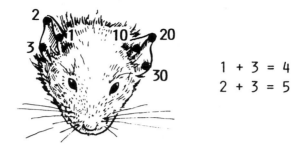

Fig. A.1.1. A system of earclips for animal identification.

Fur dyes include picric acid and gentian violet. Aqueous solutions of the dyes should be diluted with alcohol to decrease the drying time. Six positions are convenient to use-shoulder, flank and rump on the right and left sides. The dyes are best applied with cotton tipped applicators, which should be inserted under the outer fur and rolled so as to dye the inner fur.

A.1.3.2. Restraint

Mice should be picked up by the tail, near the base, and placed on a grid. When the tail is pulled gently, the animal holds onto the grid with its feet, and it can then be picked up by grasping the loose skin over the shoulders with the thumb and forefinger, while the tail is held with the little finger (Fig. A.1.2). For intravenous injection or for bleeding from the tail, a restraint consisting of a wire mesh tube closed at one end is used (Fig. A.1.3). When the mouse's head is put into the tube, it will enter it and can then be confined there by a bung with a notch in one side through which the tail protrudes.

A.1.3.3. Anaesthesia

For anaesthetising animals for short periods of time, ether is usually satisfactory. The ether jar should be arranged with a grid over the cotton wool soaked in ether, so that the animal only breathes the fumes,

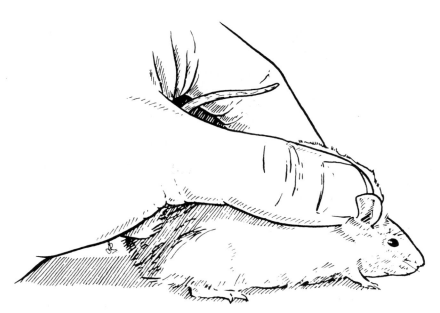

Fig. A.1.2. How to pick up a mouse.

but does not come in contact with the ether which will irritate the skin. The animal is sufficiently anaesthetised when the breathing is regular and slow, and when it does not twitch if a foot is gently pinched. Additional ether may be administered during the course of an operation by placing a small beaker with ether-soaked cotton wool in the bottom, over the animal's head.

A.1.3.4. Euthanasia

Animals may be quickly killed with CO_2 either from a cylinder or in the form of frozen pellets. The vapour is heavy, so the animal should be at the bottom of the container into which the gas is introduced.

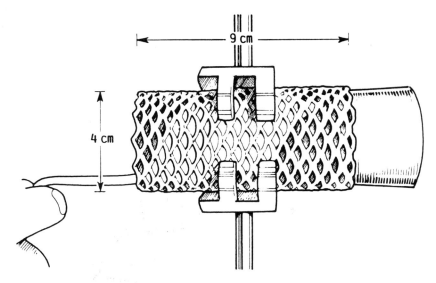

Fig. A.1.3. Tube restraint for mouse. Most mice will hold onto the mesh in the tubing with their claws. An uncooperative animal is restrained with a grooved bung in the rear end of the tube, so that only the tail is visible.

A.1.4. Immunisation

A.1.4.1. Intraperitoneal

Needle size: 23G or 25G.

Maximum amount to be injected: up to 2 ml in large mouse, up to 1 ml in smaller strains.

The mouse is held by grasping the loose skin over the shoulders with the thumb and forefinger, and holding the base of the tail with the little finger, belly upwards, the needle is inserted to a depth of approximately 5 mm, to one side of the midline, between the lower two nipples (Fig. A.1.4). Injections at the midline may enter the urinary bladder, and an injection too high in the peritoneal cavity may damage liver or spleen. The inoculum should be injected slowly, and there should be a brief pause before the needle is withdrawn, to allow the

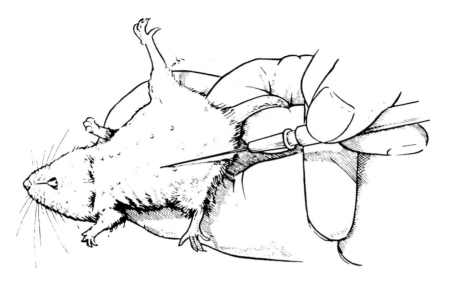

Fig. A.1.4. Intraperitoneal injection.

inoculum to disseminate. If there is a swelling at the injection site, the injection has been subcutaneous, not intraperitoneal.

A.1.4.2. Subcutaneous

Needle size: 23G or 25G.
Maximum amount: 0.2 ml.

The mouse is placed on a grid, and the loose skin and tail held as before. The animal should be left on the grid and gently held down by the backs of the third and fourth fingers on the left hand. The needle is inserted through the skin at the back of the neck, and pointing posteriorly, so that the point is below the fingers holding the skin. The point should be moved in a short arc to check that it moves freely between skin and body. The inoculum is injected, and the fingers should then be moved to grasp the site of needle penetration as the needle is withdrawn, to prevent the loss of inoculum through the hole in the skin.

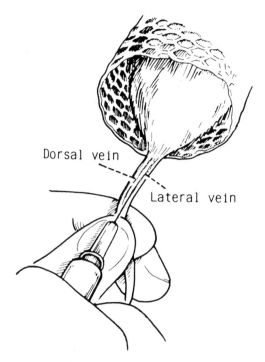

Fig. A.1.5. Intravenous injection.

A.1.4.3. Intravenous

Needle size: 25G or 26G.

   Maximum amount: 0.2 ml.

Intravenous injections in mice are neither quick nor easy, and practice is needed before the necessary skill can be acquired. It should be attempted first on albino mice, as their veins are easy to see. Some people prefer using an all-glass syringe, because the plunger moves more easily than in a plastic syringe. Great care should be taken that all air bubbles are expelled from the syringe, hub and needle before injection. The mouse should be restrained in a wire mesh tube with the tail protruding, as described above. Vasodilation should be induced either by warming the mouse with a desk lamp, or by warming the tail with cotton wool dipped in warm water. It is best to use the lateral tail veins, and to make the first injection distally, as the second attempt can then be made in a more proximal position. The mouse's tail should be held over the forefinger of the left hand, and the needle inserted into the vein on the straight part of the tail just over the finger (Fig. A.1.5). As the inoculum is injected, there should be no resistance and the vein should be seen to clear. If there is resistance as the plunger is pushed, and if the tail blanches, the injection has been sub-cutaneous.

A.1.4.4. Intramuscular

Needle size: 25G.
   Maximum amount: 0.05 ml.
   An assistant is required to hold the mouse while the experimenter extends the hind leg and makes the injection into the thigh muscle above the femur. The needle should approach from behind the animal and be pointed along the femur toward the body.

A.1.4.5. Intradermal

Needle size: 25G or 26G.
   Maximum amount: 0.05 ml.
   The skin should be shaved over a site on the back of a mouse. A fold of skin is pinched up between thumb and forefinger, and the needle inserted just below the surface of the skin, along the fold. The needle should be visible below the surface of the skin. When the inoculum is injected, the skin should blanche, and a pea-like swelling should appear, just below the surface.

A.1.4.6. Footpad

Needle size: 25G or 26G.
   Maximum amount: 0.0255 ml.

Because of the discomfort to the animal, this site should only be used if the draining lymph node is required. Only a hind foot should be used, as mice manipulate with the forepaws. An assistant is needed to hold the mouse, while the experimenter extends the hind leg and injects the inoculum just below the surface of the footpad.

A.1.4.7. Oral

Maximum amount: 2 ml.

Two kinds of fitting are used for oral dosage of mice. One is a cannula with a Luer fitting and a rounded metal end (Fig. A.1.6). The other apparatus is made by cleanly cutting and fire-polishing a short piece of narrow polythene tubing and then fitting it over a 19G or 21G needle. The mouse should be held by an assistant with its head back so that the throat and oesophagus are lined up as straight as possible. The cannula is slid gently down the throat as far as the stomach. If resistance is encountered before the cannula has penetrated as far as the stomach, the cannula may have entered the trachea. The cannula should then be withdrawn, and a second attempt made.

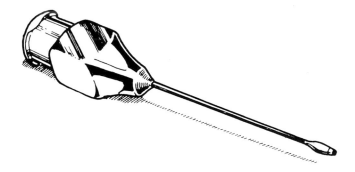

Fig. A.1.6. Fitting for oral immunisation of mice.

A.1.5. Serum collection

A.1.5.1. Bleeding from the tail

Two methods may be used to obtain blood from the tail of a mouse. Firstly, a sharp scalpel or razor blade may be used to cut a small piece off the end of the tail, and the drops of blood can be collected with a capillary tube or pasteur pipette. When sufficient blood has been collected (not more than 100 μl if the animal is to be bled repeatedly) the bleeding should be stopped by pressure of the fingers.

Alternatively, a sharp scalpel blade may be used to make a slanting cut in one of the lateral tail veins, and the blood collected and the bleeding stopped as before (Fig. A.1.7).

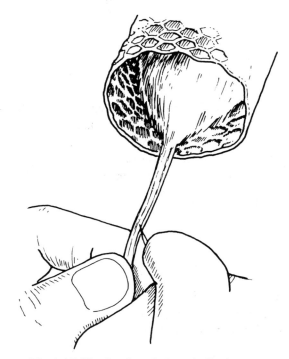

Fig. A.1.7. Bleeding from the lateral tail vein.

A.1.5.2. Serum separation

The blood should be collected into narrow glass or plastic tubes (e.g., Sarstedt 0.4 ml polythene tubes). If a large volume of blood has been collected, e.g., at exsanguination, a wooden toothpick may be put in the tube. However, the use of a toothpick is not advisable with small volumes of blood (50–100 μl). Mouse blood is rather subject to haemolysis, so the clot should be allowed to form at room temperature (rather than at 37°C) for 30–40 min. The clot should then be detached from the side of the tube by flicking the tube vigorously, and the tube left at 4°C overnight to allow the clot to retract. The serum may then be removed with a fine tipped micropipette.

A.1.6. Removal of tissues at sacrifice

A.1.6.1. Exsanguination

A.1.6.1.1. Cardiac puncture   This method is often used if the sterile removal of the spleen is to follow the collection of the blood. The mouse is killed with CO_2 and immediately after breathing has stopped the thoracic cavity is carefully opened by cutting the ribs to one side of the sternum. A 21G needle is inserted into the right ventricle and blood is slowly withdrawn from the heart, which is still beating.

A.1.6.1.2. Inferior vena cava   This is the method of choice when the maximum amount of blood is required. As soon as breathing has stopped the peritoneal cavity is opened and the gut is reflected. A 21G needle is inserted just proximal to the kidneys into the inferior vena cava (arrowed in Fig. A.1.8).

The blood is drawn slowly into the syringe, allowing time for the blood to drain into the vein, and making sure that the bevel of the needle is not blocked against the vein wall.

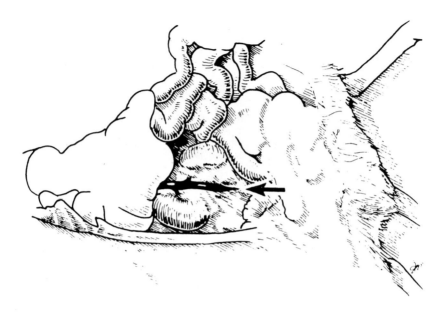

Fig. A.1.8. Inferior vena cava.

A.1.6.2. *Tissues containing immune cells*

A.1.6.2.1. Spleen   If the cells are needed for culture, the tissues must be sterilely removed from the animal. Two pairs of forceps and two scissors are required. They should be clean, dipped in 70% ethanol, and flamed before use. The mouse should be killed with CO_2, placed on its back for dissection, and soaked in 70% alcohol. The first set of scissors and forceps should be used to cut and reflect the skin over the abdomen. The second set of scissors and forceps should then be used to make a cut in the peritoneal wall on the mouse's left side. The spleen lies on the left side (from the mouse's point of view) of the peritoneal cavity just below the stomach (Fig. A.1.9). The veins and connective tissue by which it is attached all lie on the side of the organ toward the peritoneal cavity.

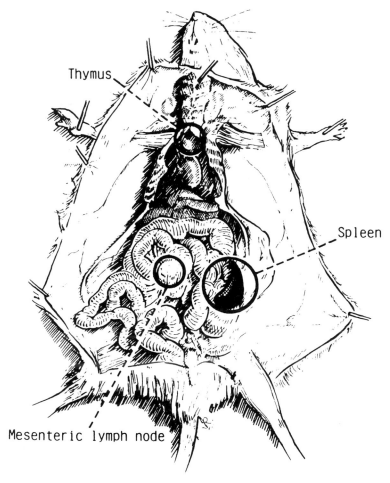

Fig. A.1.9. Spleen, thymus and mesenteric lymph nodes.

A.1.6.2.2. Lymph nodes For the sterile removal of lymph nodes the mouse should be treated for the removal of the spleen. The lymph nodes yield only small numbers of cells, and several may be required to get a sufficient cell yield. They do yield lymphocytes uncontaminated by red blood cells. In the mouse, the cervical, brachial, axillary and

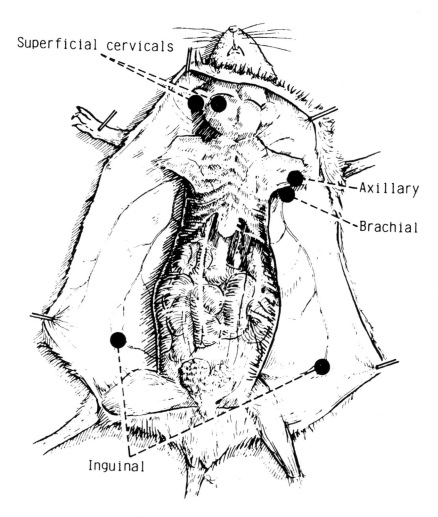

Fig. A.1.10. Some easily located lymph nodes.

inguinal nodes are easily found, and drain different areas of the body (Fig. A.1.10). The mesenteric node, which is attached to the large intestine, is a bigger node (Fig. A.1.9). It drains the gut wall, but not antigen injected intraperitoneally.

A.1.6.2.3. Thymus   The thymus is a bilobed, soft tissue which is ventral, and just anterior, to the heart (Fig. A.1.9). It is reached by first reflecting the skin and muscle layer over the sternum, along most of its length. The thymus is a greyish mass at the top of the thoracic cavity. It is attached at its anterior aspect. If a suspension of pure thymocytes is required, the two parathymic lymph nodes must be removed before teasing the tissue to obtain cells.

A.1.6.2.4. Peritoneal cells   The cells which can be washed from the peritoneal cavity consist of a mixture of macrophages (activated or normal), lymphocytes, polymorphonuclear cells, mast cells and eosinophils. The proportions of these types of cells varies with the health of the animal and its experimental treatment. The use of inducing agents alters the proportion and state of the cell types present and the timing of peritoneal lavage after the use of inducing agents is important if particular cell types are required. To obtain peritoneal cells, the dead mouse should be placed on its back on a dissecting board or tray

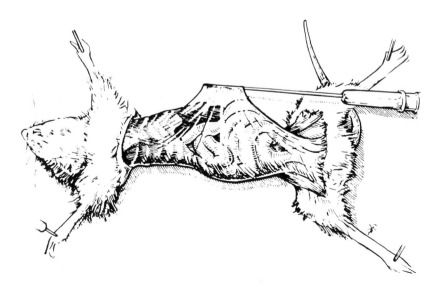

Fig. A.1.11. Peritoneal lavage.

and soaked in 70% alcohol as before. A cut should be made in the abdominal skin and the skin pulled away with the fingers towards the animal's head and tail, so that the whole peritoneal wall is exposed. Approximately 2–3 ml of medium should then be injected at the midline with a 25G needle. The mouse carcass is then massaged to disperse the medium throughout the peritoneal cavity. A 21G needle is then inserted through the peritoneal wall, pointing anteriorly, and with the point lying beside the spleen, and the fluid is slowly drawn into the syringe, allowing time for more fluid to seep into the pocket, and avoiding the needle being clogged by the nearby fat (Fig. A.1.11).

A.1.7. Ascites fluid

A.1.7.1. Introduction

Suspensions of cells may be grown in ascites fluid in mice (Chapter 10). The mouse to be used should be primed by the intraperitoneal injection of 0.5 ml Pristane (2,6,10,14-tetramethyl pentadecane) using a 21G needle. 10–20 days after priming, the washed myeloma cells in active logarithmic growth are injected (Protocol 10.1).

A.1.7.2. Tapping of ascites fluid

Two methods may be used. For either method the mouse must be lightly anaesthetised with ether. The first method is to hold the anaesthetised mouse over a beaker, use a 21G needle to make a hole in the abdominal skin and peritoneal wall, and allow the ascites fluid to drip through the hole and into the beaker. Sterile collection of the ascitic fluid may alternatively be done by a method similar to that used for peritoneal lavage. The anaesthetised mouse is placed on its back, and a 21G needle is inserted into the peritoneum at the animal's left side, with the needle pointing anteriorly and with point to one side of the spleen. The fluid is then drawn slowly into the syringe.

Appendix 2

Addresses of Suppliers and Manufacturers

Inevitably, these have the author's U.K. and, indeed, Scottish bias and better local firms may be available. The main reference texts for supplies are the Laboratory Equipment Directory (Morgan-Grampian Book Co Ltd., 48 Beresford St., London SE19 6BQ, U.K.) or International Laboratory, 30 Controls Drive, P.O. Box 870, Shelton, CT 06484–0870, U.S.A.

Abbot Laboratories Limited, Moorbridge Road, Maidenhead, Bucks, U.K.

Aldrich Chemical Company, New Road, Gillingham, Dorset, SP8 4BR, U.K.

American BioOrganics, N. Tonawanda, New York, NY, U.S.A.

American Type Culture Collection (ATCC), Rockville, MD 20852, U.S.A.

Amersham International plc, Amersham Place, Little Chlafont, Amersham, Bucks, U.K.

Amicon Ltd., Upper Mill, Stonehouse, Gloucestershire GL102 BJ, U.K.

Amicon Corp., 21 Hartwell Ave, Lexington, MA 02173, U.S.A.

Anderman & Co Ltd., London Road, Kingston-upon Thames, Surrey KT2 6NH, U.K.

Beckman Instruments, Progess Rd, Sands Industrial Estate, High Wycombe, Bucks HP12 3BR, U.K.

Beckman Instruments, P.O. Box 10200, Palo Alto, CA 94304, U.S.A.

Becton-Dickinson U.K., Between Towns Road, Cowley, Oxford OX4 3LY, U.K.

Becton-Dickinson, 2375 Galveia Ave, Mountain View, CA 94043, U.S.A.

Belmont Laboratories Europe, P.O. Box 62, 17K Westside Industrial Estate, Jackson St, St Helens, Merseyside WA9 3AJ, U.K.

Bibby Scientific Products, Stone, Staffordshire ST15 0SA, U.K.

Bioproducts for Science Inc., P.O. Box 29176, Indianapolis, IN 46229, U.S.A.

Bio-Rad Laboratories Ltd., Maylands Ave, Hemel Hampstead, Herts HP2 7TD, U.K.

Boehringer-Mannheim U.K., Bell Lane, Lewes, East Sussex BN7 1LG, U.K.

British Biotechnology Ltd., Watlington Rd, Cowley, Oxford OX4 5LY, U.K.

British Drug Houses Ltd., Poole, Dorset BH12 4NN, U.K.

Calbiochem, Novabiochem, 3, Heathcoat Building, Highfields Science Park, University Boulevard, Nottingham NG7 2QJ, U.K.

Cambridge Bioscience, 25 Signet Court, Stourbridge Common Business Centre, Swann's Road, Cambridge CB5 8LA, U.K.

Collaborative Research, Lexington, MA, U.S.A.

Costar: see Northumbria Biologicals

Coulter Electronics Ltd., Northwell Dr, Luton, Beds LU3 3RH, U.K.

Coulter Corporation, 440 W.20th St, Hialeah, FL 33010, U.S.A.

Dako Ltd., 16 Manor Courtyard, Hughenden Ave, Bucks HP13 5RE, U.K.

Dynal (U.K.) Ltd., Station House, 26 Grove St, Wirral, Merseyside L62 2AB, U.K.

European Collection of Animal Cell Cultures (ECACC), PHLS Centre for Applied Microbiology and Research, Porton Down, Salisbury, Wilts SP4 0SG, U.K.

Evans Medical Supplies Ltd., Ruislip, London, U.K.

Flow Laboratories, Woodcock Hill, Harefield Rd, Rickmansworth, Herts WD3 1PQ, U.K.

Fluka Chemicals Ltd., Peakdale Rd, Glossop, Derbyshire SK13 9XE, U.K.

Gallenkamp Ltd., Belton Road West, Loughborough LE11 0TR, U.K.

Gibco Ltd., 3175 Staley Rd, Grand Island, NY 14072, U.S.A.

Gibco Ltd., P.O. Box 35, Trident House, Paisley, Scotland, U.K.

Glaxo Laboratories Lts, Greenford, Middlesex, U.K.

Hana Biologicals, Berkeley, CA, U.S.A.

ICN Biomedicals Ltd., Lincoln Road, Cressex Industrial Estate, High Wycombe, Bucks HP12 3XJ, U.K.

Koch-Light Ltd., Rookwodd Way, Haverhill, Suffolk CB9 8PB, U.K.

May&Baker Laboratory Products, Liverpool Road, Eccles, Manchester M30 7RT, U.K.

Millipore Corporation, 80 Ashby Road, Bedford, MA 01730, U.S.A.

Millipore (U.K.) Ltd., The Boulevard, Ascot Rd, Croxley Green, Watford WD1 8WD, U.K.

New Brunswick Scientific (U.K.), Edison House, 163 Dixons Hill Road, North Mymms, Hatfield, AL9 7JE, U.K.

Northumbria Biologicals Ltd., South Nelson Industrial Estate, Cramlington, Northumberland NE23 9HL, U.K.

Olympus. See Gallenkamp.

Peninsula Laboratories, 611, Taylor Way, Belmont, CA 94002, U.S.A.

Pharmacia LKB, Biotechnology AB, S-751 82 Uppsala, Sweden

Pharmacia Ltd., Pharmacia House, Midsummer Boulevard, Central Milton Keynes, Bucks MK9 3HP, U.K.

Pierce, P.O.Box 117, Rockford, IL 61105, U.S.A.

Pierce Europe, P.O. Box 1512, 3260 BA Oud Beijerland, Holland

Promega Corp, 2800 Woods Hollow Road, Madison, WI 53711, U.S.A.

Scotlab, Unit 15, Earn Ave, Righead Industrial Estate, Bellshill ML4 3JQ, Scotland, U.K.

Sigma Chemical Co, St Louis, MO, U.S.A.

Sigma Chemical Co, Fancy Road, Poole, Dorset BH17 7NH, U.K.

Serotec, 22 Bankside, Station Approach, Kidlington, Oxford OX5 1JE, U.K.

Sterilin Ltd., Clockhouse Lane, Feltham, Middlesex, U.K.

Stratagene Cloning Systems, 11099 North Torrey Pines Road, La Jolla, CA 92037, U.S.A.

Stratagene U.K., Cambridge Innovation Centre, Cambridge Science Park, Milton Road, Cambridge CB4 4GF, U.K.

Technicon, Bayer Diagnostics U.K. Ltd., Evans House, Hamilton Close, Basingstoke, Hants RG21 2YE, U.K.

Vector Laboratories Inc., 30 Ingold Road, Burlingame, CA 94010, U.S.A.

Vector Laboratories, 16 Wulfric Square, Bretton, Peterborough PE3 8RF, U.K.

Ventrex BioVentures Group, Portland, ME, U.S.A.

Appendix 3 – Protocols for polyacrylamide gel electrophoresis (PAGE)

A.3.1. Introduction

Whole volumes in this series have been written on the electrophoretic separation of proteins and standard immunological or biochemical methods texts give much greater detail than is supplied here. The information below relates to the techniques most commonly employed in hybridoma technology and is largely for convenience to the reader.

Polyacrylamide gel electrophoresis is widely used in the characterisation of both a monoclonal antibody and its antigen. In the case of the Mab itself, it is used in particular for determination of the rate of synthesis and secretion of antibody (e.g., Fig. 3.6), particularly where the Mab has been reintroduced in recombinant systems (Chapter 9). In the case of the antigen, it is used for immunoblotting (Section 11.5). In both cases, slab gels are necessary and min-gel apparatus is less suitable.

A.3.2. Slab gel apparatus

Slab gels are poured into two glass plates, typically 18 cm × 13 cm clamped vertically together with spacers holding the plates apart. Spacers are made of plexiglas and are of thickness 1–5 mm. Thin gels are generally more suitable for autoradiographic procedures. Thicker gels hold more protein and may be suitable for immunoblotting of minor proteins. One of the glass plates has a groove 2 cm deep and approximately 14 cm long on the long (18 cm) side. When the gel has been poured, a 'comb' made of plexiglas of the same thickness as the spacers is inserted into this groove while the gel sets. The comb is removed before sample application into the slots it creates in the gel. The number of teeth in the comb is a matter of choice relating to the number of samples to be run, their volume, and the expertise of the operator.

The gel is poured in liquid form and will obviously leak out of the bottom of the apparatus unless great care is taken. Leakage can be stopped by using a third spacer along the bottom of the gel, greasing the spacers with petroleum jelly, and sealing the possible leakage points with a small amount of fast setting 1.5% agar at the edges. It is also effectively stopped by running a length of flexible 2 mm diameter silicone tubing round the edge of the plates outside the spacers. A third method involves the use of thin, plastic backed sticky tape around the outside of the glass plates. The two plates are firmly clamped together with foldback office clips.

There have been considerable advances in the quality of commercial equipment supplied and it is possible to buy leakproof equipment, gel cassettes, and even pre-set gels from several firms.

A.3.3. SDS-PAGE (sodium dodecyl sulphate– polyacrylamide gel electrophoresis)

SDS-PAGE separates proteins on the basis of size. The SDS denatures the proteins to give a uniform tertiary structure and binds to most proteins to the same extent (exceptions are highly charged proteins such as histones, and extensively glycosylated proteins such as glycoproteins or mucins). The PAGE has a molecular sieving effect so that small proteins move more readily through the gel. Gel concentrations are usually in the region of 10–12%. Lower percentages are used for larger proteins and higher percentages for smaller proteins. Gels of 5% polyacrylamide and below are extremely hard to handle and agarose is probably better.

The gel mould is prepared and the ingredients for the main gel are made up according to the information in Table A.3.1. Acrylamide and bis-acrylamide are neurotoxins and should be handled with gloves. The gel is degassed *before* the addition of SDS, ammonium persulphate and TEMED (Table A.3.1).

TABLE A.3.1
Composition of SDS-PAGE gels (50 ml)

	5%	7.5%	10%	12.5%
Stock acrylamide solution (48.75% (w/v) acrylamide, 1.25% (w/v) N,N'-methylenebisacrylamide)	5	7.5	10	12.5
1.5 M Tris-HCl, pH 8.7	12.5	12.5	12.5	12.5
Distilled water	30.8	28.3	25.3	23.3
10% (w/v) SDS in distilled water	0.5	0.5	0.5	0.5
1% Ammonium persulphate in distilled water (fresh)	1.2	1.2	1.2	1.2
TEMED (N,N,N',N'-tetramethyl-ethylaminediamine)	0.02	0.02	0.02	0.02

The TEMED catalyses the polymerisation and consequently its concentration affects the speed with which the gel sets. Too high a concentrations leads to the gel setting before it is properly poured and too low to very slow setting. The ammonium persulphate must be made up *immediately* before use. The gel is pouted into the mould to 3–4 cm from the top, immediately overlaid with water saturated butanol or propanol, and allowed to set. Usually, this is at room temperature but the gel may also be set in a 37°C oven to accelerate the polymerisation.

When the main gel has polymerised the butanol or propanol overlay is removed and the top of the gel is gently rinsed with the buffer to be used for the stacking gel. The stacking gel is then prepared according to Table A.3.2. A 5% stacking gel is generally used as a 3% one is harder to handle but 3% stacking gels are necessary where the main gel is 5% or lower. The stacking gel is then poured and the comb is inserted so that the teeth are 0.5–1 cm above the main gel. The stacking gel should polymerise in 30 min. The side spacers remain in

TABLE A.3.2
Composition of stacking gel for SDS-PAGE (10 ml)

	3%	5%
Stock acrylamide solution (48.75% (w/v) acrylamide, 1.25% (w/v) N,N'-methylenebisacrylamide)	0.6	1.0
1.5 M Tris-HCl, pH 8.7	1.25	1.25
Distilled water	7.5	7.1
10% (w/v) SDS in distilled water	0.1	0.1
1% Ammonium persulphate in distilled water (fresh)	0.5	0.5
TEMED (N,N,N',N'-tetramethyl-ethylaminediamine)	0.01	0.01

place but the bottom spaces, tape, or tubing is then removed and the gel is placed vertically in the electrophoresis apparatus with the bottom of the comb notch level with the lip of the top of the electrophoresis chamber. Vaseline or petroleum jelly are generally employed to seal the two. Both chambers are filled with the electrophoresis buffer (0.025 M Tris, 0.192 M glycine, 0.1% (w/v) SDS, pH 8.3) and the comb is then carefully removed.

The samples are prepared by mixing an equal volume of $2 \times$ sample buffer (0.125 M Tris-HCl, pH 6.8, 5% (w/v) SDS, 10% (v/v) 2-mercaptoethanol, 20% (v/v) glycerol plus 0.005% (w/v) bromophenol blue, pH 6.8) and heating in a boiling water bath for 2 min. Standard proteins of known molecular weight are also prepared for running in a separate track of the gel. The samples are loaded carefully with a micropipette. The exact volume depends on the size of the teeth of the comb but is usually 5–25 μl.

The electrodes are connected so that the sample runs down the gel towards the anode and the gel is run at constant current of 20–30 mA for the size of slab described. The progress may be monitored by the bromophenol blue. At the end of the electrophoresis the gel is carefully removed and either used for Western blotting (Section 11.5) or stained. The staining solution can be the generally employed Coomassie blue (0.25% (w/v) in methanol/acetic acid/distilled water, 5:1:5) which is more effective if warmed to 37°C and shaken slowly with the gel for 45–60 min. This is then destained with methanol/acetic acid/distilled water, 5:1:5, with several changes until the bands become visible above the background. The gel can then be vaccuum-dried and preserved.

An alternative stain is the use of 0.3 M copper chloride (Lee et al., 1987) which has equal or greater sensitivity to Coomassie blue and has the advantage that the gel stains immediately so that bands can be visualised 5 min after the gel has been removed from the electrophoresis apparatus. The protein bands are opaque/white against the green background of the gel. The protein is not further denatured as it is with the acetic acid method of staining and can be electroeluted and used for immunisation (Chapter 4). The gel can be photographed but not preserved by vacuum drying as the copper chloride will precipitate.

The most sensitive staining of a gel is by silver staining (Wray et al., 1981; Tsai and Frasch, 1982). The gel is generally fixed overnight in 40% ethanol, 5% glacial acetic acid, 55% double deionised water and the carbohydrate groups are oxidised with 0.7 (w/v)% periodic acid in fixing solution for 5 minutes, although this step is not essential. Staining is achieved by placing the gel in a solution containing 0.8 g silver nitrate in 4 ml deionised water which has been added dropwise with vigorous stirring to a solution containing 21 ml of 0.36% (w/v) NaOH and 1.4 ml of 14.8 M ammonia, and then made up to 100 ml with deionised water. The gel is stained with gentle shaking for 15–20 min and then washed with deionised water with three changes. The bands are then visualised with a developing reagent which contains 2.5 ml of 1% (w/v) citric acid and 250 μl of 38% formaldehyde made up to 500 ml with deionised water, again for 15–20 min. The reaction is stopped by placing the gel in 50% methanol.

A.3.4. Isoelectric focussing of immunoglobulins

This technique has its main application in hybridoma technology in the demonstration of antibody homogeneity. It is, however, not suitable for use with IgM molecules as polyacrylamide is used and agarose gels are generally employed in such cases (Rosen et al., 1979). The type of agarose employed is critical and special material is marketed by Pharmacia and LKB for this purpose.

Isoelectric focussing equipment may be obtained from most commercial suppliers and, again, preformed gels may also be purchased. These are probably worth the cost as the technique is quite tricky.

With home made gels, one plate is usually removed after the gel has been poured and consequently this is usually siliconised prior to the pouring of the gel. The other plate on which the gel is run, is frequently coated with a protein solution such as chromium-hardened gelatin to avoid tearing and distortion of the gel. Alternatively, the polyacrylamide may be covalently attached to specially coated plates (Nicoletti et al., 1980). The gel is poured vertically and can be run vertically but it is more commonly run in a flatbed electrophoresis tank. Spacers are usually 10-mm thickness because of gel fragility but thinner gels may be used.

The acrylamide gel solution is 5% (w/v) acrylamide and 0.25% (w/v) N,N'-methylenebisacrylamide together with the stock ampholines. For antibody solutions, they usually contain 3 M urea which is only necessary if the sample has been reduced. The stock ampholines are purchased at 40% and used at 2%. Ampholines cover a variety of pH ranges and it is usually best to mix two sets covering the pH range 5–7 and 7–9 each at a concentration of 2%. Polymerisation is by the addition of riboflavin (0.1 mg/ml) and TEMED (30 μl/100 ml of solution) just before the gel is poured followed by fluorescent illumination of the gel for 3–4 hours. A sample comb may be used if a vertical gel is to be run. However, it is more usual to remove the siliconised plate gently from the top of the polymerised gel and lay the gel on the bottom plate on a flatbed electrophoresis tank.

Samples are usually reduced to allow for resolution of both light

and heavy chain and are prepared in 6 M urea, 5% (v/v) 2-mercap-
toethanol, 0.1 M phosphate buffer, pH 8. They are warmed to 37°C
for 30 min and then applied directly to 0.5 cm × 3 cm strips of Whatman 3-mm filter paper for flatbed electrophoresis. The strips are
placed on the gel about 1 cm from the anode.

The anode buffer is 5% phosphoric acid and the cathode one 5%
ethylene diamine. Close contact between the gel and the electrodes is
helpful and this may be performed by placing the gel directly onto
graphite electrodes with the sample on the anodic side but not touch-
ing the anode. Alternatively, the electrodes may be placed on the gel.
If the plate on which the gel lies is not coated with gelatin to hold the
gel the latter process is essential. Whatman 3-mm paper wicks are
used to form contacts between the anodic and cathodic buffers and
the gel surface. Focussing is approached gradually starting at a current of 5 mA/plate and increasing the voltage stepwise over a period
of 2 hours. The plate is then focussed overnight at 450 V for a 20 cm
gel. In the morning, the voltage may be further increased to 600 V
for a 20 cm gel for another hour.

The apparatus is then switched off and the pH gradient is measured
with a flat membrane electrode. The gel is then fixed with 3.5% (w/v)
sulphosalicylic acid, 11.5% (w/v) trichloroacetic acid, and autoradio-
graphed and/or stained and destained as in Section A.3.3.

A.3.5. Electrophoresis of DNA on agarose

This is much simpler than protein electrophoresis as the nucleic acids
already carry their own charge. It is usually performed on flatbed
equipment which can be purchased at low cost. The agarose (0.8–1%)
is prepared in 0.04 M Tris acetate, 0.001 M EDTA, pH 8, and poured
onto a flat glass or perspex slab where it is held in a block by spacers.
The vertical comb is inserted as the gel sets. The block in the electrophoresis tank is then overlaid with the same Tris-acetate EDTA
buffer and the samples are inserted in the slots in loading buffer containing 10% glycerol and the dye markers bromophenol blue (0.04%)

and xylene cyanol FF (0.04%) which serve to show the progress of the fast (bromophenol blue) and slower (xylene cyanol FF) fragments. Electrophoresis is towards the anode at 1–5 V/cm. The gel is then stained with 0.5 μg/ml ethidium bromide which is a mutagen and must be handled and disposed of with great care. Detailed protocols may be found in Sambrook et al. (1989).

A.3.6. Autoradiography or fluorography of gels

In autoradiography the direct emission from the isotope is measured. In fluorography the energy from the isotope is converted into light which is more efficient in exposing X-ray film. Fluorography is essential for weak beta emitting isotopes.

For autoradiography the gel is dried down by vacuum in a special apparatus (Pharmacia, Bio-Rad). The gel is placed on a rubber sheet and overlaid with 3-mm Whatman filter paper, a second perforated rubber sheet, and a nylon sinter. The fluid is then drawn out by a vacuum pump.

The dried gel is then placed (in the dark) onto a sheet of Kodak X-Omat S film and the two are clamped between glass plates or in a customised cassette and secured in several layers of black plastic. Intensifying screens are generally used for high-energy isotopes. Exposure is for 2 days at $-70°C$ to prolong the half life of the silver atoms. The gel can be exposed to fresh film for a longer or shorter time period if this is unsuitable.

In fluorography, the gel is photographed after destaining, since the stain will be removed by the fluorography. It is then soaked in pure dimethyl sulphoxide (DMSO) for 1 hour and then incubated in 17% 2,5-diphenyloxazole (PPO) in DMSO for a further 4 hours in the dark. It is washed with water and dried as for autoradiography. Exposure is with a light sensitive film such as Fuji RX and is for a shorter time than that required for autoradiography but also at $-70°C$.

References

Adams, R.L.P. (1990) Cell Culture for Biochemists, 2nd Edn. In: Laboratory Techniques in Biochemistry and Molecular Biology. Elsevier, Amsterdam.

Ahkong, Q.F., Fisher, D., Tampion, W. and Lucy, J.A. (1973) Biochem. J. *136*, 147.

Aizawa, M. (1987) Immunosensors Phil. Trans. Roy. Soc Lond B *316*, 121–134.

Akerstrom, B. and Bjorck, L. (1986) J. Biol. Chem. *261*, 10240.

Al-Kaissi, E. and Mostratos, A. (1983) J. Immunol. Methods *58*, 127.

Alt, F.W., Blackwell, T.K., DePinho, R.D., Reth, M.G. and Yancopoulos, G.D. (1986) Immunol. Rev. *89*, 5.

Altschuler, G.L., Dziewulski, D.M., Sowek, J. and Belfort, G. (1986) Biotechnol. Bioeng. *28*, 646.

Andrade, J.D., Van Wagenen, R.A., Gregonis, D.E., Newby, K. and Lin, J.N. (1985) IEEE Trans. Electron Devices ED 32, 1175–1179.

Arnold, B., Battye, F.L. and Miller, J.F.A.P. (1979) J. Immunol. Methods *29*, 353.

Atchison, M.L. (1988) Annu. Rev. Cell Biol. *4*, 127.

Avreamas, S. (1969) Immunochemistry *6*, 43.

Azim, T., Allday, M.J. and Crawford, D.H. (1990) J. Gen. Virol. *71*, 665–671.

Badley, R.A., Drake, R.A.L., Shanks, I.A., Smith, A.M. and Stephenson, P.R. (1987) Phil. Trans. R. Soc. Lond. B *316*, 143–160.

Baldwin, T.O., Johnson, T.C. and Swanson, R. (1984) In: Flavins and Flavoproteins (Bray, R.C., Engle, P.C. and Mayhew, S.G., eds.), De Gruyter, Berlin. pp.345–358.

Barker, S.A. (1987) In: Biosensors: Fundamentals and Applications (Turner, A.P.F., Karube, I. and Wilson, G.S., eds), Oxford University Press, pp. 85–99.

Bator, J.M. and Reading, C.M. (1989) J. Immunol. Methods *125*, 167.

Bayer, E.A. and Wilchek, M. (1980) Methods. Biochem. Anal. *26*, 1.

Bazin, H., Beckers, A., Deckers, C. and Heremans, J.F. (1972) Eur. J. Cancer *10*, 568.

Bazin, H., Beckers, A., Deckers, C. and Heremans, J.F. (1973) J. Natl. Cancer Inst. *51*, 1359.

Bazin, H. (ed.)(1990) Rat hybridomas and Rat Mabs. CRC Press, Boca Raton, FL, 480pp.

Baldwin, E. and Schultz, P.G. (1989) Science *245*, 1104.

Bayer, E.A. and Wilcheck, M. (1980) Methods. Biochem. Anal. *26*, 1.

Beezley, B., Ruddle, N.H. (1982) J. Immunol. Methods *52*, 269.

Benkovic, S.J., Adams, J.A., Borders, C.L., Janda, K.D. and Lerner, R.A. (1990) Science *250*, 1135.

Bentley, G.A., Boulot, G., Riottot, M.M. and Poljak, R.J. (1990) Nature *348*, 254.

Bergmeyer, H.-U. (1974) Methods of Enzymatic Analysis, Vol. 1–4. Academic Press, New York.

Berkowitz, D.B. and Webert, D.W. (1981) J. Immunol. Methods *47*, 121.

Better, M. and Horwitz, A.H. (1989) Methods Enzymol. *178*, 476.

Bhat, T.N., Bentley, G.A., Fischmann, T.O., Boulot, G. and Poljak, R.J. (1990) Nature *347*, 483.

401

Birch, J.R., Boraston, R. and Wood, L. (1985) Trends Biotechnol. *3*, 162.

Bischoff, R., Eisert, R.M., Schedel, I., Vienken, J. and Zimmerman, U. (1982) FEBS Lett. *147*, 64.

Bjorkman, P.J., Saper, M.A., Samraoui, B., Bennett, W.S., Strominger, K.L. and Wiley, D.C. (1987) Nature *329*, 512.

Bjorck, L. and Kronvall, G (1984) J. Immunol. *133*, 969.

Bjorkman, P.J., Saper, M.A., Samraoui, B., Bennett, W.S., Strominger, J.L. and Wiley, D.C. (1987) Nature *329*, 506 and 512.

Blackwell, T.K. and Alt, F.W. (1988) In: Molecular Immunology (Hames, B.D. and Glover, D.M., eds.) IRL Press, Oxford. pp. 1–46.

Blanchard, G.C., Taylor, C.G., Busey, B.R. and Williamson, M.L. (1990) J. Immunol. Methods *130*, 263.

Bloom, A.D. and Nakamura, F.T. (1974) Proc. Natl. Acad. Sci. USA *71*, 2689.

Bolognesi, D.P. (1989) Nature *340*, 431.

Borrebaeck, C.A.L. (1989) J. Immunol. Methods *123*, 157 .

Borrebaeck, C.A.K. (1990) (ed.) Electromanipulation in Hybridoma Technology. Macmillan, New York.

Bothwell, G.D., Yancopoulos, G.D. and Alt, F.W. (1990) Methods for Cloning and Analysis of Eukaryotic Genes. Jones & Bartlett, Boston.

Boyd, J.E., James, K. and McClelland, D.B.L. (1984) Trends Biotechnol. *2*, 70.

Brodin, T., Olsson, L. and Sjogren, H. (1983) J. Immunol. Methods *60*, 1.

Brown, J.H., Jardetzky, T., Saper, M.A., Samraoui, B., Bjorkman, P.J. and Wiley, D.C. (1988) Nature *332*, 845.

Bruins, S.C., Ingwer, I., Zeckel, M.I. and White, A.C. (1978) Infect. Immunol. *21*, 721.

Burrows, P.D., Beck-Engeser, G.B. and Wable, M.R. (1983) Nature *306*, 243.

Campbell, A.M., Whitford, P. and Leake, R.E. (1987) Br. J. Cancer *56*, 709.

Campbell, A.M. and Leake, R.E. (1990) Cancer J. *3*, 40.

Campbell, A.K. and Patel, A. (1983) Biochem. J. *216*, 185.

Capon, D.J., Chamow, S.M., Mordenti, J., Martsers, S.A., Gregory, T., Mitsuya, H. Byrn, R.A., Lucas, C., Wurm, F.M., Groopman, J.E., Broder, S. and Smith, D.H. (1989) Nature *337*, 525.

Cardosi, M.F. and Turner, A.P.F. (1987). In: Biosensors Fundamentals and Applications (Turner, A.P.F., Karube, I. and Wilson, G.S., eds.) Oxford University Press, London.

Casali, P. and Notkins, A.L. (1989) Annu. Rev. Immunol. *7*, 513.

Cass, A.E.G., Francis, D.G., Hill, H.A.O., Aston, W.J., Higgins, I.J., Plotkin, E.V., Scott, L.D.L. and Turner, A.P.F. (1984). Anal. Chem. *56*, 667.

Cattermole, J.A., Crosier, P.S., Leung, E., Overell, R.W., Gillis, S. and Watson, J.D. (1989) J. Immunol. *142*, 3746.

Chard, T. (1990) An Introduction to Radioimmunoassay and Related Techniques. Laboratory Techniques in Biochemistry and Molecular Biology. Elsevier, Amsterdam.

Chatelier, R.C., Ashcroft, R.G., Lloyd, C.J., Nice, E.C., Whitehead, R.H., Sawyer, W.H. and Burgess, A.W. (1986) EMBO J. *5*, 1181.

Clackson, T., Hoogenboom, H.R., Griffiths, A.D. and Winter, G (1991) Nature *352*, 624.

Chiang, Y.L., Sheng-Dong, R., Brow, M.A. and Larrick, J. (1989) Biotechniques 7, 360–366.

Civin, C.I. and Banquerigo, M.L. (1983) J. Immunol. Methods 61, 1.

Claflin, L. and Williams, K. (1978) Curr. Top. Micro. Immunol. 81, 107.

Cleveland, D.W., Fischer, S.G., Kirschner, M.W. and Laemmli, U.K. (1977). J. Biol. Chem. 252, 1102.

Coleman, P.M., Laver, W.G., Varghese, J.N., Baker, A.T., Tulloch, P.A., Air, G.M. and Webster, R.G. (1987) Nature 326, 358.

Colwell, D.E., Michalek, S.M. and McGhee, J.R. (1986) In: Methods in Enzymology 121 (Langone, J.J. and Van Vanukis, H., eds.), Academic Press, New York. pp. 42–51.

Cordosi, M.F. and Turner, APR (1987) In: Biosensors (Turner A.P.F., Karube, I. and Wilson, G.F., eds.), Oxford University Press, London. pp. 60.

Cote, R.J., Morrisey, D.M., Houghton, A.N., Beattie, E.J., Oettgen, H.F. and Old, R.J. (1983) Proc. Natl. Acad. Sci. USA 80, 2026.

Croce, C.M. and Koprowski, H. (1974) J. Exp. Med. 139, 1350.

Croce, C.M., Linnenbach, A., Hall, W., Steplewski, Z. and Koprwoski, H. (1980) Nature 288, 488.

Cox, R. and Masson, W. (1978) Nature 276, 629.

Damato, B.E., Campbell, A.M., McGuire, B.J., Lee, W.R. and Foulds, W.S. (1988) Br. J. Cancer 58, 182.

Dangl, J.L. and Herzenberg, L.A. (1982) J. Immunol. Methods 52, 1.

Danilov, V.S. and Ismailov, A.D. (1989) In: Applied Biosensors (Wise, D.L., ed.), Butterworths, London. p. 39.

Davidson, R.L., O'Malley, K.A. and Wheeler, T.B. (1976) Somat. Cell. Genet. 2, 271.

Davies, D.R. and Padlan, E.A. (1990) Annu. Rev. Biochem. 59, 439.

Davis, M.M. (1988) In: Molecular Immunology (Hames, B.D. and Glover, D.M., eds.), IRL Press, Oxford.

Dean, C.J., Gyure, L.A., Hall, J.G. and Styles, J.M. (1986) Methods Enzymol. 121, 52–59.

De Leij, L., Schwander, E. and The, T.H. (1987) Methods in Hybridoma Formation (Bartal, A.H. and Hirshaut, Y., eds.), Humana Press, Clifton, NJ. p. 419.

Doyle, A., Jones, T.J., Bidwell, J.L. and Bradley, B.A. (1985) Human Immunol. 13, 199.

Doyle, M.J., Halsall, H.B. and Heineman, W.R. (1982) Anal. Chem. 54, 2318.

D'Souza, S.F., Melo, J.S., Deshpande, A. and Nadkarni, G. (1986) Biotech. Lett. 8, 643.

Duff, R.G. (1985) Trends Biotechnol. 3, 167.

Duhamel, R.C., Schurr, P.H., Brendel, K. and Meezan, E. (1979) J. Immunol. Methods 31, 211.

Duncan, A.R., Woof, J.M., Partridge, L.J., Burton, D.R. and Winter, G. (1988) Nature 332, 563.

Duncan, A.R. and Winter, G. (1988) Nature 332, 563.

Eddowes, M.J. (1988) Biosensors 3, 1.

Edwards, , P.A.W., Smith, C.M., Munro-Neville, A. and O'Hare, M.J. (1982) Eur. J. Immunol. *12*, 641.

Ehrlich, P., Moyle, W.R., Moustafa, Z.A. and Canfield, R.E. (1982) J. Immunol. *128*, 2709.

Eilat, D. (1986) Clin. Exp. Immunol. *65*, 215.

Ekins, R., Chiu, F. and Micallef, J. (1989) J. Bioluminescence Chemiluminscence *4*, 59–78.

Ekins, R. (1989) Nature *340*, 256.

Ekins, R., Chu, F. and Micallef, J. (1989) J. Bioluminescence Chemiluminescence *4*, 59.

Ekins, R. (1990) Nature Commentary *347*, 118.

Elwing, H. and Stenberg, M. (1981) J. Immunol. Methods *44*, 343–349.

Engvall, E. and Perlman, P. (1971) Immunochemistry *8*, 871.

Engvall, E. and Pesce, A.I. (1978) Quantitative Immunoassay Scand. J. Immunol. Suppl. 7.

Engvall, E. (1981) Methods Enzymol. *70*.

Erlich, P.H., Moustafa, Z.A., Justice, J.C., Harfeldt, E., Gadl, I.K., Sclorra, L.J., Uhl, F.P., Isaacson, C. and Ostberg, L. (1988) Clin. Chem. *34*, 1681. European Patent Handbook (2nd edn., 1989), Longman.

Evans, H.J. and Vijayalaxmi (1981) Nature *292*, 601.

Ey, P.L., Prowse, S.J. and Jenkin, C.R. (1978) Immunochemistry *15*, 429.

Farquhar, M.G. (1985) Annu. Rev. Cell Biol. *1*, 447.

Fazekas de St. Groth, S.J. and Scheidegger, D. (1980) J. Immunol. Methods *35*, 1.

Fernley, H.N. (1971) The Enzymes (Boyer, P.D., ed.), Vol. 4, Academic Press, New York. p. 417.

Festing, M.F.W. (1979) Inbred Strains in Biomedical Research. Macmillan, London.

Finkelman, F.D., Holmes, J., Katona, I.M., Urban, J.F., Beckmann, M.P., Park, L.S., Schooley, K.A., Coffman, R.L., Mosmann, T.R. and Paul, W.E. (1990) Ann. Rev. Immunol. *8*, 303.

Fogh, J. and Fogh, H. (1968) Proc. Soc. Exp. Biol. Med. *117*, 899.

Fonong, T. and Reichnitz, G.A. (1984) Anal. Chem. *65*, 2586.

Foon, K.A. (1989) Cancer Res. *49*, 1621.

Foung, S.K.H., Saski, D.T., Groumet, F.C. and Engleman, E.G. (1982) Proc. Natl. Acad. Sci. USA *79*, 484.

Foung, S.K.H., Blunt, J.A., Wu, P.S., Ahearn, P., Winn, L.C., Engleman, E.G. and Grumet, F.C. (1987) Vox. Sang. *53*, 44.

Fox, R.M., Tripp, E.H. and Tattersall, M.H.N. (1980) Cancer Res. *40*, 1718.

Freudenberg, M.A., Better, M. and Horwitz, A.H. (1989) Methods Enzymol. *178*, 476.

Freund, J. and McDermott, K. (1942) Proc. Soc. Exp. Biol. Med. *49*, 548.

Freund, J. (1956) Adv. Tuberc. Res. *7* 130.

Freund, Y.R. and Blair, P.B. (1982) J. Immunol. *129*, 2826.

Friguet, B., Djavadi-Ohaniance, L., Pages, J. Bussard, A. and Goldberg, M. (1983) J. Immunol. Methods *60*, 351.

Friguet, B., Chaffotte, A.F., Djavadi-Ohaniance, L. and Goldberg, M. (1985) J. Immunol. Methods *77*, 305.

Fulop, G.M. and Phillips, R.A. (1990) Nature *347*, 479–482.

Galfre, G., Milstein, C. and Wright, B. (1979) Nature *277*, 131.
Galfre, G. and Milstein, C. (1981) Methods Enzymol. *73*, 1.
Gebauer, C.R. and Reichnitz, G.A. (1982) Anal. Biochem. *124*, 338.
Gefter, M.L., Margulies, D.H. and Scharf, M.D. (1977) Somat. Cell Genet. *3*, 231.
Ghosh, S. and Campbell, A.M. (1986) Immunol. Today *7*, 217.
Ghosh, S. Cannon, C.A. and Campbell, A.M. (1987) J. Lab. Clin. Immunol. *23*, 129.
Giallongo, G., Kochoumina, L. and King, T.P. (1982) J. Immunol. Methods *52*, 379.
Glenney, J. (1986) Anal. Biochem. *156*, 315.
Gutmann, G.A., Werner, N.C., Harris, A.W. and Bowles, A. (1978) J. Immunol. Methods *21*, 101.
Goosens, D., Champomier, F., Rouger, P. and Salmon, C. (1987) J. Immunol. Methods *101*, 193.
Gorny, M.K., Gianakakos, V., Sharpe, S. and Zolla-Pazner, S. (1989) Proc. Natl. Acad. Sci. USA *86*, 1624.
Greaves, M. (1982) J. Cell. Physiol. Suppl. *1*, 113–127.
Greaves, M.F. and Brown, G. (1974) J. Immunol. *112*, 420.
Green, H.E. and Duft, B.J. (1990) Nature *347*, 117.
Green, M.J. (1987a) Electrochem. Immunoassays Phil. Trans. R. Soc. London B *316*, 135–142.
Green, M.J. (1987b) In: Biosensors: Fundamentals and Applications (Turner, A.P.F., Karube, I. and Wilson, G.S., eds.), Oxford University Press, London. pp. 60–70.
Griswold, W.R. (1987) Hybridoma *6*, 191.
Gritzmacher, C.A. (1989) Crit. Rev. Immunol. *9*, 173–200.
Guilbault, G.G. and Jordan, J. (1988) CRC Crit Rev. Anal. Chem. *19*, 1.
Guilbault, G.G. (1989) Biotechnology *7*, 349.
Goding, J.W. (1980) J. Immunol. Methods *39*, 285.

Haas, W. and Von Boehmer, H. (1982) J. Immunol. Methods *52*, 137.
Hale, G., Clark, M.R., Marcus, R., Winter, G., Dyer, M.J.S., Phillips, J.M., Riechmann, L. and Waldmann, H. (1988) Lancet *ii*, 1394–1399.
Hames, B.D. and Glover, D.M. (1988) Molecular Immunology. IRL Press, Oxford.
Hardman, N., Gill, L.L., De Winter, R.F.J., Wagner, K., Hollis, M., Businger, F., Ammaturo, A., Buchegger, F., Mach, J.-P. and Huesser, C. (1989) Int. J. Cancer *44*, 424.
Hardy, R.R.(1986) In: Handbook of Experimental Immunology, 4th Edn. (Weir, D.M., Herzenberg, L.A., Blackwell, C. and Herzenberg, L.A., eds.), Chapter 31. Blackwell, Oxford.
Harlow, E. and Lane, D. (1988) Antibodies: a Laboratory Manual. Cold Spring Harbor Press, Cold Spring Harbor, NY.
Harris, H. (1970) Cell Fusion. The Dunham Lectures. Oxford University Press, London.
Harris, H. and Watkins, J.F. (1965) Nature *205*, 640.
Hasemann, C.A. and Capra, J.D. (1990) Proc. Natl. Acad. Sci. USA *87*, 3942.
Haugland, R.P. (1989) Handbook of Fluorescent Probes and Research Chemicals. Molecular Probes Inc., Eugene, OR 97402.

Hawkes, R. (1986) Methods Enzymol. *121*, 484.

Hendry, R.M. and Herrman, J.E. (1980) J. Immunol. Methods *35*, 285.

Herbert, W.J. (1973) Laboratory Animal Techniques for Immunologists. In: Handbook of Experimental Immunology, Vol. 3 (Weir, D.M., ed.), 2nd Edn., Blackwell, Oxford.

Heusser, C.H., Stocker, J.W. and Gisler, R.H. (1981) Methods Enzymol. *73*, 406.

Hiatt, A., Cafferkey, R. and Bowdish, K. (1989) Nature *342*, 76.

Hilfiker, M.L., Morre, R.N. and Farrar, J.J. (1981) J. Immunol. *127*, 1983.

Hilvert, D., Carpenter, S.H., Nared, K.D. and Auditor, M.M. (1988) Proc. Natl. Acad. Sci. USA *85*, 4953.

Hilwig, I. and Gropp, A. (1972) Exp. Cell. Res. *78*, 122.

Horibata, K. and Harris, A.W. (1970) Exp. Cell. Res. *60*, 61.

Hornick, C.L. and Karush, F. (1972) Immunochemistry *9*, 325.

Horwitz, A.H., Chang, C.P., Better, M., Hellstrom, K.E. and Robinson, R.R. (1988) Proc. Natl. Acad. Sci. USA *85*, 8678.

Huse, W.D., Sastry, L., Iverson, S.A., Kang, A.S., Alting-Mees, M., Burton, D.R., Benkovic, S.J. and Lerner, A.R. (1989) Science *246*, 1275.

Huston, J.S., Levinson, D., Mudgett-Hunter, M., Tai, N., Novotny, J., Margolies, M.N., Ridge, R.J., Bruccoleri, R.E., Haber, E., Crea, R. and Opperman, H. (1988) Proc. Natl. Acd. Sci. USA *85*, 5879.

Hyman, R. and Stallings, V. (1974) J. Natl. Cancer Inst. *52*, 429.

Innis, M.A., Gelfand, D.H., Sninsky, J.J. and White, T.J. (eds.) (1990) PCR Protocols: a Guide to Methods and Applications. Academic Press, New York.

Iversen, B.L., Iversen, S.A., Roberts, V.A., Getzoff, E.D., Tainer, J.A., Benkovic, S.J. and Lerner, R.A. (1990) Science *249*, 659.

James, K. and Bell, G.T. (1987) J. Immunol. Methods *100*, 5–40 .

Johansson, K.E. and Bolske, J. (1989) J. Biochem. Biophys. Methods *19*, 185.

Johnson, G.D. and Holborow, E.J. (1986) In: Handbook of Experimental Immunology, 4th Edn. (Weir, D.M., Herzenberg, L.A., Blackwell, C. and Herzenberg, L.A., eds.), Chapter 28, Blackwell, Oxford.

Johnstone, A. and Thorpe, R. (1987) Immunochemistry in Practice, 2nd Edn. Blackwell, Oxford.

Jones, P.T., Dear, P.H., Foote, J., Neuberger, M.S. and Winter, G. (1986) Nature *321*, 523.

Junghans, R.P., Waldmann, T.A., Landolfi, N.F., Avdalovic, N.M., Schneider, W.P. and Queen, C. (1990) Cancer Res. *50*, 1495.

Kaneshima, H., Baum, C., Chen, B., Namikawa, R., Outzen, H., Rabin, L., Tsukamoto, A. and McCune, J.M. (1990) Nature *348*, 561.

Kaplan, M.E. and Clark, C. (1974) J. Immunol. Methods *5*, 131.

Kaplan, R.S., Pratt, R.D. and Pedersen, P.L. (1986) J. Biol. Chem. *261*, 12767.

Karube, I. and Gotoh, M. (1987) NATO Advanced Workshop on Analytical Uses of Immobilised Biological Compounds. Reidel Press, Amsterdam. p. 187.

Kawamoto, T., Sato, J.D., McClure, D.B. and Sato, G.H. (1986) Methods Enzymol. *121*, 266.

Kearney, J.F., Radbruch, A., Leisganag, B. and Rajewsky, K. (1979) J. Immunol. *123*, 1548.

Keating, M.Y. and Rechnitz, G.A.(1984) Anal. Chem. *56*, 801.

Keating, M.Y. and Rechnitz, G.A. (1985) Anal. Lett. *18*, (B1) 1–10.

King, T.P. and Kochoumian, L. (1979) J. Immunol. Methods *78*, 201.

Kints, J.P., Manouvriez, P. and Bazin, H. (1979) J. Immunol. Methods *119*, 241.

Klebe, R.J. and Mancuso, M.G. (1981) Somat. Cell. Genet. *7*, 473.

Klein, J., Figueroa, F. and David, C.S. (1983) Immunogenetics *17*, 553.

Knapp, W., Rieber, P., Dorken, B., Schmidt, R.E., Stein, H. and Borne, A.E.G. (1989) Immunology Today *10*, 253.

Knox, J.P. and Galfre, G. (1986) Anal. Biochem. *155*, 92.

Knutton, S. and Pasternak, C.A. (1979) Trends Biochem. Sci. *4*, 220 .

Kohler, G and Milstein, C. (1975) Nature *256*, 495.

Kohler, G. and Milstein, C. (1976) Eur. J. Immunol. *6*, 511.

Komisar, J.L., Fuhrman, J.A. and Cebra, J.J. (1982) J. Immunol. *128*, 2376.

Kovar, J. and Franek, F. (1986) Methods Enzymol. *121*, 277.

Kozbor, D. and Roder, J.C. (1981) J. Immunol. *127*, 1275.

Kozbor, D., Triputti, P., Roder, J.C. and Coroce, C.M. (1984) J. Immunol. *133*, 3001.

Kricka, L.J. and Thorpe, G.H.G. (1986) Parasitol. Today *2*, 123.

Kumpel, B.M., Wiener, E., Urbaniak, S.J. and Bradley, B.A. (1989) Br. J. Haematol. *71*, 415.

Kumpel, B.M., Poole, G.D. and Bradley, B.A. (1989) Br. J. Haematol. *71*, 125.

Kunkel, T.A., Roberts, J.D. and Zakour, R.A. (1987) Methods Enzymol. *154*, 367.

Kurie, J.M., Morese, H.C., Principato, M.A., Wax, J.S., Troppmair, J., Ropp, P., Potter, M. and Mushinski, J.F. (1990) Oncogene *5*, 577.

Kyhse-Andersen, J. (1984) J. Biochem. Biophys. Methods *10*, 203.

Lachmann, P.J., Olroyd, R.G., Milstein, C. and Wright, B.W. (1980) Immunology *43*, 503.

Laing, P. (1986) J. Immunol. Methods *92*, 161.

Lanzavecchia, A. (1985) Nature *314*, 537.

Laver, W.G., Hir, G.M., Webster, R.G. and Smith-Gill, S.J. (1990) Cell *61*, 553.

Lee, C., Levin, A. and Branton, D. (1987) Anal. Biochem. *166*, 308–312.

Lehtonen, O. and Viljanen, M.K. (1980a) J. Immunol. Methods *34*, 61.

Lehtonen, O. and Viljanen, M.K. (1980b) J. Immunol. Methods *36*, 63.

Lifson, J.D., Feinberg, M.B., Reyes, G.R., Rabin, L., Banapour, B., Chakrabarti, S., Moss, B., Wong-Staal, F., Steimer, K.S. and Engleman, E.G. (1986) Nature *323*, 725.

Littlefield, J.W. (1983) Proc. Natl. Acad. Sci. USA *50*, 568.

Liu, Y, Joshua, D.E., Williams, G.T. Smith, C.A., Gordon, J. and MacLennan, I.C.M. (1989) Nature *342*, 929–931.

Lo Buiglio, A.F., Wheeler, R.H., Trang, J., Haynes, A., Rogers, K., Harvey, E.B., Sun, L., Ghrayeb, J. and Khazaeli, M.B. (1989) Proc. Natl. Acad. Sci. USA *86*, 4220.

Loh, E.H., Elliott, J.F., Cwirla, S., Lanier, L.L. and Davis, M.M. (1989) Science *243*, 217–220.

Riechmann, L., Clark, M., Waldmann, H. and Winter, G. (1988) Nature *332*, 323..

Roberts, S, Cheetham, J.C. and Rees, A.R. (1987) Nature *328*, 731.

Robinson, W.E., Kawamura, T., Gorry, M.K., Lake, D., Xu, J.Y., Matsumoto, Y., Mitchell, W.M., Hersh, E. and Zolla, Pazner, S., (1990) Proc. Natl. Acad. Sci. USA *87*, 3185.

Roitt, I., Brostoff, J. and Male, D. (1989) Immunology, 2nd Edn. Churchill Livingstone, Edinburgh.

Rosen, A., Ek, K. and Aman, P. (1979) J. Immunol. Methods *28*, 1.

Roth, M.A. and Pierce, S.B. (1987) Biochemistry *26*, 4179.

Rousseaux, J., Picque, M.T., Bazin, H. and Biserte, G. (1981) Mol. Immunol. *18*, 639.

Ruddle, F.H. and Kucherlapali, R.S. (1974) Sci. Am. *231*, 36.

Russ, C., Callegaro, I., Lanza, B. and Ferrone, S. (1983) J. Immunol. Methods *65*, 269.

Russel, W.C., Newman, C. and Williamson, D.H. (1975) Nature *253*, 461.

Saiki, R.K., Sharf, S., Faloona, F., Mullis, K.B., Horn, G.T., Erlich, H.A. and Arnhein, N. (1985) Science *230*, 1350.

Saltvedt, E. and Harboe, M. (1976) Scand. J. Immunol. *5*, 1103.

Sambrook, J., Fritsch, E.F. and Maniatis, T. (1989) Molecular Cloning, 2nd Edn. Cold Spring Harbour Laboratory Press, Cold Spring Harbor.

Samoilovich, S.R., Dugan, C.B. and Macario, A.J.L. (1987) J. Immunol. Methods *101*, 153.

Sanchez-Madrid, F. and Springer, T.A. (1986) Methods Enzymol. *121*, 239.

Sastry, L., Alting-Mees, M., Huse, W.D., Short, J.M., Sorge, J.A., Hay, B.N., Janda, K.D., Benkovic, S.J. and Lerner, R.A. (1989) Proc. Natl. Acad. Sci. USA *86*, 5728.

Schlager, S.I. (1980) Methods Enzymol. *70*, 252.

Schekman, R. (1985) Annu. Rev. Cell Biol. *1*, 115.

Scheppenheim, R. and Rautenberg, P. (1987) Eur. J. Clin. Microbiol. *6*, 49.

Schimmelpfeng, L., Langenberg, U. and Peters, J.H. (1980) Nature *285*, 661.

Schmidtt, K., Daeubener, W., Bitter-Suermann, G. and Hadding, U. (1988) J. Immunol. Methods *109*, 17.

Schneider, C., Newman, R.A., Sutherland, D.R., Asser, U. and Greaves, M.F. (1982) J. Biol. Chem. *257*, 10766.

Schultz, J.S. (1987) Ann NY Acad Sci *506*, 406–414.

Schultz, J.H. (1987) In: Biosensors: Fundamentals and Applications (Turner, A.P.F., Karube, I. and Wilson, G.S., eds.), Oxford University Press, London. pp. 638–654.

Schwaber, J. and Cohen, E.P. (1974) Proc. Natl. Acad. Sci. USA *71*, 2203.

Secher, D.S. and Burke, D.C. (1980) Nature *285*, 446.

Seitz, W.R. (1987) In: Biosensors. Fundamentals and Applications (Turner, A.P.F., Karube, I. and Wilson, G.S.,eds.), Oxford University Press, London. pp. 599–616.

Sharon, J., Kabat, E.A. and Morrison, S.L. (1982) Mol. Immunol. *19*, 389.

Shin, S. and Morrison, S.L. (1989) Methods Enzymol. *178*, 459.

Shokat, K.M. and Schultz, P.G. (1990) Annu. Rev. Immunol. *8*, 335.

Shons, A. (1972) J. Biomed. Mater. Res. *6*, 565.

Shulman, M. Wilde, C.D. and Kohler, G. (1978)Nature *276*, 269.

Sinha, A.A., Lopez, M.T. and McDevitt, H.O. (1990) Science *248*, 1380.

Sklar, L.A. and Finney, D.A.(1982) Cytometry 3, 161.

Sklar, L.A., Finney, D.A., Oades, Z.G., Jesiatis, A.J., Painter, R.G. and Cochrane, C.G. (1984) J. Biol. Chem. 259, 5661.

Smith, P.F. (1971) The Biology of Mycoplasmas. Academic Press, New York.

Southern, E. (1965) J. Mol. Biol. 98, 503.

Spitz, M. (1986) Methods Enzymol. 121, 33.

Springer, T.A. (1990) Nature 346, 425.

Sternberger, L.A. (1979) Immunochemistry, 2nd Edn., John Wiley & Sons, New York.

Steward, M.W. (1986) In: Handbook of Experimental Immunology, 4th Edn. (Weir, D.M., Herzenberg, L.A., Blackwell, C. and Herzenberg, L.A., eds.), Chapter 25. Blackwell, Oxford.

Stewart, F., Callander, A. and Garwes, D.J. (1989) J. Immunol. Methods 119, 269.

Stollar, B.D., Zon, G. and Pastor, R. (1986) Proc. Natl. Acad. Sci. USA 83, 4469.

Stott, D.I. and McLearie, J. (1986) Immunol. Invest. 15, 113.

Stott, D.I. (1989) (Review) J. Immunol. Methods 119, 153.

Sutherland, R.M. and Dahne, C. (1987) In: Biosensors: Fundamentals and Applications (Turner, A.P.F., Karube, I. and Wilson, G.S., eds.), Oxford University Press, London. pp. 655–678.

Taggart, R.T. and Samloff, I.M. (1982) Science 219, 1228.

Tanaguchi, M. and Miller, J.F.A.P. (1978) J. Exp. Med. 148, 373.

Talmage, D.W.(1959) Science 129, 1643.

Thomson, A., Contreras, M., Gorick, B., Kumpel, B., Chapman, G.E., Lane, R.S., Teesdale, P., Hughes-Jones, N.C. and Mollison, P.L. (1990) Lancet i, 1147.

Tiebout, R.F., Stricker, E.A.M., Hagenaars, R. and Zeijlmaker, W.P. (1984) Eur. J. Immunol 14, 399.

Tijssen, P. (1985) Practice and Theory of Immunoassays. Laboratory Techniques in Biochemistry, Vol. 15. Elsevier, Amsterdam

Tor, R., Rosen, I, Rishpon, J. and Freeman, A. (1989)In: Applied Biosensors (Wise, D.L., ed.), Butterworths, London. p. 79.

Towbin, H., Staehelin, T. and Gordon, J. (1979) Proc. Natl. Acad. Sci. USA 76, 4350.

Tramontano, A., Janda, K.D. and Lerner, R.A. (1986) Science 234, 1566.

Tramontano, A. and Schloeder, D. (1989) Methods Enzymol. 178, 531.

Traub, R., Gould, R.J., Garsky, V.M., Ciccarone, T.M., Huxie, J., Friedman, P.A. and Shattil, S.J. (1989) J. Biol. Chem. 264, 259.

Tsai, B. and Frasch, C.E. (1982) Anal. Biochem. 119, 115.

Underwood, P.A., Kelly, J.F., Harman, D.F. and MacMillan, H.M. (1983) J. Immunol. Methods 60, 33.

Van Meel, F.C.M., Steenbakers, P.G.A. and Oomen, J.C.H. (1985) J. Immunol. Methods 80, 267.

Van Meurs, G.J.E. and Jonker, M. (1986) J. Immunol. Methods 95, 123.

Van Oss, C.J., Good, R.J. and Chaudry, M.K. (1987) J. Chromatogr. 391, 53.

Vindelov, L.L., Christensen, J. and Nissen, N.I., (1983) Cytometry 3, 323.

Voyta, J.C., Edwards, B. and Bronstein, I. (1988) Clin. Chem. *34*, 1157.

Ward, E.S., Gussow, D., Griffiths, A.D., Jones, P.T. and Winter, G. (1989) Nature *341*, 544.

Weber, G. (1975) Adv. Protein Chem. *29*, 1.

Weber, S.G. and Purdy, W.C. (1982) Anal. Lett. *12*, 1–9.

Wehmeyer, K.L., Halsall, H.B. and Heineman, W.R. (1982) Clin. Chem. *28*, 1968–1972.

Weir, D.M., Herzenberg, L.A., Blackwell, C. and Herzenberg, L.A. (1986) Handbook of Experimental Immunology, 4th Edn. Blackwell, Oxford.

Wen, L., Hanvanich, M., Werner-Favre, C., Brouwers, N., Perrin, L.H. and Zubler, R.H. (1987) Eur. J. Immunol. *17*, 887.

White, T.J., Arnheim, N. and Erlich, H.A. (1989) Trends Genet. *5*, 185.

Whitehead, T.P., Thorpe, G.H., Carter, T.J., Groucutt, C. and Kricka, L.J. (1983) Nature *305*, 158.

Williams, C.A. and Chase, M.W. (1967) Methods in Immunology and Immunochemistry, Vol 1. Academic Press, New York.

Williams, W.V., Moss, D.A., Kieber-Emmons, T., Cohen, J.A., Myers, J.N., Weiner, D.B. and Greene, M.I. (1989) Proc. Natl. Acad. Sci. USA *86*, 5537.

Wilson, M.B. and Nakane, P.K. (1978) In: Fluorescence and Related Techniques. (Knapp, W., Holubar, H. and Wick, G.,eds.), Elsevier, Amsterdam. p.215.

Winger, L., Winger, C., Shastry, P., Russell, A. and Longnecker, M. (1983) Proc. Natl. Acad. Sci. USA *80*, 4484.

Winter, G. and Milstein, C. (1991) (Review) Nature *349*, 293.

Wohlrab, H., Kolbe, H.V.J. and Collins, A. (1986) Methods Enzymol. *125*, 697.

Wray, W., Boulikas, T., Wray, V.P. and Hancock, R. (1981) Anal. Biochem. *118*, 197.

Ziola, B.R., Matikainen, M.T. and Salmi, A. (1977) J. Immunol. Methods *17*, 309.

Zubler, R.H., Werner-Favre, C., Wen, L., Sekita, K. and Straub, C. (1987) Immunol. Rev. *99*, 281.

ZuPulitz, J.Z., Kubasek, W.L., Duchene, M., Marget, M., Specht, B.V.S. and Domdey, H. (1990) Biotechnology *8*, 651.

Zwickl, M., Zaninetta, D., McMaster, G.K. and Hardman, N. (1990) J. Immunol. Methods *130*, 49.

Subject index